RADIATION THERAPY FOR HEAD AND NECK NEOPLASMS

RADIATION THERAPY FOR HEAD AND NECK NEOPLASMS

Third Edition

C. C. WANG, M.D., F.A.C.R.
Clinical Head and Professor, Division of Clinical Services
Department of Radiation Oncology
Massachusetts General Hospital
Boston, Massachusetts

⊗ **WILEY-LISS**
A JOHN WILEY & SONS, INC., PUBLICATION
New York / Chichester / Brisbane / Toronto / Singapore / Weinheim

Copyright © 1997 by Wiley-Liss, Inc.

Published simultaneously in Canada.

While the authors, editors, and publisher believe that drug selection and dosage and the specification and usage of equipment and devices, as set forth in this book, are in accord with current recommendations and practice at the time of publication, they accept no legal responsibility for any errors or omissions, and make no warranty, express or implied, with respect to material contained herein. In view of ongoing research, equipment modifications, changes in governmental regulations and the constant flow of information relating to drug therapy, drug reactions, and the use of equipment and devices, the reader is urged to review and evaluate the information provided in the package insert or instructions for each drug, piece of equipment, or device for, among other things, any changes in the instructions or indication of dosage or usage and for added warnings and precautions.

Library of Congress Cataloging-in-Publication Data

Wang, C. C. (Chiu-Chen)
    Radiation therapy for head and neck neoplasms / by C.C. Wang.—
3rd ed.
        p.   cm.
    Includes bibliographical references and index.
    ISBN 0-471-14971-3 (cloth : alk. paper)
    1. Head—Cancer—Radiotherapy.   2. Neck—Cancer—Radiotherapy.
I. Title.
        [DNLM: 1. Head and Neck Neoplasms—radiotherapy.   WE 707 W246r
1997]
    RC280.H4W36   1997
    616.99'4910642—dc20
    DNLM/DLC
    for Library of Congress   96-16482
                                                                  CIP

Printed in the United States of America

10 9 8 7 6 5 4 3 2 1

To my most excellent wife Pauline, my dear daughter Janice,
and my Zin-Jin

CONTENTS

PREFACE

Since the publication of the second edition of *Radiation Therapy for Head and Neck Neoplasms* in 1990, radiation therapy for these diseases of the head and neck has undergone significant changes in the treatment techniques, use of modalities, and concepts of management of early and advanced tumors. The need for a new edition was inevitable.

This book presents new information, treatment diagrams, techniques, and up-to-date data regarding treatment results. Since the data on accelerated hyperfractionated radiation therapy for head and neck tumors have matured, results of treatment with this approach are presented in detail and compared with conventional once-daily radiation therapy. Most of these data have not been published elsewhere.

I wish to thank my professional and technical associates, who have provided me with frequent discussions on the management of these tumors. Special thanks are due to Jimmy Efird, who set up the head and neck database program, and Patricia Martins, who performed the statistical analysis for this book. The secretarial assistance provided by Claire Hunt and Jeannine Park is greatly appreciated. The treatment plans, isodose distribution, and diagrams from Karen Doppke and her assistants are gratefully acknowledged. The medical artwork provided by Bob Galla and the photographic prints by Kathy Grady and her assistants are deeply appreciated. My close affiliation with Dr. Herman Suit and Dr. Edward Epp in the Department of Radiation Oncology made preparation of this edition possible and less painful. Any errors in this text are my own. Finally, my gratitude goes to the staff at John Wiley & Sons for their cooperation in undertaking this project.

C. C. WANG, M.D.

Boston, Massachusetts
August 1996

CHAPTER 1

BASIC CONCEPTS OF RADIATION THERAPY FOR HEAD AND NECK CANCER

Cancer of the head and neck constitutes a major anatomic group of tumors with respect to morbidity and mortality. In the United States approximately 53,650 new patients were diagnosed in 1995[1] or 4.3% of all newly diagnosed cases annually. Of these, 13,490 patients or 25% inflicted with mortalities.

Malignant tumors originating from the upper aerodigestive tract are predominantly squamous cell carcinoma of varying degrees of differentiation. They constitute approximately 85% of the head and neck malignancies, and the remaining 15% are tumors of the salivary gland, thyroid gland, and lymph nodes, and bone and soft tissue sarcomas.

Squamous cell carcinomas of the head and neck commonly are the diseases of middle and old age, occurring especially in patients having long-standing habits of cigarette smoking, alcoholism, and poor oral hygiene. Males are more often involved, although the incidence of female patients is rapidly increasing due to change in the life-style of American women.

Evaluation of the extent of the lesion prior to decision-making for treatment is extremely important, including careful inspection and palpation of the primary site and neck areas whenever possible. Indirect laryngoscopy and fiberoptic endoscopy are highly informative in assessing the extent of the tumor of the pharynx, larynx, and nasopharynx as well as the mobility of the involved parts. Direct laryngoscopy and multiple biopsies to define mucosal and submucosal extension of tumor and/or to rule out a second primary cancer should be carried out prior to any definitive therapeutic program. Appropriate radiographic examinations, for example, soft tissue films of the lateral pharynx or larynx, nasopharynx, and base of tongue, are extremely useful in identifying various anatomic structures, shown in Figure 1.1, and to assess the extent of the lesions. In certain tumor sites, computed tomography (CT) and magnetic resonance (MR) scans have been found

1

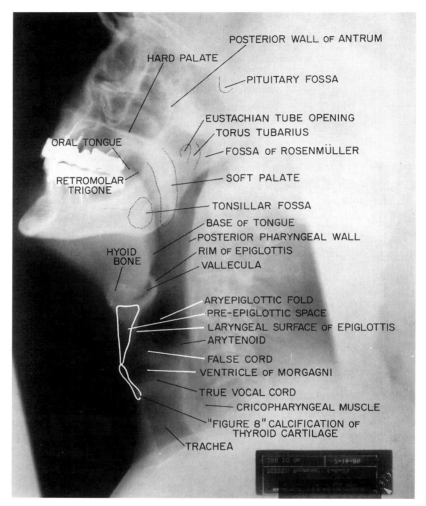

FIGURE 1.1   Radiograph of lateral neck showing various anatomic structures and their locations, useful to the radiation oncologist for placement of treatment portals.

necessary in obtaining information such as bone and muscle invasion, which otherwise may not be shown by conventional radiography. As part of the medical work-up, a general physical examination, chest radiographs, and a basic liver profile are necessary to assess the medical condition of the patient. Since hemoglobin level may affect local control of head and neck tumors,[2,3] anemia found to be present should be corrected.

Carcinomas arising from various anatomic sites of the head and neck, such as the oral cavity, oropharynx, hypopharynx, larynx, nasopharynx, nasal cavity and paranasal sinuses, and salivary gland, possess different tumor characteristics. Each has its own natural history, different biological behavior, and separate mode of tumor growth and spread. The therapeutic management and results may differ greatly.

A variety of therapeutic measures are available for the management of cancers of the head and neck. These include surgery, radiation therapy, and chemotherapy. The choice of treatment modalities depends on many factors such as (1) cell type and degree of differentiation, (2) site and extent of the primary lesion, (3) metastatic nodal status, (4) gross characteristics of the tumor (i.e., exophytic, superficial versus endophytic, infiltrative), (5) presence or absence and extent of bone and muscle involvement, (6) the possibility of preservation of speech and/or swallowing mechanisms, (7) the physical condition, social status, and occupation of the patient, (8) the experience and skill of both the surgeon and radiation oncologist, and (9) last, but not least, the cooperation and wishes of the afflicted, the patient.

COMBINED THERAPIES

The Rationale

Radiobiologically, it is known that an approximately exponential relationship exists between the dose of ionizing radiations administered to a cell population and the surviving fraction of the cells.[4-7] Experimental studies have demonstrated that relatively low doses will inactivate a vast number of cells in a tumor. D_{37}, which is related to the dose required to reduce the surviving cell population to the original 37%, ranges from 1 to 2.5 Gy in most biological systems.[4,7,8] Other factors influencing cell survival include the ability to repair sublethal damage after radiation injury, the environment of oxygenation[9,10] or hypoxia, total dose and fraction size, and the quality of radiations. Clinical observation indicates that small microscopic aggregates of tumor cells, so-called subclinical disease, which cannot be palpated on physical examination and yet by previous experience are microscopically and histopathologically detectable, can be controlled by conventional once-daily radiation therapy with a dose of 45–50 Gy in 5 weeks in more than 90% of cases.[11,12] However, for grossly palpable tumors much higher doses, such as 60–70 Gy in 7 weeks, are required for inactivation or eradication of the entire cell population to maximize the possibility of local control. For large, extensive advanced tumors, a dose of 80–85 Gy is needed for local control; therefore radiation therapy is handicapped not only by excessive tumor cell population but also by the presence of a large number of radioresistant hypoxic cells.[13] In such situations, the radiation dose level often exceeds the limits of tolerance of the normal vasculoconnective tissues, thus resulting in radiation necrosis. Therefore eradication of an advanced, massive tumor by conventional or common once-daily radiation therapy is highly improbable.

Surgery and radiation therapy are presently known to be effective in eradicating cancers of the head and neck region. Each of these modalities has its own merits, indications, and limitations. Radiation therapy has the advantage of being able to control the disease in situ, thus avoiding removal of a useful and necessary part as well as preserving speech and/or swallowing functions. Therefore radiation therapy must be considered as the best "tissue- and organ-sparing procedure" presently available and, in certain lesions, particularly the early tumors, is the procedure of choice. On the other hand, for certain early lesions situated in less cosmetically strategic locations, surgery can be carried out expediently and effectively without functional and cosmetic mutilation and is therefore preferred.

The cure rates for advanced squamous cell carcinoma are less than satisfactory, whether treated by radiation therapy or surgery alone. In these extensive lesions, failures from surgical treatment are usually the result of marginal recurrences, and failures from radiation therapy are primarily due to inability to control either the tumor core at the primary site or the nodal disease, and these central tumor cells are hypoxic and are resistant to radiations.[13]

Based on the presently available radiobiologic knowledge and the mechanisms of treatment failures, the major strength of radiation therapy is to eradicate the radiosensitive, actively growing, well nourished and oxygenated cells in the periphery of the tumor, or the subclinical disease implanted in the wound or in the lymph nodes. The strength of surgery, on the other hand, is to remove the central tumor core containing radioresistant hypoxic cells. Therefore for the advanced, extensive carcinomas, which are rarely curable by either method alone, the logical approach is a combination of radiation therapy and surgery.[14]

There are two basic approaches to combined therapies: preoperative and postoperative radiation therapy.

Preoperative Radiation Therapy

The aims of preoperative radiotherapy are to prevent marginal recurrences and wound implant, to control subclinical disease at the primary site or in the nodes, or to convert technically inoperable tumors into operable ones. Theoretically, preoperative radiation therapy performed with the cancer cells in their maximum stage of oxygenation possesses a possible advantage over irradiation in the postoperative hypoxic condition. This form of combined approach has been found to decrease both local recurrence and the incidence of distant metastases.

The disadvantages of preoperative radiation therapy are obscuration of exact tumor extent at the time of surgery, delay of surgery, and an increase in postoperative complications. The dosage employed in the preoperative program is subcancericidal, consisting of 45 Gy in one month. This is followed in 3–4 weeks by radical surgery encompassing all possible areas of disease, as though radiation therapy has not been given. The program is applicable to operable and resectable medium-sized or advanced tumors with poor radiotherapeutic or surgical cure rates, including tumors of the oral cavity, oropharynx, and hypopharynx, and is not commonly associated with significant postoperative functional morbidity.

Postoperative Radiation Therapy

The theoretical advantage of postoperative radiation therapy is that a higher dose of radiation can be delivered according to the known sites of residual disease and the extent of pathologic involvement. The aim therefore is to eradicate residual cancer in the wound or in the neck nodes. The clinical indications for postoperative radiation therapy consist of (1) positive or close tumor resection margins, (2) perineural tumor spread, (3) extensive primary tumor, and (4) more than three positive nodes and/or extracapsular spread.[15,16,17]

The procedure usually is carried out approximately 3–4 weeks after surgery, when the wound is healed. A dose of 55–60 Gy in 5–6 weeks[18] generally is given if the surgery is radical in extent. On the other hand, if the surgery is primarily a de-bulking procedure, higher-dose radiation therapy for gross residual disease must be given, that is, 65–70 Gy in 7 weeks.

Whether radiation therapy should be used preoperatively or postoperatively has been the subject of a great deal of discussion. In certain tumors with exophytic component, good tumor response following a modest dose of preoperative radiation has encouraged additional irradiation for cure, thus eliminating the need for muti-lating surgical procedures. The decision therefore should be made individually, on the basis of personal preference and experience.

The randomized prospective and retrospective trial indicated better loco-regional control by postoperative radiation therapy as compared to preoperative radiation therapy. There was a higher incidence of distant metastases in the postoperative group; whether this finding is due to selection of the lesions or iatrogenic dissemi-nation of unirradiated cancer cells at surgery is a matter of conjecture. The im-proved local control, however, did not translate into improved survival, due to the increased distant metastases and death from second primaries.[19,20,21]

In spite of such disappointing data, for the past 15 years, postoperative radiation therapy is often preferred at Massachusetts General Hospital (MGH) and Massa-chusetts Eye and Ear Infirmary (MEEI).

In order to improve loco-regional control for head and neck cancer in the post-operative setting, prospective trials of accelerated (BID) radiation therapy[23,23] indi-cated some improvement in local control of fast growing lesions as compared to conventional (QD) radiation therapy. A phase III prospective randomized trial is on-going.

Fractionated Radiation Therapy

Radiobiologically, the radiation effects produced by a single dose of x-rays or gamma rays are more pronounced than those produced by the same amount deliv-ered in divided daily fractionated doses over a longer period of time. The decreased response with reduced daily fraction sizes and prolonged treatment course is due to cell recovery and repair from sublethal damage occurring between radiation expo-sures,[24] somewhat fully often in 4–6 hours,[5,24] and accounts for most of the in-creased doses necessary with fractionated radiation therapy. Repair of sublethal damage is less pronounced in densely ionizing radiations such as neutrons. The shoulder of the cell survival curve is therefore duplicated (at least in part) at each fraction. This type of recovery or sublethal repair occurs predominantly in oxygenated normal tissues, both acute and late responding tissues, and is possibly less marked or absent in some chronically hypoxic tumor cells.[25]

After radiation injuries, the regenerative process is followed by the resumption of mitotic activity of normal cells and repopulation of the stem cells.[26] The malignant cells may exhibit similar regenerative capability but it is less than normal oxygenated cells. Fractionation therefore spares normal cells and results in more damage to tumor cell population from radiations. During fractionation and protraction of radiation therapy, the radiosensitive oxygenated cancer cells are destroyed with subsequent reduction of tumor size and the radioresistant hypoxic cells, originally distant from functional vasculature, will become closer to the blood supply and become reoxygenated and therefore radiosensitive. The result is a transfer of hypoxic cells to a more oxygenated compartment and the overall radiosensitivity and radiocurability of the entire tumor are enhanced, leading to eventual complete sterilization of the entire tumor without significant injury to the adjacent normal tissues. This concept is routinely applied to daily clinical radiation therapy.

The altered fractionated radiation therapy given twice (BID) or three times daily (TID) is based on the concepts of differential repair of sublethal damage between normal and cancerous tissues. It is a novel approach, with considerable promise, used for the past 15–20 years in the treatment of advanced carcinoma of the head and neck. For detailed information see Chapter 4 on the Principles and Practice of Altered Fractionation Radiation Therapy.

Shrinking Field and Mixed Beam Therapy

It is generally recognized that the larger the tumor mass, the larger the radiation therapy portals required and the lower the total dose that can be tolerated, with subsequently lower tumor control. The peripheral subclinical microscopic tumor masses can be controlled by a relatively lower dose of radiation, that is, 50 Gy in 5 weeks. After this dose level is reached, with shrinkage of the oxygenated elements, the residual macroscopic mass can be irradiated with reduced fields at higher dose level without undue damage to the adjacent normal tissues. The initial radiation therapy portals therefore always include the gross tumor mass with generous margins and its microscopic extension. After 50 Gy, the treatment portal is reduced only to include the gross tumor with smaller margins, on the assumption that the peripheral microscopic subclinical disease is controlled, and the total dose is carried to 65–70 Gy.

If the residual tumor remains large, an additional boost of radiation therapy is given through further field reduction to a total of 70–75 Gy if needed. Frequently, during the entire treatment course, repeated field reductions are made in order to spare the peripheral tissues; and radiation therapy is administered through multiple portals of entry and/or with interstitial or cone down boost techniques. In some instances, surgical excision of the residual disease (i.e., nidusectomy) is carried out,

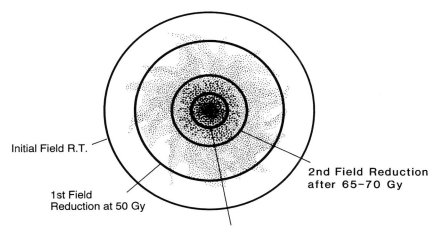

Initial Field R.T.

1st Field
Reduction at 50 Gy

2nd Field Reduction
after 65–70 Gy

Final Boost to 75–80 Gy or Nidusectomy

FIGURE 1.2   Diagram showing shrinking field radiation therapy with various components of a solid tumor with microscopic disease at the periphery requiring 50 Gy in 5 weeks for eradication; gross disease requiring 65–70 Gy; and residual disease treated by nidusectomy or highest dose by interstitial implant or intraoral cone.

being considered as a surgical boost. This concept, diagrammed in Figure 1.2, is routinely applied in the treatment of most head and neck cancers with improved local tumor control and decrease in complications.

With the availability of a variety of radiation equipment, various photon and electron energies may be applied for radiation therapy of a single tumor, for example, 10 MV and 4 MV photons or 9–18 MV electrons. Commonly, a combined approach employing photons and electrons is used in order to deliver maximal dose to the tumor with minimal radiation complications.

Therapeutic Ratio

The probability of tumor control and probability of normal tissue complications versus radiation dose are both related by a sigmoid curve, but with different slopes. The relative position of these curves or their differential is termed *therapeutic ratio*.[27] This ratio is the foundation of clinical radiation oncology and determines whether any particular tumor related to the adjacent normal tissue or tumor bed can be treated easily, with difficulty, or not at all. As the tumor control probability curve is located further to the left of that for normal tissue complications, there is increased or favorable therapeutic ratio. To the contrary, any tumors with control probability curve situated to the right of the normal tissue complications curve have negative therapeutic ratio and are rarely treatable by radiation therapy alone with success. All therapeutic techniques must exploit this differential between tumor control and normal tissue complications versus dose. No improved therapeutic results can be expected by shifting both sigmoid curves in the same direction and to the same degree. Methods of increasing tumor control probability without affecting normal tissue complication probability are urgently needed to achieve further therapeutic gain.

In clinical practice, the level of total dose to any particular tumor and anatomic site must be scrutinized carefully. Generally, the incidence of tumor control probability is increased with increase in dose. The level of maximum limit of dose increases is closely related to the incidence of late radiation complications, as shown in Figure 1.3. Dose A is associated with a 90% probability of local tumor control and a 5% probability of complications. A further small increase of dose (from A to B) is accompanied by much higher complications, that is, 50%, and yet the percentage of local control is not proportionately increased. This concept is supported by published clinical observations, which indicate that the dose–response curve is very shallow in the range of 70–75 Gy.[30] Therefore the definition of an "optimum" tumor control dose is different for each individual radiation oncologist. Only by his/her clinical experience and expertise can a valid judgment be made as to what dose level and normal tissue complication are acceptable in return for improved probability of tumor control—that is, the reward/risk ratio. In certain instances, the increased risk of complications such as transverse myelitis or temporal bone necrosis is totally unacceptable and should be avoided. On the other hand, the risks of soft tissue necrosis, osteoradionecrosis of the mandible, or radiation pneumonitis of limited extent, which can be corrected by surgery or are relatively asymptomatic, are worth taking if significant tumor control can be achieved with higher doses of radiation therapy.

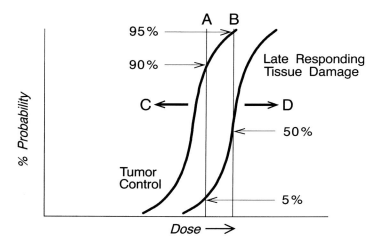

FIGURE 1.3 Definition of optimal tumor control dose. (A) shows 90% tumor control probability and 5% complications. With further increase of dose, tumor control probability is increased to 95% (5% improvement) with 50% complications. (B) Methods to shift tumor control curve to the left (C) or complication curve to the right (D) may improve the therapeutic ratio.

RADIATION DOSES, FRACTIONS, AND COMPLICATIONS

Time–Dose–Fraction (TDF) Concept

The biologic effects for tumor control and radiation injuries of the adjacent normal tissues are closely related to the total dose of radiations, total treatment time, dose per fraction per day, and the number of daily fractions.[28,29] It is the tolerance of the vasculoconnective tissues of the tumor bed that determines the success or failure of radiation therapy. Ellis[30] proposed the tolerance dose of normal tissue related to the overall treatment time and number of fractions. This expression of dose of the normal tissue tolerance is known as nominal standard dose (NSD) in RET.[30] Similarly, by using the time–dose–fractionation (TDF) factor, a value of the isobioeffect dose can be calculated and the results of these expressions can be used to compare various radiation therapy schemes.[29] There are published tables or nomograms to estimate doses that yield comparable radiobiologic response. These isobioeffect values are being refined and modified so as to employ exponents more appropriate to the normal tissue of concern.

The published tables of TDF values, for instance, should not be used to estimate the tolerance of central nervous system (CNS) tissues. Likewise, large daily fractions delivered 3 or 4 days a week even with identical TDF may result in serious complications. This is due to dissociation of acute and late effects from large fraction size. Various mathematical formulas are available for clinicians.[29,30,31,32] These can only be used as a general guideline for the acute responding tissue, such as the tumors for conventional radiation therapy. For the late responding tissues and CNS tissues or large daily fractions, or identical NSD or TDF, the results may vary greatly with severe late complications.

It is therefore important to recognize the limitations of NSD or TDF isoeffect formulas, which must be used only as guidelines, not rules, for treatment planning for normal tissue tolerance involving small deviation from established practice, that is, 1.8–2 Gy per fraction.

In daily radiation practice, combined external beam radiation therapy and interstitial or intracavitary implant are commonly carried out. In such instances, combined TDF values may be calculated,[9] which are useful to the experienced clinician who has a clear understanding of the limitations of the isobioeffect formulations. The TDF values for twice-daily radiation therapy have not been worked out satisfactorily.

The radiation dosage is determined by the tumor site, size of the lesion, irradiated volume, number of fractions of treatment, fraction size, and total time, as well as by the various techniques of radiation delivery and also by the patient's tolerance and the tumor's response. In general, a dose of 50–55 Gy in 5–6 weeks is considered adequate for sterilization of microscopic or occult disease[13] and 65–70 Gy in 7 weeks for control of gross squamous cell carcinoma. Such a dosage is usually given initially as 45 Gy wide field comprehensive irradiation, including the primary lesion and the first echelon regional nodal drainage areas for overt or occult metastases. A further dose to the primary site is given by reduced portal toward completion.

For the highest level of local control, radiation complications may occur in a small percentage of patients treated by curative radiation therapy. If one is unduly concerned with complications at all times, the radiation oncologist may timidly reduce the dose level and this, in turn, could result in decrease of local control and patient survival. However, frequent and repeated occurrences of severe complications (i.e., greater than 10%) are not regarded as good radiation therapy and should prompt review of dose calculations, treatment policy, and radiation techniques and modalities. Not infrequently, severe complications are the result of an unrealistic and unjustifiable enthusiasm on the part of the radiation oncologist to treat a biologically radioinsensitive tumor too vigorously or to retreat recurrences in previously irradiated areas with high radiation doses.

In clinical radiation therapy, the fraction size is related to late complications and must be scrutinized carefully during the entire treatment course. For a standard radiation therapy program for patients with curable tumors or patients with incurable tumors but with the prospect of prolonged survival, fractions of 2.5–3 Gy per daily treatment should not be exceeded due to the high likelihood of late complications in long-term survivors. A larger fraction size, that is, from 2 to 2.5 Gy per fraction per day, delivered to the optic nerve or chiasm may significantly increase the incidence of optic neuropathy. Likewise, the treatment of head and neck tumors, such as oropharyngeal carcinoma, with large fraction size, that is, 3–4 Gy per fraction per day and/or reduced number of fractions from 5 to 4 per week with the same total dose achieved by increasing fraction sizes, results in marked increase in late complications such as severe subcutaneous fibrosis, skin necrosis, or osteoradionecrosis of the mandible.[30] The exception to this rule is the treatment of small cancers of the skin (1–2 cm in diameter) for which a daily fraction of 5 or 9 Gy is a common practice in our institution.

Radiation Dose Determination

Epithelial Malignancies   For squamous cell carcinomas or adenocarcinomas, the "conventional" radiation therapy program consists of daily fractions of 1.8–2 Gy per fraction, 5 fractions per week for a total dose of approximately 65–66 Gy in 6.5–7 weeks. For certain tumor sites, higher dosages are required; for example, the dose for a nasopharynx site would be 70–72 Gy; for oral tongue and base of tongue, 72–75 Gy; for skin and lip, 60 Gy in 4 weeks or the isobiological equivalent (TDF value = 115–120). For subclinical disease, a dose of 50–55 Gy in 5–6 weeks is used.

Nonepithelial Tumors   Lymphomas and myelomas are occasionally seen in the head and neck area. The doses for these tumors generally are modest, ranging between 45 and 50 Gy with a conventional fractionation scheme. For gross mesenchymal tumors, higher doses are required, that is, 70–75 Gy in 6–7 weeks.

Importance of Daily Multifield Treatment

The biologic effects and radiation injuries to the adjacent normal tissues from radiation therapy of deep-seated tumors are well recognized. When parallel opposing portals or a wedge pair technique is used, it is important that all fields are treated every day.[33] This is particularly true for patients with field separation greater than 15 cm when treated by low megavoltage radiations. Severe subcutaneous fibrosis and/or greater injury to the superficial peripheral normal tissue may result from the higher isobioeffect due to increase of physical and isobiological doses with a single field alternate-day treatment than daily treatment of all fields. This phenomenon, designated *edge effect,* is magnified by treating 4 days or 3 days a week instead of 5 days a week due to the necessity of increased fraction size to deliver the same total weekly dose as the conventional 5-day fractions. On the contrary, for smaller field separation, less than 6 cm, for example, in carcinoma of the vocal cord, the isobioeffect between the midline tumor and the peripheral normal tissues is not significantly increased, and therefore it would not be absolutely necessary to treat all fields each day as in wider field separation.[34]

MANAGEMENT OF NECK NODAL DISEASE

The management of metastatic nodes in the neck from a primary arising from the head and neck region depends on the size and location of the primary, cell type, and number of nodes and bilaterality (N stage) and consists of surgery, irradiation, and a combination of both modalities. Radiation therapy is effective for controlling the small metastatic nodes (N1–2) or nodes less than 3 cm in diameter. Therefore the patient with clinically positive nodes should receive radiation therapy both to the primary site and the neck. If the metastatic nodes become nonpalpable after radiation therapy and this is confirmed by CT scans, careful follow-up without radical neck dissection (RND) is justified. On the other hand, if the metastatic nodes persist or reappear, therapeutic radical or functional neck dissection is carried out without jeopardizing the ultimate control of the disease and the survival of the patient. For the extensive nodal disease, N2A and N3 with advanced primary lesions arising from the oral cavity, hypopharynx, and larynx, a combination of radiation therapy and surgery is the treatment of choice, that is, preoperative radiation therapy with a dose of 60–65 Gy to both sides of the neck for any residual nodes 4–6 weeks to be followed by radical surgery. Such adjuvant radiation therapy is not only able to reduce the incidence of recurrent disease in the dissected neck but is also highly effective in preventing the development of nodal metastases in the contralateral neck. Thus the necessity for bilateral radical neck dissection can be eliminated. For inoperable metastatic nodes in the neck, high-dose radiation therapy is necessary for local control with a dose of 70–75 Gy, which may result in painful fibrosis of the neck.

The management of the N0 neck is controversial. In patients with advanced primary lesions with high risk of occult metastases, elective neck treatment should be considered. Elective radical neck dissection (RND) is effective in controlling ipsilateral neck disease. Experience indicates that over one-half of the resected specimens failed to show tumors in the nodes. Another option is delayed therapeutic RND after clinical appearance of nodes. Comparative analysis of results of an elective RND group with microscopic positive nodes and a delayed RND group indicates no significant difference in disease-free survival between these two groups.[35] Thus the elective RND offers no real advantage over a careful watchful approach in most patients; however, it may be offered to patients in whom the nodes are demonstrated on CT scan of the neck[38] or to those patients with aggressive tumors who can not be relied on to observe a regimen of frequent and thorough follow-up examinations. On the other hand, studies by Fletcher[36] and others indicate that 50–55 Gy in 5 weeks is effective in controlling 90% of occult metastases. These results would further argue against the routine use of elective RND (i.e., radical or functional neck dissection) for the N0 neck, and elective irradiation should provide a viable option in managing patients with N0 neck.

In general, primary tumors arising from various anatomic sites present different risks of occult metastases in patients with N0 neck. Likewise, different cell types carry various risk factors; for example, poorly differentiated, lymphoepithelioma cell types have a higher incidence of occult metastases as compared to the well differentiated or verrucous carcinomas. The management of N0 neck should be made according to the various risk factors of the lesions as follows:

1. *High-Risk Group (>50%)*. Includes T1–3 lesions of Waldeyer's ring, that is, nasopharynx, tonsil, base of tongue, and hypopharynx; T3 lesions of the supraglottis; and all T3–4 lesions of the oral cavity.
2. *Intermediate-Risk Group (20–30%)*. Includes T1–2 lesions of the supraglottic larynx and oral tongue, and T2 lesions of the soft palate, floor of mouth (FOM), buccal mucosa, gingival ridge, hard palate, and pharyngeal wall.
3. *Low-Risk Group (<15%)*. Includes T1 lesions of the FOM, buccal mucosa, gingival ridge, hard palate, glottis, paranasal sinuses, nasal cavity, salivary gland, skin, and temporal bone.

Metastatic squamous cell carcinomas generally follow orderly and predictable patterns.[37] The well lateralized lesions generally spread to the ipsilateral neck nodes; the midline lesions may spread to both sides and contralateral side of the neck. The involvement of the posterior cervical triangle by metastases is uncommon and usually seen in patients with carcinomas arising from Waldeyer's ring, that is, nasopharyngeal, tonsil, and base of tongue carcinomas. With these exceptions, elective radiation therapy for the N0 neck routinely including the posterior cervical nodes is not indicated. Likewise, involvement of the submandibular and submental nodes by N0 pharyngeal and laryngeal carcinomas is most uncommon, and therefore these group of nodes should not be included in the elective radiation fields.

RECURRENCES AFTER PRIMARY RADIATION THERAPY

In radiation therapy as in surgery, the first choice of treatment must be the correct one. If the lesion recurs after radiation therapy, it may have acquired resistance to further irradiation because of impairment of local blood supply and/or formation of more radioresistant hypoxic cells usually due to changes in cellular component and increased fibrosis and other factors in or about the tumor. Consequently, with a few exceptions, after a full course of previous irradiation, re-irradiation generally is of little value and is less likely to be successful. If the lesion is operable, such recurrences would best be managed by surgical resection. Unfortunately, certain recurrences are often unresectable due to their strategic locations, such as the nasopharynx and posterior pharyngeal wall. Thus re-irradiation is looked upon as a last curative measure.[38]

When assessing the role of re-irradiation of carcinoma of the head and neck region, a distinction must be made between recurrent disease preceded by a period of local control, and overt persistent disease at the primary site following irradiation. Additional distinction must also be made between in-field recurrence and marginal recurrence. Experience has shown that re-irradiation for overt persistent cancer after radical radiation therapy is destined to failure and would make a bad matter worse. In-field recurrence or relapse after an elapsed period of freedom from disease may be either a true recurrence or a new primary. The distinction between these two is a subject of academic discussion and the management is exactly the same.

For successful re-irradiation for in-field recurrence, a detailed evaluation of the extent of the recurrence is mandatory, including complete physical examination, appropriate radiographs, and, in some instances, CT or MR scans and others. In general, the lesions must be small and superficial and/or those previously treated with low doses of irradiation. As a rule, the earlier the local recurrence is detected, the smaller the irradiated portal used, the higher the radiation dose that can be delivered, and the higher the cure rate and the lower the complication rate.

The radiotherapeutic techniques must carefully be planned to tailor-fit an individual lesion. Only high dose re-irradiation, that is, 60 Gy in 6 weeks, can result in satisfactory control of the disease and occasional cures. Intermediate doses, that is, 40 Gy or less, are ineffective in controlling local recurrence and often worthwhile palliation cannot be achieved.

Extensive in-field recurrences are rarely curable by re-irradiation. If the disease is not amenable to salvage surgery, chemotherapy may be used to slow down the neoplastic process; otherwise, symptomatic treatment and supportive care should be offered to the patient for a comfortable and useful life.

Small marginal recurrences may be re-irradiated by external beam or implant, for example, carcinomas of the eyelid or skin and small lesions of the oral cavity. Due to unavoidable overlapping with previous fields during re-irradiation, radiation ulcers may result. The small radiation ulcers may heal without lasting consequences or can be managed by excision.

Cervical nodal recurrence after a curative dose of radiation therapy should be dealt with by neck dissection if resectable. High-dose re-irradiation of cervical nodal recurrences may be possible and occasionally is curative, but the procedure frequently results in painful, wood-like fibrosis and therefore is ill advised.

CARE OF PATIENTS UNDERGOING RADIATION THERAPY

Before Radiation Therapy

After radiation therapy is elected, treatment should carefully be planned according to the nature, size, and location of the tumor, the volume of tissue to be encompassed, the normal organs to be spared, and the intent of treatment—curative or palliative. All work-ups should be complete, and the extent of the primary lesion and its nodal status should be known and staged. The patients must be apprised of the treatment, side effects, and potential complications and benefits from the proposed therapies. Other options, including surgery and chemotherapy, should also be explained. When the patient agrees to the proposed radiation therapy, an informed consent must be signed prior to initiation of radiation therapy.

During Radiation Therapy

While receiving radiation therapy, the patient should carefully be monitored as to extent of mucosal reaction and tumor regression. In lesions in the pharynx and larynx, indirect laryngoscopy should be done at least once weekly to assess tumor response and/or the development of edema of the laryngeal structures, and more often if complications are pending. Our experience has shown that examination of the oral cavity, oropharynx, and larynx after a dose of approximately 20 Gy in 2 weeks with 1.8–2 Gy per fraction may clearly delineate the true extent of the tumor by the development of tumoritis (Figure 1.4). This provides an opportunity to evaluate the superficial spread of the tumor and its margins. Such an earlier tumor reaction is due to the differential response to radiation between normal and pathologic tissues. Once the radiation dose reaches 40 Gy, the confluent mucositis and tumoritis make such distinction impossible.

Symptomatic mucosal reactions in the form of pain, sore throat, or dysphagia are often associated with treatment to the oropharynx and/or oral cavity. These may vary in degree and can be minimized by analgesics and topical anesthetics, such as 0.5–1.0% dyclonine hydrochloride (Dyclone) mouthwash, or by a small treatment break. Silver or gold fillings or dental appliances in the mouth emit secondary electrons when they are in the path of the external radiation beam. These contaminated electrons may produce pinpoint painful mucosal reaction to the adjacent tongue or buccal mucosa commonly described by patients as a "thumb-tack" pain. Such localized painful reaction can be lessened or eliminated by "capping" the teeth fillings with a sheet of 0.5 mm thick tinfoil, which will absorb the symptom-producing electrons from the metals before reaching the adjacent tongue or buccal mucosa during radiation exposure (Figure 1.5). Most of the exophytic component of the tumor and acute mucositis should regress at the end of the treatment course. Experience has shown that the last anatomic site of tumoritis often represents the origin of the tumor.

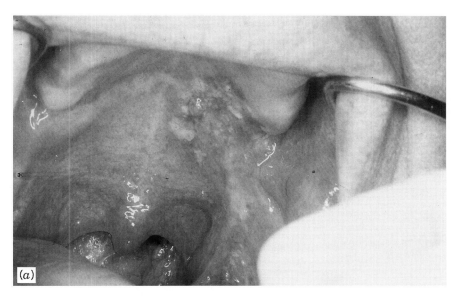

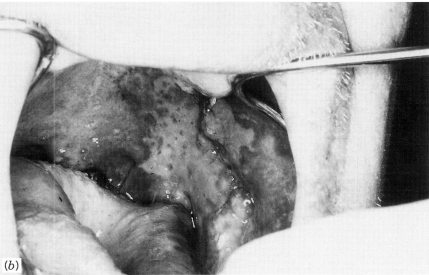

FIGURE 1.4   (a) Photograph of a seemingly small, limited carcinoma of the left retromolar trigone and palate before radiation therapy. (b) Photograph showing a much more extensive lesion demonstrated by the development of tumoritis after treatment with 21 Gy in 2 weeks.

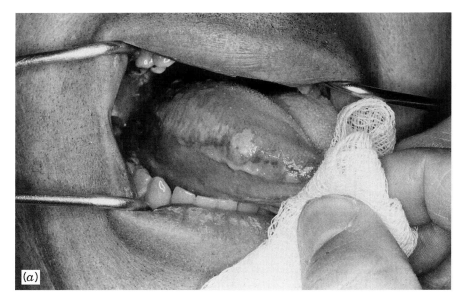

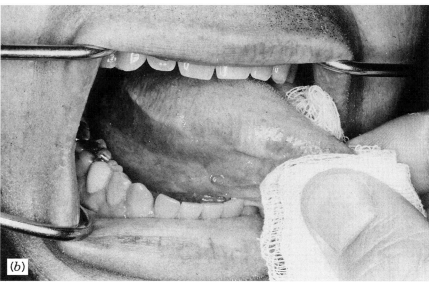

FIGURE 1.5 (a) Photograph of lateral border of tongue showing localized "pinpoint" mucositis from secondary electrons originating from the silver fillings in the teeth during irradiation. (b) Photograph showing subsidence of localized mucositis, after capping of the teeth with tinfoil, despite continuation of radiation therapy.

After Radiation Therapy

After the treatment is completed, patients should be followed regularly by both the radiation oncologist and the referral physician for evidence of residual disease, recurrence, and/or complications. The irradiated part should be smooth and pliable without tumefaction or ulceration. To simply biopsy the previous tumor site with a relatively normal anatomic part would invite complications and the yield is low. On the other hand, if residual tumor is suspected, it should be biopsied for tissue confirmation to be followed by appropriate treatment. Most patients with head and neck carcinoma must be followed regularly for a lifetime, due to the propensity for multiple primaries arising from the upper air and food passages.

REFERENCES

1. American Cancer Society: *CA Cancer J Clin* 1995;45:11–13.
2. Blitzer PH, Wang CC, Suit HD: Blood pressure and hemoglobin concentration: multivariate analysis of local control after irradiation for head and neck cancer. *Int J Radiat Oncol Biol Phys* 1984;10:98.
3. Overgaard J, Hansen HS, Jorgensen K, et al: Primary radiotherapy of larynx and cancer carcinoma: an analysis of some factors influencing local control and survival. *Int J Radiat Oncol Biol Phys* 1986;12:515–521.
4. Hewitt HB, Wilson CW: Survival curve for mammalian leukemia cells irradiated in vivo. *Br J Cancer* 1959;13:69–75.
5. Elkind MM, Whitmore GF: *The radiobiology of cultured mammalian cells.* New York: Gordon and Breach, 1967;7–143.
6. Fowler JF: Differences in survival curve shapes for formal multi-target and multi-hit models. *Phys Med Biol* 1964;9:177–188.
7. Puck TT, Marcus PI: Actions of x-rays on mammalian cells. *J Exp Med* 1956;103: 653–666.
8. Suit HD, Urano M: Radiation biology for radiation therapy. In: Wang CC, ed. *Clinical radiation oncology—indications, techniques and results.* Littleton, MA: PSG Inc, 1988.
9. Gray LH, Conger AD, Ebert M, et al: The concubation of oxygen dissolved in tissues at the time of irradiation as a factor in radiotherapy. *Br J Radiol* 1953;26:638–648.
10. Glassburn JR, Brady LW, Plenk HP: Hyperbaric oxygen in radiation therapy. *Cancer* 1977;39(suppl):751–765.
11. Fletcher GH: Elective irradiation of subclinical disease in cancers of the head and neck. *Cancer* 1972;29:1450–1454.
12. Fletcher GH: Lucy Wortham James lecture: subclinical disease. *Cancer* 1984;53: 1274–1284.
13. Thomlinson RH, Gray LH: The histological structure of some human lung cancers and the possible implications for radiotherapy. *Br J Cancer* 1955;9:539–549.
14. Powers WE, Palmer LA: Biologic basis of preoperative radiation treatment. *Am J Roentgenol* 1968;102:176–192.

15. Carter RL, Tanner NS, Clifford P, Shaw HJ: Perineural spread in squamous cell carcinoma of the head and neck: a clinicopathological study. *Clin Otolaryngol* 1979;4: 271–281.

16. Looser KJ, Shah JP, Strong EW: The significance of "positive" margins in surgically resected epidermoid carcinomas. *Head Neck Surg* 1978;1:107–111.

17. Johnson JT, Barnes EL, Myers EN, Schramm L, Borochovitz D, Sigler BA: The extracapsular spread of tumors in cervical node metastasis. *Arch Otolaryngol* 1981;107: 725–729.

18. Peters LJ, Ang KK: The role of altered fractionation in head and neck cancers. *Semin Radiat Oncol* 1992;2(3):180–194.

19. Kramer S, Gelber RD, Snow JB, Marcial VA, Lowry LD, Davis LW, Chandler R: Combined radiation therapy and surgery in the management of advanced head and neck cancer: final report of 73-03 of the radiation therapy oncology group. *Head Neck Surg* 1987;10:19–30.

20. Tupchong L, Scott CB, Blitzer PH, et al: Randomized study of preoperative versus postoperative radiation therapy in advanced head and neck carcinoma: long-term follow-up of RTOG study 73-03. *Int J Radiat Oncol Biol Phys* 1991;20:21–28.

21. Vandenbrouck C, Sancho H, Le Fur R: Results of randomized clinical trial of preoperative irradiation versus postoperative in treatment of tumors of the hypopharynx. *Cancer* 1977;39:1445–1449.

22. Awwad HK, Khafagy Y, Barsoum M, et al: Accelerated versus conventional fractionation in the postoperative irradiation of locally advanced head and neck cancer: influence of tumor proliferation. *Radiother Oncol* 1992;25:261–266.

23. Trotti A, Klotch D, Endicott J, Ridley M, Greenberg H: A prospective trial of accelerated radiotherapy in the postoperative treatment of high-risk squamous cell carcinoma of the head and neck. *Int J Radiat Oncol Biol Phys* 1993;26:13–21.

24. Elkind MM, Sutton-Gilbert H, Moses WB, et al: Sub-lethal and lethal radiation damage. *Nature* 1967;214:1088–1092.

25. Suit HD, Urano M: Repair of sublethal radiation injury in hypoxic cells of a C3H mouse mammary carcinoma. *Radiat Res* 1969;37:422–434.

26. Withers HR: The four "R's" of radiotherapy. In: Lett JT, Adler H, eds. *Advances in radiation biology,* vol 5. New York: Academic Press, 1975.

27. Paterson R: *The treatment of malignant disease by radiotherapy,* 2nd ed. Baltimore: Williams & Wilkins, 1963.

28. Goitein M: The computation of time, dose and fractionation factors for irregular treatment schedules. *Br J Radiol* 1974;47:665–669.

29. Orton CG, Ellis F: A simplification of the use of NSD concept in practical radiotherapy. *Br J Radiol* 1973;46:529–537.

30. Ellis F: Nominal standard dose and the RET. *Br J Radiol* 1971;44:101–108.

31. Goitein M: Review of parameters characterizing response of normal connective tissues to radiation. *Clin Radiol* 1976;27:389–404.

32. Ellis F: Dose-time and fractionation: a clinical hypothesis. *Clin Radiol* 1969;20:1–7.

33. Wilson CS, Hall EJ: On the advisability of treating all fields at each radiotherapy session. *Radiology* 1971;98:419.

34. Gitterman M, Littman P, Doppke K, et al: Rethinking the necessity of treating all fields in each radiotherapy session. *Radiology* 1975;117:419–424.

35. Khafif RA, Gelbfish GA, Tepper P, Attie JN: Elective radical neck dissection in epidermoid cancer of the head and neck cancer. A retrospective analysis of 853 cases of mouth, pharynx, and larynx cancer. *Cancer* 1991;67:67–71.

36. Fletcher, FH: Elective irradiation of subclinical disease in cancers of the head and neck. *Cancer* 1972,29:1450.

37. Friedman M, Shelton VK, Mafee M, Belity P, Grybauskas V, Skolnik E: Metastatic neck disease—evaluation by computed tomography. *Arch Otolaryngol* 1984;110:443–447.

38. Wang CC: Re-irradiation of recurrent nasopharyngeal carcinoma: treatment techniques and results. *Int J Radiat Oncol Biol Phys* 1987;413:953–956.

CHAPTER 2

TECHNICAL CONSIDERATIONS OF RADIATION THERAPY OF HEAD AND NECK TUMORS*

RADIOTHERAPEUTIC MODALITIES

Kilovoltage Radiations

Ionizing x-radiations of low penetration from 50 to 250 kV can be generated by relatively simple machines. Except for treatment of superficial tumors, such as cancers of the skin and eyelids and in selective instances through an intraoral cone (IOC) for superficial cancers of the oral cavity, these kilovoltage radiations have no place in the primary management of deep-seated head and neck tumors. As a matter of fact, the kilovoltage machines, except for the 50-kV Phillips contact skin unit, are no longer available in modern radiation oncology centers and their use is largely replaced by low megavoltage electron beam therapy.

Megavoltage X-Radiations or Photons

The commonly available megavoltage radiations used for the treatment of head and neck cancers are from a cobalt-60 machine. This device, though technically not an x-ray machine, is used in the same manner as a megavoltage x-ray machine. The radiations possess the physical advantages of skin- and bone-sparing properties of megavoltage radiations and yet deliver optimum irradiation to the primary site as well as to the cervical lymph nodes. It is therefore a practical machine for clinical radiation therapy for head and neck tumors; unfortunately, the machine is out of

*The author acknowledges contributions by Karen Doppke, M.S., and the staff of the Division of Biophysics, Department of Radiation Oncology, Massachusetts General Hospital.

vogue and is rapidly being replaced by 4–10 MV linear accelerators, commonly known as Clinac, which provide a compact source of x-rays in the range of 4–10 MV.

A characteristic feature of these high-energy radiations is an increase of depth dose in tissues, which is a function of the energy of the beam in terms of megavolts. As shown in Figure 2.1, with a percent depth dose normalized at 7.5 cm, the higher the energy of the photons, the better the depth dose and the lower the entrance skin dose. Figure 2.2 shows the build-up region for various energies of radiation; surface doses are low in the higher energy beam. Due to these physical features, with the energy at or above 4 MV, there are considerable skin- and node-sparing properties. Therefore, in using megavoltage radiation energies from 6 to 10 MV to irradiate head and neck tumors, there is a high risk of underdosing the superficial lesions and metastatic nodes. In order to correct this physical disadvantage, a beam "spoiler" may be placed between the patient and the collimator to bring the skin dose to levels comparable to that of cobalt-60 radiations[1] or a thin layer of bolus may be placed over the lesions.

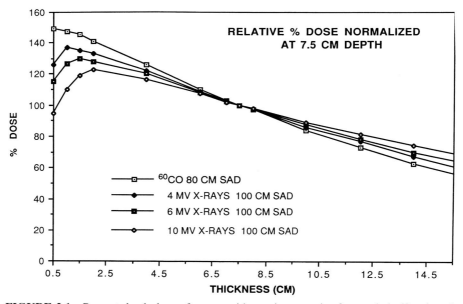

FIGURE 2.1   Percent depth dose of x-rays with varying energies from cobalt-60 unit and Clinac 4, 6, and 10 MV x-rays, 10×10 cm^2 portal. Note relative increase of percentage of dose at depth and decrease of entrance skin dose in higher energies.

With cobalt-60 or 4–6 MV x-rays, employing parallel opposing portals, the dose to the peripheral tissues is always higher than the midline dose, by approximately 8–10% if the field separation is greater than 15 cm, and 3–4% in lesser separation, as shown in Figure 2.3. Likewise, the width of the effective treatment beam (90–95% line) at the isocenter or within the target volume is affected by the sepa-

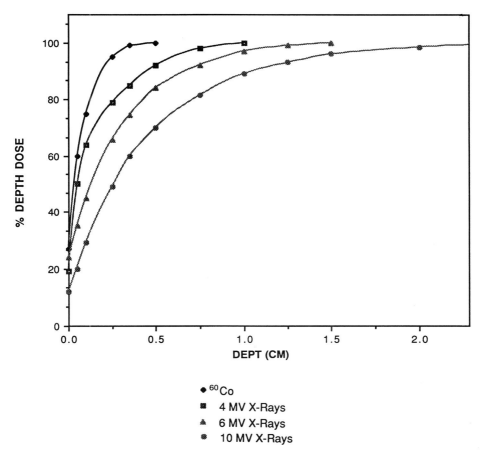

FIGURE 2.2   Diagram showing the doses in the build-up region for ^{60}Co, 4 MV x-rays, 6 MV x-rays, and 10 MV x-rays.

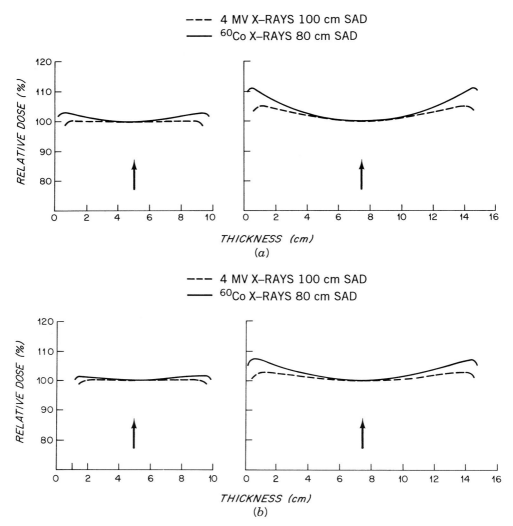

FIGURE 2.3   Diagrams showing central axis dose distribution in 10 cm and 15 cm separations irradiated through opposing lateral portal techniques. The peripheral dose is higher in ^{60}Co, 80 cm SAD radiation than 4 MV 100 cm SAD x-rays. (a) 5×5 cm^2. (b) 10×8 cm^2.

ration and the size of the photon beam portal; that is, the smaller the beam, the narrower the effective treatment beam at midplane ($D_{1/2}$). As shown in Figure 2.4a, in 15 cm separation with a collimator setting of 4 cm wide on 6 MV x-rays, the width of the 95% isodose beam at midline ($D_{1/2}$) is reduced to 2.8 cm and for 4 MV, it is reduced to 2.6 cm (Figure 2.4b). The difference is more exaggerated with the Theratron 780 Cobalt-60 unit, showing only 2.3 cm (Figure 2.4c).

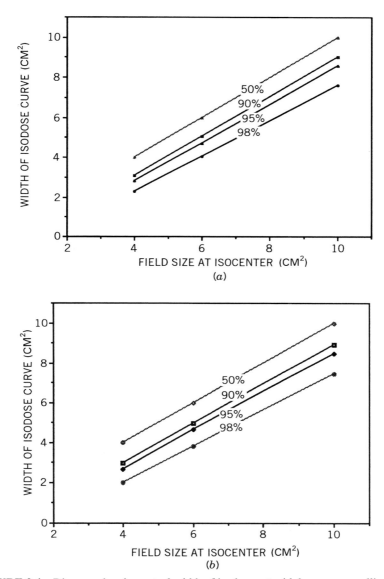

FIGURE 2.4 Diagram showing actual width of isodoses at midplane versus collimator setting with 15 cm separation through parallel opposing portals on 50%, 90%, 95%, and 98%
lines: (a) 6 MV x-rays, 100 cm SAD; (b) 4 MV x-rays, 100 cm SAD; and (c) Cobalt-60 unit,
80 cm SAD.

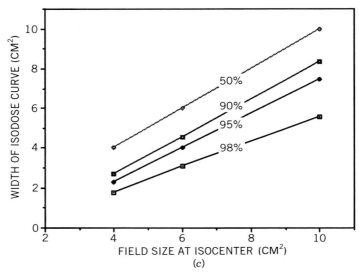

FIGURE 2.4 *Continued*

Other physical features to be considered are the shape and depth of the isodose distribution to the irradiated volume with wedge beam therapy. It is related to the hinge angles and the thickness of the wedges, field size, and so on. As shown in Figure 2.5a–c, 4 MV x-rays, 6×6 cm^2 and 100 cm SAD, the isodoses vary with the angle of the wedge from $30°–60°$ and the angle of wedge separation from $45°$ to $120°$.

During radiation therapy, normal tissues must be spared from the high-dose volume by shielding and shaped portals of high Z material, such as lead. The required thicknesses of lead or Cerrobend materials are shown in Table 2.1.

Megavoltage Electrons

Energetic electrons can be generated by a linear accelerator. The characteristics of an electron beam are rapid dose buildup and sharp dose fall-off, dependent on the specified energy applied. Thus the tissues or organs beyond the treatment volume receive relatively less radiation. Figure 2.6a shows the percent depth dose in phantom of various energies of electrons from 4 to 18 MV. The other feature of electrons is constriction of the isodose at depth, as shown in Figure 2.6b. The width constrictions of the 80% and 90% isodoses are related to various energies of the electron beam and are much narrower than the width indicated at the surface of entrance, shown in Figure 2.6c.

Electron beams can be shaped and shielded by high atomic weight materials such as lead. The selection of the thickness of the lead depends on the electron energies used, as shown in Table 2.2. As a general rule, for clinical application, it requires 0.5 mm of lead to reduce 1 MV. To protect normal tissues or organs from the electron beam, a piece of waxed lead can be sandwiched between the tumor and normal tissue, for example, behind the lip, buccal mucosa, or pinna of the ear.

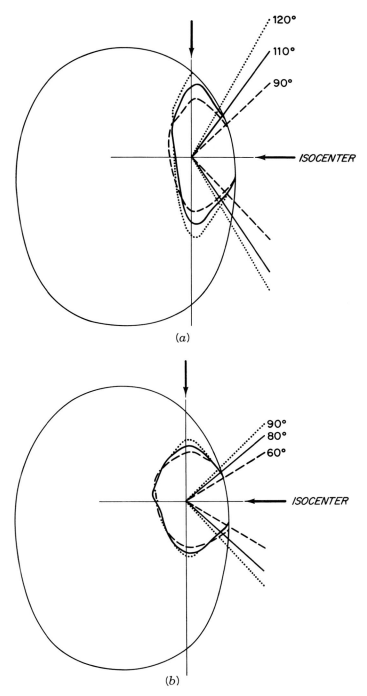

FIGURE 2.5 Diagram showing size and shapes of dose distribution (95% isodose) related to hinge angles and thicknesses of wedges with 4 MV x-rays: (a) 30° wedge, (b) 45° wedge, and (c) 60° wedge.

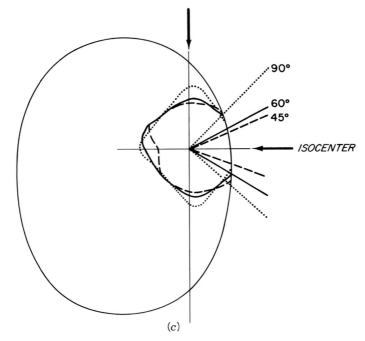

(c)

FIGURE 2.5 *Continued*

The dose to the skin from low-energy electrons can be quite small and can have some skin-sparing features. For treatment of cancer of the skin, for instance, it is necessary to "bolus" the lesions with at least 5 mm tissue equivalent material or more to obtain full equilibrium on the skin (Figure 2.7).

The air-containing organ or bone may affect the dose distribution of traversing electrons; thus the problem of dose inhomogeneity in heterogeneous tissue occurs. These effects must be taken into consideration in planning treatment using an electron beam for lesions lying within or behind a complex organ. For dose calculations, 1 cm of compact bone is equivalent to 1.65 cm of soft tissue.[2,3]

The relative biologic effectiveness (RBE) of electrons ranges from unity to below unity, that is, 0.85–0.90, as compared to cobalt-60 radiations.[3] Because the contribu-

TABLE 2.1 Thickness of Cerrobend Required to Attenuate the Photons of Various Energies to Approximately 5% of Incidence

Energy of Photons	Lead Thickness (cm)
^{60}Co	6.1
4 MV	7.3
6 MV	7.9
10 MV	8.5

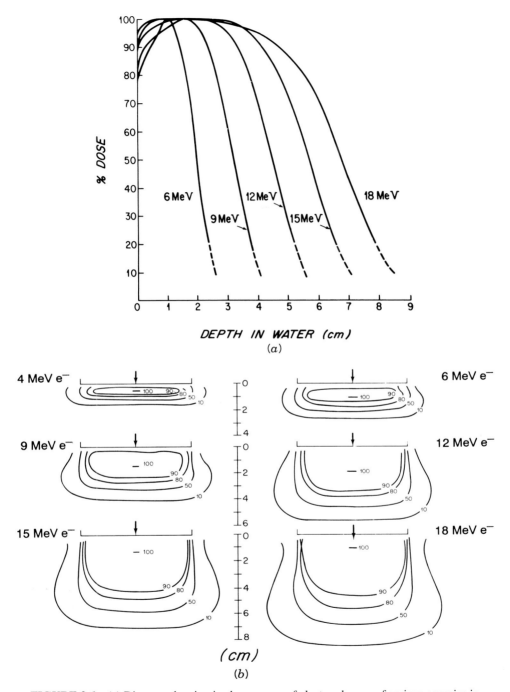

FIGURE 2.6 (a) Diagram showing isodose curves of electron beams of various energies in phantom. (b) Diagram showing constriction of isodose at depth with decreased width of therapeutic beam (electrons, 100 cm SSD, 8×8 cm^2 fields). (c) Diagrams showing constriction and reduction (80% and 90%) of the width of isodoses in comparison to electron beam entrance sizes; both are more marked in smaller fields.

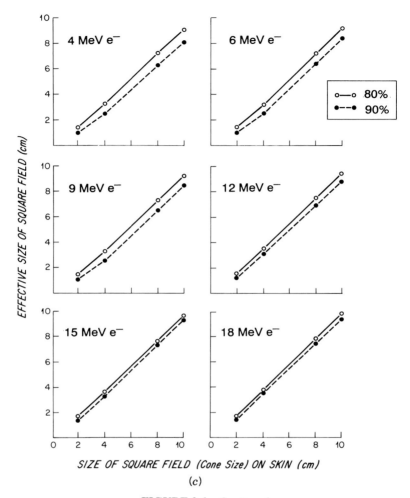

FIGURE 2.6   *Continued*

TABLE 2.2   Thickness of Lead Required to Attenuate the Electron Beam Energy to Approximately 5% of Incidence

Energy of Electrons (MeV)	Lead Thickness (mm)
6	2
9	4
12	5
15	6[a]
18	8[a]

[a]Add 7% photon contamination (machine specific).

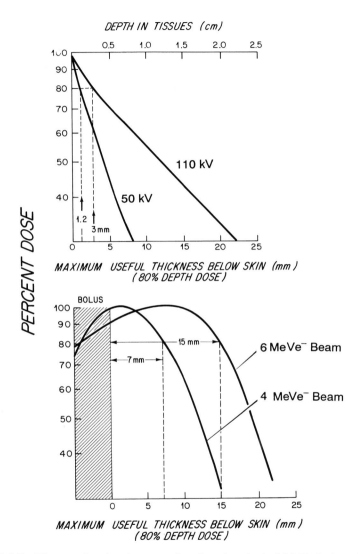

FIGURE 2.7   Diagram showing decrease of surface dose in 4–6 MeV electron. For radiation therapy of skin carcinoma, 5 mm of bolus is needed to create D$_{max}$ on the skin and tumor.

tion of electron beam dose in daily radiation therapy is only one-third or one-quarter of the total dose, the value of RBE as 1 (unity) is used in dose calculation.

The principal areas of clinical application of the electron beam include irradiation of lesions of the skin and lip and eccentrically located tumors 2–5 cm deep below the skin, such as the parotid gland, temporal bone, tracheal stoma, some intraoral lesions, and metastatic cervical nodes.[3] It is often used as a "boost" dose to tumors following external beam radiation therapy.[2] Commonly, 6–18 MeV electrons are used. When bilateral metastatic cervical nodes are treated simultaneously with a crossfiring technique, it is most important to determine the dose to the midline structures of the neck—namely, the spinal cord. In a relatively thin neck, higher energy electron beams from both sides of the neck may overdose the cervical cord unknowingly, due to summation of the "tails" of the beams. Figure 2.8 shows the dose to the midline structures (i.e., the spinal cord) related to the energies of the opposing electron beams impacting the neck.

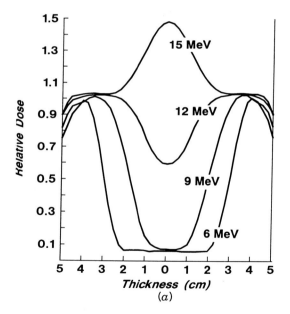

FIGURE 2.8 Composite electron beam dose at midline structures using opposed lateral technique versus energies of electrons in neck: (a) 10 cm in diameter.

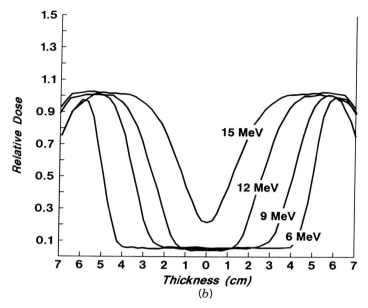

FIGURE 2.8 Composite electron beam dose at midline structures using opposed lateral technique versus energies of electrons in neck: (b) 14 cm in diameter.

Intraoral Cone (IOC) Electron Beam Radiation Therapy

The electron beam may be delivered per orally for treatment of oral cancers, sparing the lips or teeth and mandible, by adapting a specially made apparatus to the linear accelerator, as shown in Figure 2.9a. A detachable telescoping mirror (Figure 2.9b) is essential for visualization of the lesion and daily setup. A series of cones of various sizes and shapes (Figure 2.9c) are made to accommodate the various lesions of the oral cavity. Electron beam energies of 9–12 MeV are used.

For eccentrically situated lesions of the oral cavity, such as in the buccal mucosa, in which use of the IOC is not possible, en face electrons may be used, sparing the mandible as much as possible.

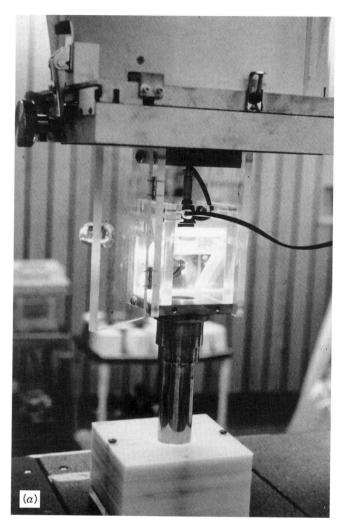

FIGURE 2.9   (a) Mechanical setup of IOC apparatus attached to Clinac 18 linear accelerator. (b) and (c) appear on the next page.

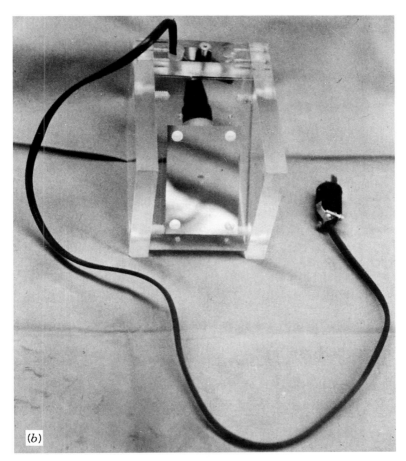

(b)

FIGURE 2.9 (b) Photograph showing detachable telescopic mirror placed between electron beam window and cone for visualization of lesions during setup.

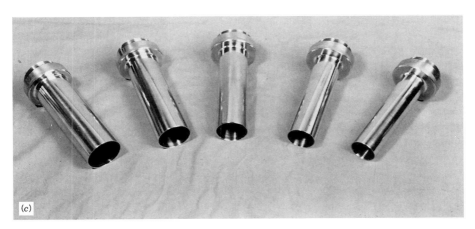

(c)

FIGURE 2.9 (c) Photograph showing a set of cones of various sizes and shapes for IOC irradiation.

Radioactive Isotopes

Radium-226 was an important gamma-ray source for brachytherapy of head and neck neoplasms. It has a half-life of approximately 1600 years and 1.65 MV gamma rays. Because of its relative rigidity and the highly energetic gamma rays, it possesses a few disadvantages, such as the necessity of "preload" techniques and the unnecessary radiation exposure to the therapy staff. Radium-226 is therefore no longer used and has been replaced by other isotopes, primarily iridium-192, which has a half-life of 74 days with 0.38 MV gamma rays. It is used primarily for interstitial implants. An afterloading technique using angiocaths and ^{192}Ir seeds[4] and/or hollow needles has been developed at the Massachusetts General Hospital (MGH), as shown in Figure 2.10, and found to be practical and satisfactory.

In the head and neck area the intracavitary implants are primarily used for treatment of carcinoma of the nasopharynx. Cesium-137 slugs with a half-life of 30 years and 0.66 MV gamma rays, afterloaded into pediatric endotracheal tubes, are used in lieu of radium sources.[5] This method also has been found satisfactory. (See Chapter 10 on Carcinoma of the Nasopharynx.)

For the past few years, a high dose rate (HDR) apparatus using a large amount of [192]Ir (i.e., 10 curies) has been available for use in a boosting proce-

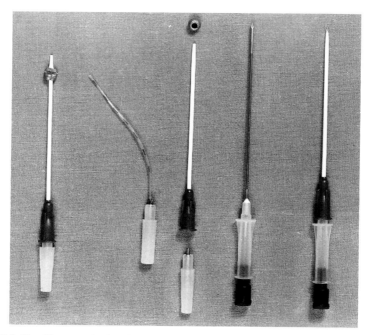

FIGURE 2.10   Photograph showing angiocatheters, lead shot, and ^{192}Ir seeds in plastic ribbon for interstitial implant.

dure in lieu of low dose rate sources; this apparatus has been found to be accept-able.

Radiation therapy delivered by interstitial implant with radioactive isotopes with a dose rate of 40–50 cGy per hour may be considered an approach to accelerated hyperfractionation. A total dose of approximately 70 Gy is thought of as a sum of numerous fractions of small fraction sizes. For a standard implant for squamous cell carcinoma, a daily dose of 10 Gy for 6–7 days is generally given and is well toler-ated. In spite of unavoidable inhomogeneity of dose distribution from the interstitial implant, the effects are generally minimal and the local control rates, as well as the cosmetic and functional results, are often superior to conventional once-a-day radia-tion therapy. In order to minimize the extent of the inhomogeneous dose distribution, interstitial implants are often done in combination with external beam irradiation.

GENERAL CONCEPT OF RADIOTHERAPEUTIC TECHNIQUES

Immobilization and Simulation

It is most important that the irradiated part be immobilized during radiation therapy. Many devices have been developed such as a face mask, cast, bite block, or tapes. With the availability of Thermoplastic, or Aquaplast, a face mask can readily be made and used for daily treatment setup. After the leveling of the face and neck, the face mask is made prior to simulation. Simulation is carried out with the mask in place, and the isocenter and portals are clearly marked on the mask for daily setup (Figure 2.11).

For immobilization of the tongue, a bite block is used, which is made of a cold-cured acrylic material and has a notched upper surface allowing placement of in-cisors and a smooth lower plate surface that sits flatly on the dorsum of the tongue. The specially made acrylic bite block offers reproducible treatment setup with con-sistent position of the tongue and separation of the mandible and maxilla; in addi-tion, it is disposable. When the bite block is used, a segment of the face mask is cut out to accommodate the block (Figure 2.12).

A treatment planning session with a simulator is necessary for precise localiza-tion of the tumor volume and target volume to be irradiated. If accessible, the extent of the tumor margins in the oral cavity and oropharynx are outlined by radio-opaque gold seeds and the neck nodes are outlined by lead wire. For most lesions of the head and neck, the patients are treated in the supine position with cross-tabletop photon or electron beams. For leveling of the head, the right and left tragi of the ears are used for reference. After the target volumes are localized isocentrically, the entrance and exit points of the portals on the skin are tattooed and radiographed for permanent record. The simulation radiographs are the "key" for daily treatment setup and future field modification. It is seldom necessary to simulate the head and neck patients more than once during the entire course of radiation therapy, except when oblique portals or marked changes of the treatment plans are needed. Contour making, Cerrobend shaped blocks, and computerized treatment plans are made prior to initiation of radiation therapy.

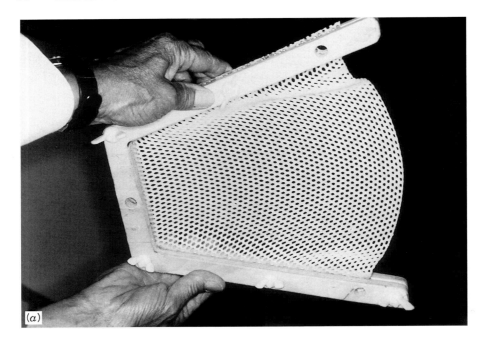

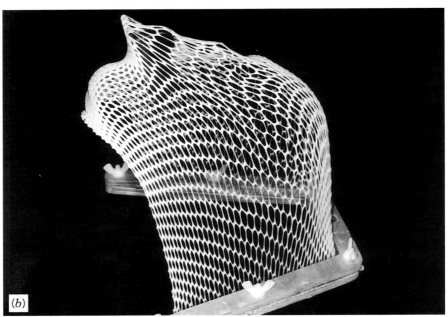

FIGURE 2.11   Photographs of face mask for immobilization. The Aquaplast is available commercially. (a) Sheet of material mounted on a frame, softened in water of 160°F and 2 mm in thickness. (b) It can be molded on patient's face instantly and a face mask made.

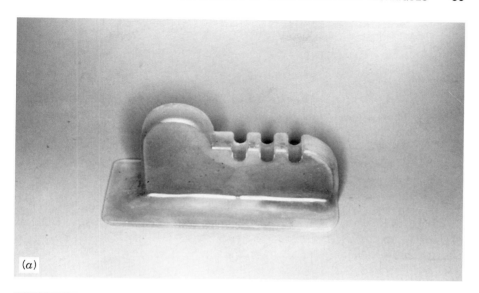

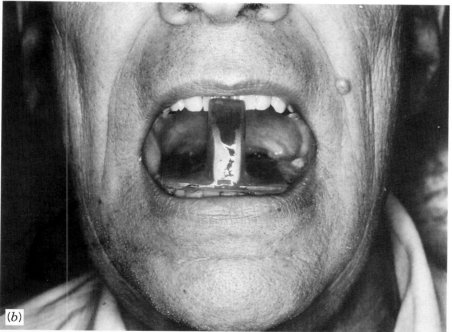

FIGURE 2.12   (a) Biteblock or tongue depressor. (b) Apparatus positioned in patient during irradiation.

BASIC TREATMENT PLANS

The radiotherapeutic techniques are determined by the location and extent of the lesion as well as by the cervical nodal status. In general, the basic treatment plans include (1) parallel opposing portals, (2) wedged parallel opposing and anterior portal three-field approach, (3) ipsilateral oblique wedge pair or AP and lateral wedge pair, (4) arc rotation, (5) intraoral cone or submental boost, and (6) interstitial or intracavitary implant. Frequently, two or more plans are used during the entire treatment course. A few treatment plans are shown below using 4 MV photon radiation.

Parallel Opposing Portal

This technique is commonly used for treatment of large lesions and/or midline lesions associated with bilateral lymph node metastases, such as carcinoma of the nasopharynx, soft palate, base of tongue, hypopharynx, and larynx among others. The distribution of radiation is relatively uniform throughout the en bloc irradiated volume but without specific localization. The primary and lymph nodes are irradiated by the same portals. This technique is frequently used up to 45 Gy to the midline structures, such as the nasopharynx, oropharynx, and larynx, and is followed by "off-cord" to 60–65 Gy. Additional doses are given to the primary lesions by boosting techniques to a final total dose of 70–72 Gy. In using this technique, care must be exercised to avoid overdosing the peripheral normal tissues (i.e., the mandible) or underdosing the target at the midline (Figure 2.13a).

For more localized lesions, a combination of two parallel opposing wedged and anterior portals may be used, showing isodose at midplane (Figure 2.13b) and eccentrically to one side (Figure 2.13c).

Ipsilateral Oblique Wedge Pair

This technique is often used as a major portion of radiation therapy for the eccentric lesions with low contralateral nodal metastases, that is, tumors of the parotid gland, orbit, and temporal bone, and eccentrically situated lesions of the oral cavity including the retromolar trigone, alveolar ridge, buccal mucosa, floor of mouth, or tonsil. It may also be used as a boost technique following parallel opposing portal irradiation.

The ipsilateral wedge pair technique consists of anterior and posterior oblique pairs (Figure 2.14a). If the lesions are more anteriorly situated (i.e., carcinoma of the retromolar trigone or alveolar ridge), a modified form of the wedge pair may be used, consisting of an ipsilateral and anterior wedge pair (Figure 2.14b).

A full course of radiation therapy for squamous cell carcinoma should not be given by the wedge pair technique alone because of the "hot spot" that may result in radiation complications from higher physical and biologic doses. Therefore a portion of the radiation therapy is often given by electrons or parallel opposing or arc rotation or IOC techniques to complete the treatment program. When combined parallel opposing portals and ipsilateral wedge pair techniques are used, a composite plan of the isodose distribution is necessary for evaluation of the final dose distribution within the irradiated volume.

POS: .00 cm T=1

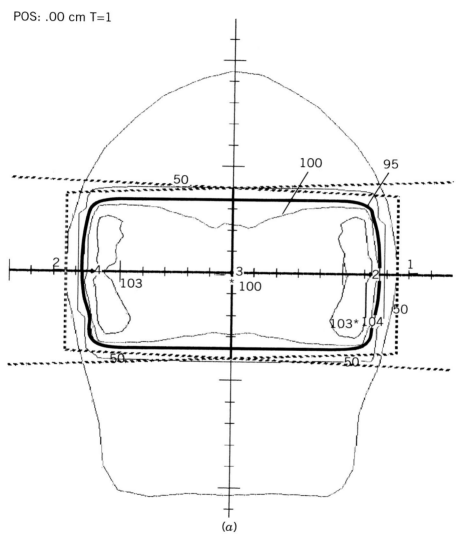

(a)

FIGURE 2.13   Representative treatment plans with various portals of entry and wedges suitable for treatment of various head and neck tumors with 4 MV radiation: (a) parallel opposing.

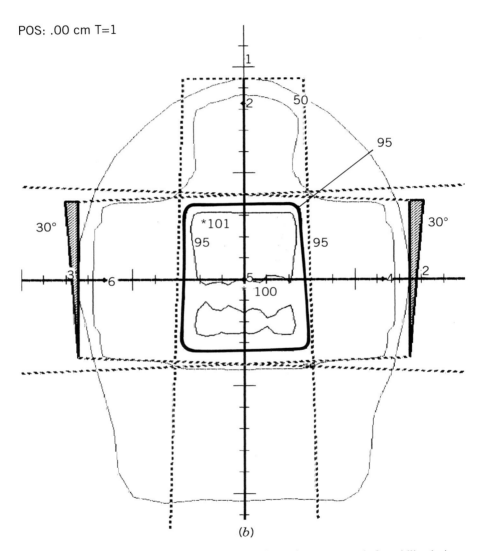

FIGURE 2.13 (b) Parallel opposing wedge and anterior open portals for midline lesion.

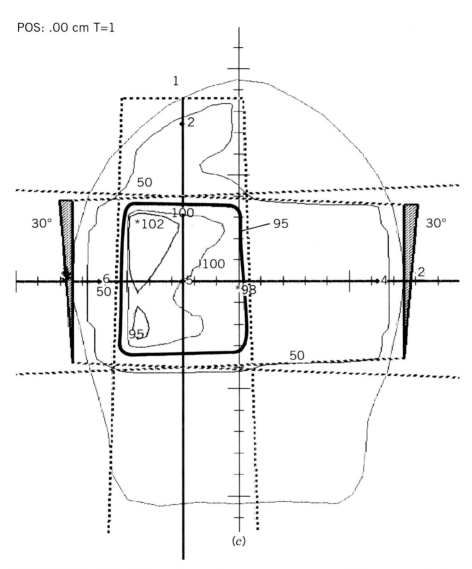

POS: .00 cm T=1

FIGURE 2.13   (c) Parallel opposing wedge and anterior open portals for eccentrically situated lesions suitable for retromolar trigone, faucial tonsil, and soft palate lesions.

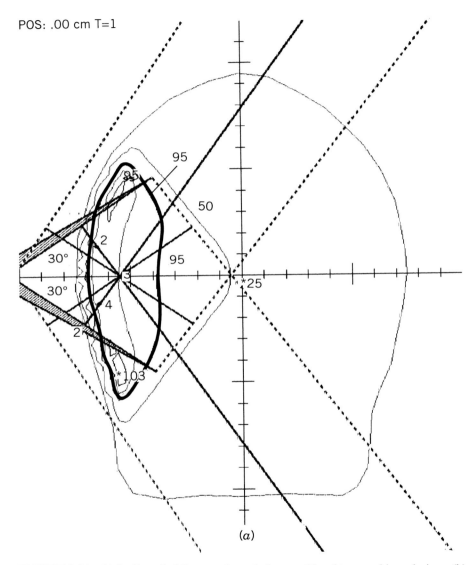

FIGURE 2.14   (a) Ipsilateral oblique wedge pair for parotid and temporal bone lesions. (b) Ipsilateral wedged and anteroposterior wedged pair portals for alveolar ridge, buccal mucosa lesions.

POS: .00 cm T=1

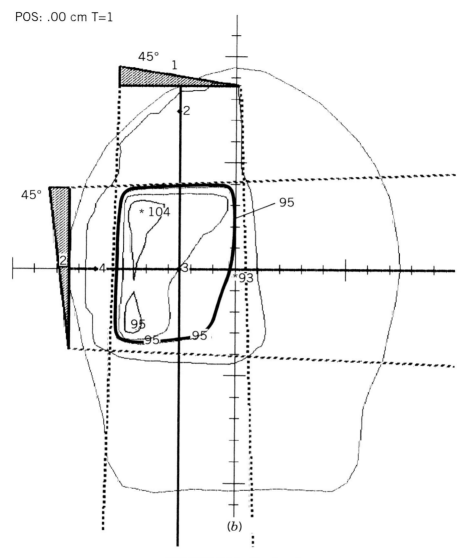

FIGURE 2.14 *Continued*

Rotation

With an isocentric machine rotation technique a 360° rotation or a 270° arc rotation may be achieved with or without wedges. It may be used as a primary method of radiation therapy or as a boost to the centrally situated primary lesions following parallel opposing or wedge pair portals, for example, carcinomas of the nasopharynx, soft palate, and uvula or pituitary tumors. For any rotational technique, sensitive organs such as the eyes must be excluded from the path of the radiation beam (Figure 2.15).

POS: .00 cm T=1

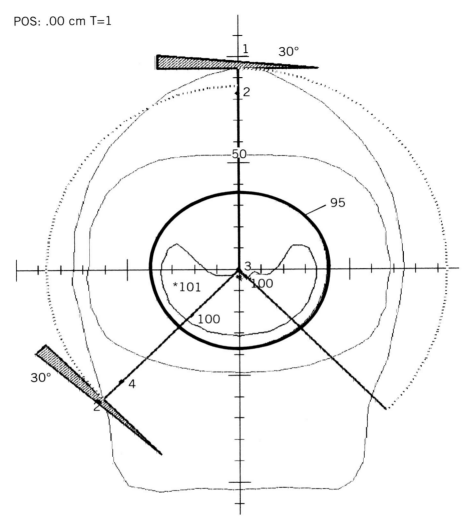

FIGURE 2.15   A 270° arc rotation with 30° wedge of lesions of the soft palate, nasopharynx, pituitary, and skull base.

Submental Boost Technique

This technique adds radiation to the primary site to a high dose without exceeding the tolerance of the mandible. It is used primarily for carcinoma of the base
of the tongue or faucial tonsil as shown in Figures 2.16a–c. For lesions inside
the mandibular arch of the oral cavity, in which use of the IOC is not possible,
electrons may be administered through the submental route, sparing the
mandible as much as possible, as a boosting procedure, as shown in Figure
2.16d on page 48.

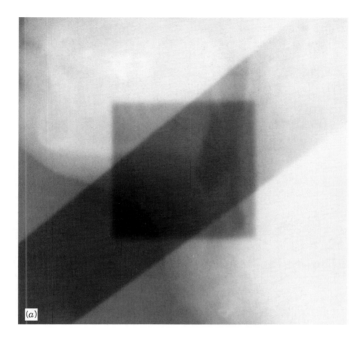

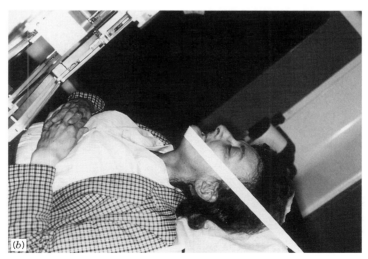

FIGURE 2.16   (a) Portal film showing submental photon boost in lateral projection, localizing the tumor volume. (b) Photograph showing patient receiving submental photon boost for base of the tongue or tonsil.

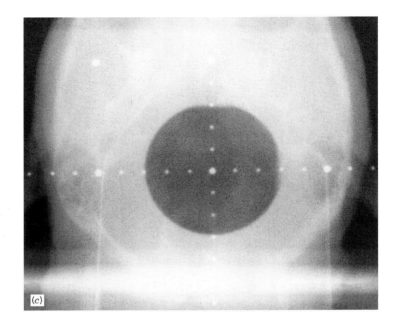

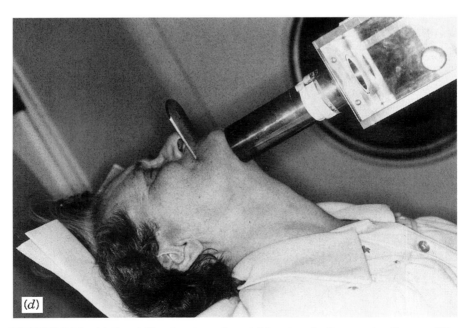

FIGURE 2.16   (c) Portal film showing submental boost projection, sparing the mandible. (d) Photograph showing submental boost projection using 18 MeV electron beam through IOC cone for carcinoma of the anterior floor of the mouth, with mouth piece used as a back pointer and shield.

Intraoral Cone (IOC)

Radiation therapy given per orally through a "cone" either by low megavoltage electrons or orthovoltage radiations is extremely effective for the treatment of early lesions of the oral cavity. This often results in good local control with excellent functional and cosmetic results[6] and minimal complications. The concept of IOC irradiation is to spare the mandible from high dose volume. The anatomic sites suitable for IOC radiation therapy include the oral tongue, floor of the mouth, retromolar trigone, buccal mucosa, and hard and soft palate.

Brachytherapy

Brachytherapy employing the interstitial implants with afterloading angiocath – ^{192}Ir technique is highly effective in delivering boost doses of radiation to small lesions of the head and neck, mainly cancers of the skin, lip, buccal mucosa, and lymph nodes. Because of the high incidence of osteoradionecrosis, brachytherapy for carcinoma of the oral tongue and floor of the mouth is rarely used at the MGH. Instead, IOC boost is commonly used in lieu of implant. Intracavitary implant is used for carcinoma of the nasopharynx as a boost to the primary site.

Three-Dimensional Treatment

Because of the recent availability of sophisticated computers, the planning of irradiation employing 3D concepts has emerged. Such a procedure is time-consuming and can only be used as a research protocol project trial with the hope of achieving better local control and fewer complications.

"Mini-mantle" for Irradiation of Larynx and Neck

Traditionally, radiation therapy for advanced carcinoma of the larynx consists of parallel opposing lateral portals, designed to include the primary lesion and the first echelon lymph nodes and a separate low anterior appositional portal to include the inferior jugular, paratracheal, and supraclavicular nodes and upper mediastinum with 0.5 cm juncture gap. The inherent hazards with this technique may involve overlapping of these three divergent beams over the esophagus and spinal cord, which could result in irreparable radiation damage, such as soft tissue ulceration, fistulization, fibrosis, esophageal stenosis, or radiation myelitis. If this technique is used without a midline cord block, the spinal cord and esophagus at the inferior posterior borders of the lateral portals must be shielded by a small cord block.

A "mini-mantle" technique for irradiation of extensive carcinoma of the larynx has been devised and found to be efficacious. The patients are treated in the supine position with hyperextension of the chin and immobilization with a face mask on the Clinac 18 linear accelerator using 10 MV photons and an isocentric technique. Opposing parallel AP open and PA portals with spinal cord block are used, including the entire neck from the mastoid tips down to the superaclavicular and upper mediastinal areas. The loading for the portals is 4:1, respectively. Both fields are treated each day. The dose reference point is at the prevertebral fascia. The physical aspects of this technique have been published elsewhere.[7] Treatment plan with iso-doses is shown in Figure 2.17.

For lesions managed by postoperative radiation therapy, the dose to the preverte-bral fascia is 45–50 Gy at 1.8–2 Gy per fraction. The tracheal stoma is boosted for 10 Gy at 2 cm depth in 5 days using 9 MV electrons with 0.5 cm bolus to the high risk area of the dissected neck. For the T3–4 lesions managed by radiation therapy alone, an additional dose of 20 Gy is given through opposing lateral off-cord portals.

SUMMARY

Modern practice of radiation therapy for head and neck tumors demands extreme technical sophistication. By using various treatment modalities and techniques planned by computer, most of the major irreparable radiation injuries of bone and soft tissue that were commonly seen in the kilovoltage era are greatly reduced, and sal-vage surgery can often be performed without significant postoperative complications.

With careful simulation and localization of the target volume, and the use of im-mobilizing devices and tattooing of the portals, most of the treatments to patients, as prescribed by the radiation oncologist, can be delivered by the well-trained thera-pist with confidence, and hopefully local control of the tumors and survival of the patients will be improved with reduced complications.

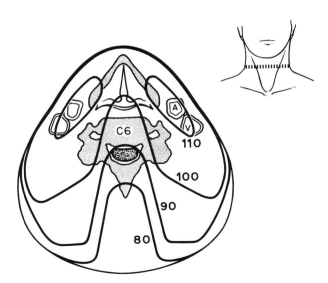

FIGURE 2.17   Diagram showing percent isodoses in treatment of larynx and neck using "mini-mantle" portal arrangement, normalized to the prevertebral fascia as a preoperative or postoperative procedure using 10 MV x-rays and AP "beam spoiler". (AP open/PA and pos-terior cord block ratio = 4 : 1.)

REFERENCES

1. Kubo H, Russel M, Wang CC: Use of 10 MV spoiled x-ray beam for treatment of head and neck tumors. *Int J Radiat Oncol Biol Phys* 1982;8:1795–1798.

2. Tapley N DuV. *Clinical applications of the electron beam.* New York: Wiley, 1976.

3. Sinclair WK, Kohn HI: The relative biological effectiveness of high-energy photons and electrons. *Radiology* 1964;82:800.

4. Wang CC, Boyer A, Mendiondo O: Afterloading interstitial radiation therapy. *Int J Radiat Biol Phys* 1976;1:365–368.

5. Wang CC, Busse J, Gitterman M: A simple afterloading applicator for intracavitary irradiation for carcinoma of the nasopharynx. *Radiology* 1975;115:737–738.

6. Wang CC, Doppke KP, Biggs PJ: Intra-oral cone radiation theapy for selected carcinomas of the oral cavity. *Int J Radiat Oncol Biol Phys* 1983;9:1185–1189.

7. Doppke K, Novak D, Wang CC: Physical considerations in the treatment of advanced carcinomas of the larynx and pyriform sinuses using 10 MV x-rays. *Int J Radiat Biol Phys* 1980;6:1251–1255.

CHAPTER 3

DENTAL CARE OF PATIENTS RECEIVING RADIATION THERAPY

In the modern practice of head and neck oncology, dentists or oral surgeons are essential members of the team. They play an important role in early recognition of oral cancer, participate in pretreatment evaluation of the oral tissue and teeth, and supervise post-treatment reconstruction of the surgical defect and postradiation dental treatment to reduce the incidence of dental caries and development of osteoradionecrosis and to maintain a healthy mouth. Patients receiving radiation therapy for head and neck cancer in and around the oral cavity therefore should undergo dental evaluation prior to treatment. Patients are advised to brush, rinse, and floss the teeth after each meal.

Preradiation evaluation includes Panorex radiographic examination of the jaw to detect infectious processes around the teeth, dental caries, retained root tips, impacted teeth, or periodontal bone absorption. For evaluation of bone involvement by the carcinoma, an occlusal radiograph of the portion of the mandible involved by the lesion or CT scans of the mandible are more informative than Panorex radiographs alone. The teeth beyond repair should be extracted, in conjunction with alveolectomy, with removal of any bony spicules and careful closure of the socket. When the state of the underlying disease allows, a healing time of 10–14 days should be granted prior to commencement of radiation therapy when the extracted socket is healed.[1,2] Pretreatment extraction of teeth does not necessarily prevent osteoradionecrosis; studies have shown that dental extractions increase its incidence, particularly at the site of extraction[3] (Figure 3.1). Most patients with good teeth receiving a dose of 50 Gy external beam radiation to the mandible do not require full mouth extraction as the dose to the mandible would not result in osteoradionecrosis even after teeth extraction. If the radiation therapy portal is sufficiently large, resulting in extreme xerostomia, it is necessary to have a special individualized dental mold made by an oral surgeon or dentist for use as a vehicle for the daily applica-

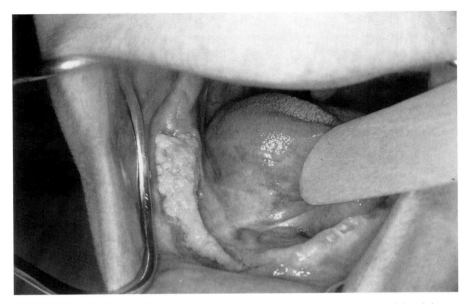

FIGURE 3.1   A 48-year-old woman with a T1N0 squamous cell carcinoma of the right anterior floor of the mouth. Prior to radiation therapy her lower teeth were extracted in an attempt to prevent osteoradionecrosis. The lesion was treated with combined external radiation therapy and interstitial implant to 70 Gy in 45 days. Six months later a small ulcer appeared and was treated conservatively. Later, osteoradionecrosis developed, which required sequestrectomy and partial mandibulectomy for control of pain. Extraction of teeth before radiation therapy did not prevent this complication.

tion of fluoride gel prophylaxis. This may be started during or after radiation therapy.

During radiation therapy, supportive care includes xylocaine viscous mouth rinse and/or Dyclone to minimize discomfort. Baking soda and salt mixed solution mouth gargle may alleviate the discomfort of stickiness of the secretion and xerostomia. Oral candidiasis is not uncommon, resulting in discomfort and dysphagia. Treatment consists of nystatin and/or ketoconazole.

Postradiation management of the oral cavity includes fluoride treatment to strengthen the teeth and prevent dental caries and restoration of missing dentition with partial plates or dentures in the edentulous jaw. Preradiation dentures generally require realignment. These dentures must fit the irradiated alveolar ridge comfortably without pain or tenderness. Extreme care must be exercised to nurse the irradiated tender tissue of the oral cavity to prevent soft tissue ulceration or osteoradionecrosis. If tooth extraction becomes necessary, the procedure should be done with full coverage with antibiotic before and after the extraction. Frequent dental check-ups are mandatory along with maintenance of good oral hygiene.

RADIATION EFFECTS ON SALIVARY GLANDS AND ORAL TISSUES

The major salivary glands are responsible for 90% of the salivary output. Histologically, these glands are differentiated tissues with rare mitoses and are therefore relatively radioresistant, yet radiation therapy that includes the major salivary glands is often followed by diminution of secretory output and thickening of saliva. The effects of radiation therapy on the salivary glands are probably due to the effects of radiation on the fine vasculature of the gland, with secondary changes in the parenchymal epithelium and interstitial and interlobular fibrosis, leading to degeneration of the functional acini. The serous acini are more responsive to radiation therapy than the mucous acini, which accounts for the tenacious character of the saliva after fractionated radiation therapy with approximately 10 Gy. The effects of reduced salivation and increased salivary viscosity are noted by the patients in the early part of the treatment course. When both parotid glands are irradiated with 50 Gy, there is marked (80%) reduction of salivary flow, and after 65–70 Gy, the secretory function of the gland ceases in 1–7 months. At the beginning of irradiation there is marked and prompt elevation of serum amylase levels and a decrease in serum immunoglobulin A (IgA), which are progressive with increasing doses.[4,5] Partial recovery is possible, but the process is slow, depending on the dose delivered.

It is therefore most important for the radiation oncologist to appreciate the changes resulting in xerostomia, and care must be taken to protect the normal salivary glands from irradiation as much as possible. Decreased salivary output and increased viscosity change the oral flora, leading to a higher risk of dental caries.[6] This is due to the lack of the cleansing mechanism of normal saliva. Microorganisms tend to accumulate on the teeth, particularly at the gum line, resulting in rapid decay of the infected teeth and amputation of the crown of the tooth (Figure 3.2). The decay may occur outside the irradiated portal. Teeth capped prior to radiation therapy are rarely affected by this decay process because of the protective barrier of the cap (Figure 3.3). The development of dental caries is a direct result of xerostomia. This complication can be prevented by observing meticulous oral hygiene and daily application of fluoride.[7]

Treatment of xerostomia is primarily palliative. Artificial saliva may be used to temporarily alleviate some discomfort. The use of pilocarpine has been tried and found to be somewhat effective in relieving the signs and symptoms of postradiation xerostomia.[8] To achieve these benefits the drug must be administered continuously. The patient should be fully informed of the effects of xerostomia after radiation therapy and most patients will cooperate with a moist and semisolid diet.

Because of the use of megavoltage radiation and a combination of external beam

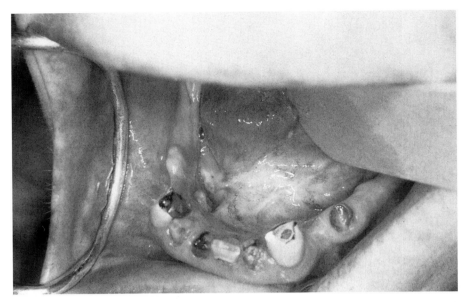

FIGURE 3.2   A 46-year-old woman with T2N0 carcinoma of the right floor of the mouth treated in May 1965 with interstitial implant to 65 Gy in 5 days followed by IOC boost to 20 Gy in three daily fractions. A tiny ulceration developed on the medial aspect of the right side of the lower gum but healed after conservative treatment. Photograph shows extensive dental caries 3 years after radiation therapy. When last seen in 1981, she was free of disease.

therapy and/or the intraoral cone boost technique, sound teeth or teeth in good repair can survive radiation therapy well and need not be sacrificed if the radiation dosages are kept within the limits of tolerance of the mandible or the major portion of the salivary gland is spared.[9]

Early response of the sensation of taste to radiation at about 20 Gy corresponds to the prominence of the circumvillate papillae. The altered taste sensations precede by a few days the development of patchy mucositis and the diminution of salivation. The sensation of taste of bitter and acid flavors is more impaired than for salty and sweet flavors.[10] Impairment of taste becomes severe after a dosage of 60 Gy. Partial to complete recovery from radiation effects on the taste buds is probable, but the process is slow; in some cases complete recovery takes months or years after doses of 60 Gy or greater.

Radiation ulceration of the soft tissues or osteoradionecrosis (Figures 3.4 and 3.5) is often due to excessive radiation therapy or extensive cancer.[11] The normal tissues fail to maintain homeostasis, with impairment of blood supply and decreased viability. These ischemic tissues generally cannot withstand trauma or irritation without breakdown. When the process occurs over or adjacent to the

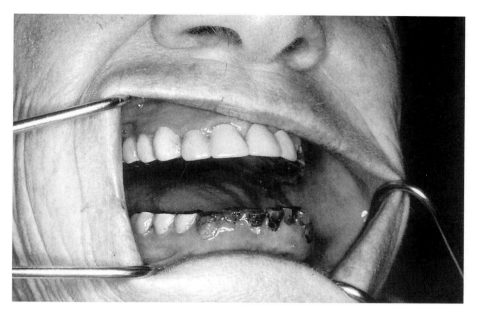

FIGURE 3.3   A 58-year-old woman with a T4N0 carcinoma of the right retromolar trigone in 1971, treated with external beam therapy to 65 Gy over 49 days on a cobalt-60 machine. She was well until 1978, when a second squamous cell carcinoma developed on the left side of the tongue. She died of this second malignancy. Photograph shows dental caries in the exposed teeth but none in the capped teeth.

mandible, infection may set in, with resultant osteoradionecrosis. If the involvement is small, the soft tissue ulceration will heal after conservative measures, but the healing process sometimes is slow. In severe cases, where ulceration is extensive, an orocutaneous fistula may result. Spontaneous healing seldom occurs, and surgical repair will have to be considered. These sequelae are prone to occur in patients with poor nutritional status and in chronic alcoholics and heavy cigarette smokers. The mucosa overlying the medial surface of the angle of the jaw is often the area of soft tissue ulceration because of its thinness. Due to the difference in vascular supply, the mandible is more prone to osteoradionecrosis than the maxilla.

Dental caries from xerostomia and osteoradionecrosis of the mandible are totally unrelated. The former is due to radiation ablation of the salivary glands, partially or preeminently, and the latter is due to excessively high-dose or large fraction size external beam therapy or interstitial implant to the floor of the mouth or tongue. Osteoradionecrosis may be caused by the proximity of the tumor infiltration and may also occur in an edentulous jaw (Figure 3.5) or in patients who had dental extractions prior to or in preparation for radiation therapy.

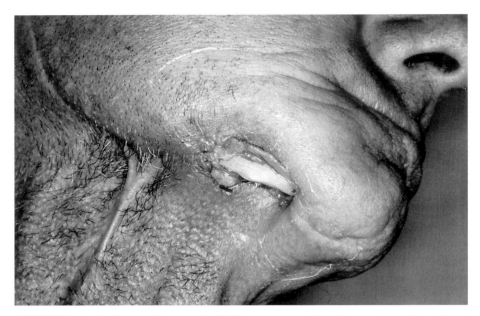

FIGURE 3.4   A 48-year-old man with T2N1 squamous cell carcinoma of the right side of the floor of the mouth. A lymph node was removed prior to radiation therapy and was found to be metastatic carcinoma. Radiation therapy was administered to 66 Gy in 45 days with a cobalt-60 unit with 1.8 Gy per fraction. After radiation therapy a right radical neck dissection was performed; seven metastatic nodes were found in the specimen. One and one-half years later, a small area of exposed bone was noted over the right mandible, associated with a small orocutaneous fistula. After conservative treatment a small sequestrum was separated from the mandible and he was entirely asymptomatic. In 1990, 20 years after his initial treatment, the patient, developed a secondary carcinoma in the base of the tongue and died of the disease. Photograph shows exposed bone and an orocutaneous fistula.

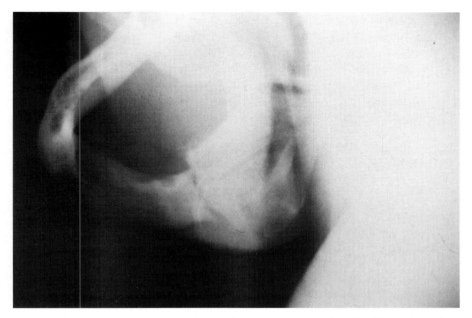

FIGURE 3.5   A 59-year-old man with T1N0 carcinoma of the right faucial tonsil received 70 Gy in 45 days through combined opposing lateral and ipsilateral wedge portals on a cobalt-60 unit. Seven years after radiation therapy, he noted a "popping" sensation on the right side of the face, without any strain or trauma. Radiographic films of the mandible revealed a fracture of the midportion of the jaw, which was apparently the result of an excessively high dose of radiation therapy. The original carcinoma was under control.

PREVENTION OF OSTEORADIONECROSIS

To keep the incidence of osteoradionecrosis of the mandible to a minimum, the following guidelines should be observed[12]:

1. Fraction size should not exceed 2.5 Gy/f.
2. Total mandibular dose is limited to 65–70 Gy over 7–8 weeks, with 1.8–2 Gy/fraction/day.
3. With further increase of mandibular doses (i.e., 72 Gy, 2 Gy/f over 7 weeks), the incidence of osteoradionecrosis is significantly increased (i.e., 25–30%).
4. Incidence of osteoradionecrosis may be reduced by mixing the external beam dose and boost dose (e.g., 20–30%) with techniques sparing the mandible.
5. If intraoral electron cone therapy is not used as the "boost" therapy, the

treatment portals must be reduced after 45 Gy for the remainder of the treatment up to a total of 65–70 Gy.

6. Brachytherapy to the carcinoma of the floor of the mouth accounts for a high incidence of osteoradionecrosis and limited surgical excision also may be considered as a boost procedure in lieu of interstitial implant.

7. Dental extraction in patients who have had prior radiation therapy to the mouth should be done with antibiotic coverage. Carious teeth outside the irradiation portals can safely be extracted, because adjacent bone does not receive the full radiation dose, as can teeth in the mandible receiving less than 50 Gy in conventional radiation therapy.

MANAGEMENT OF OSTEORADIONECROSIS

Osteoradionecrosis of the mandible is a serious complication following curative radiation therapy. Fortunately, its incidence is quite low. Once osteoradionecrosis develops, conservative treatment with good oral hygiene and patience ("hands off" policy) may suffice. The small sequestrum may fall out by itself, followed by healing. In severe cases of large areas of osteoradionecrosis with intractable pain and infection, treatment consists of good oral hygiene, saline irrigation, and debridement of dead or nonviable bone. In severe instances, partial mandibulectomy may be indicated for removal of the devitalized necrotic bone to affect a cure. Hyperbaric oxygen is recommended by several investigators with occasional success.[13–15]

Osteoradionecrosis, often confused with dental caries, is due to the high dose of radiation to the bone, while dental caries are the result of xerostomia. Low doses of radiation with resultant xerostomia rarely result in necrosis of the mandible despite dental extraction of the carious teeth. Treatment of radiation xerostomia is palliative, and pilocarpine may relieve some discomfort.[8]

SUMMARY

Oral and dental problems related to radiation therapy vary in extent and magnitude and must be accepted as a risk of treatment of malignant disease in and around the oral cavity region. The risks and benefits of radiation must be fully weighed before treatment is undertaken. Frequent follow-up of patients with carcinomas of the head and neck may detect subsequent second and third primary lesions in the upper aerodigestive tract.

Figures 3.1 through 3.5 illustrate the major dental problems related to curative radiation therapy. It is hoped that the degree and extent of these problems may be minimized with better understanding of this disease process and improvement in radiotherapeutic and surgical techniques.

REFERENCES

1. Marx RE: Osteoradionecrosis: a new concept of its pathophysiology. *J Oral Maxillofac Surg* 1983;41:283–288.
2. Marx RE, Johnson RP: Studies in the radiobiology of osteoradionecrosis and their clinical significance. *Oral Surg Oral Med Oral Pathol* 1987;64:379–390.
3. Beumer J, Harrison R, Sanders B, Kurrasch M: Preradiation dental extractions and the incidence of radionecrosis. *Head Neck Surg* 1983;5:514–521.
4. Marks JE, Davis CC, Gottsman VL, et al: The effects of radiation on parotid salivary function. *Int J Radiat Oncol Biol Phys* 1981;7:1013–1019.
5. Cheng VS, Downs J, Herbert D, et al: Function of the parotid gland following radiation therapy for head and neck cancer. *Int J Radiat Oncol Biol Phys* 1981;7:253–258.
6. del Regato JA: Dental lesions observed after roentgentherapy in cancer of the buccal cavity, pharynx and larynx. *Am J Roentgenol* 1939;42:404–410.
7. Hinds EC: Dental care and oral hygiene before and after treatment. *JAMA* 1971;215:964–966.
8. Greenspan D, Daniels TE: Effectiveness of pilocarpine in postradiation xerostomia. *Cancer* 1987;59:1123–1125.
9. Daley TE, Drane JB: Dental care for irradiated patients. In: *Neoplasia of head and neck.* Chicago: Year Book Medical Publishers, 1974;225–232.
10. Bonanni G, Perazzi F: Behavior of taste sensitivity inpatients subjected to high energy radiologic treatment for tumor of the oral cavity. *Nunt Radiol* 1965;31:383–397.
11. Bedwinek JM, Shukovsky LJ, Fletcher GH, et al: Osteonecrosis in patients treated with definitive radiotherapy for squamous cell carcinoma of the oral cavity and naso- and oropharynx. *Radiology* 1976;119:665–667.
12. Cheng VS, Wang CC: Osteoradionecrosis of the mandible resulting from external megavoltage radiation therapy. *Radiology* 1974;12:685–689.
13. Davis JC, Dunn JM, Gates GA, Heinbach RD: Hyperbaric oxygen: a new adjunct in the managements of radiation necrosis. *Arch Otolaryngol* 1979;105:58–61.
14. Hart GB, Mainous EG: The treatment of radiation necrosis with hyperbaric oxygen. *Cancer* 1976;37:2580–2585.
15. Davis JC, Dunn JM, Gates GA, Heimbach RD: Hyperbaric oxygen. A new adjunct in the management of radiation necrosis. *Arch Otolaryngol* 1979;105:58–61.

CHAPTER 4

PRINCIPLES AND PRACTICE OF ALTERED FRACTIONATION RADIATION THERAPY

ALTERED FRACTIONATION SCHEMES

"Conventional" or "standard" fractionation radiation therapy for carcinomas of the head and neck varies. In the United States, most of the treatment programs in the last few decades have consisted of 1.8–2.0 Gy/fraction/day, 5 days a week, for a total of 65–70 Gy of continuous radiation therapy in 7–8 weeks. This fractionation scheme was arrived at because of the reasonably good results for early tumors, with tolerable acute reactions and acceptable late effects. For T1–2 lesions, local tumor control rates of 80–90% have been achieved. For advanced tumors, T3–4, the success rates generally were poor, ranging from 30% to 40%. From the standpoint of modern radiobiology, this schedule of conventional fractionation radiation therapy may not be optimal in terms of maximal local tumor control of advanced tumors with minimal late complications.

One attempt to improve the therapeutic ratio—and hopefully the results—is altered fractionation. This may involve changes of fraction size, number of daily fractions, total doses, or total treatment time. The change of fraction size may be 1.2 Gy/f or 1.6 Gy/f in the hyperfractionated scheme, or 3–4 Gy/f in the hypofractionated program. Treatment may be given two or three times daily, five times or fewer than five times weekly, for a total dose equal to or higher than conventional radiation therapy, either continuous or split-course. The overall treatment course may be either much shorter or longer than conventional radiation programs.

With these possible changes and combinations, there are many altered fractionation schemes, with dose modification of fraction sizes, differing number of fractions, continuous or interrupted programs, and various overall treatment courses. At the present time, the altered fractionation schemes or programs can be divided into

(1) hypofractionation, (2) split-course radiation therapy, (3) hyperfractionation, and (4) accelerated fractionation.

Hypofractionation

Hypofractionation implies a larger dose per fraction per day (e.g., 4 or 5 Gy/f, 3 or 4 days per week), for a total dose equal to, or slightly lower than, conventional fractionation. The number of fractions per week is reduced and the overall treatment time can be shortened or unchanged. Clinical experience indicates that such an approach results in decreased tumor control[1–3] and is often associated with severe late complications on the normal tissues. The acute effects may be similar to those with the conventional five fractions per week, even with identical time–dose–fractionation (TDF) or nominal standard dose (NSD) values, yet the late complication rates are higher, indicating a dissociation of responses to large dose per fraction between acute- and late-responding tissues.

Split-Course Radiation Therapy

Split-course radiation therapy involves conventional fraction size (1.8–2.0 Gy/f/day) with a midcourse split, or rest period, of 2–3 weeks. The overall treatment time of split-course radiation therapy is lengthened, and generally the patient experiences less discomfort during the entire course of radiation therapy. Another split-course approach includes rapid fractionation of 3 Gy/f/day for 10 days with a 2-week treatment break or split, followed by 3 Gy/f/day for 10 days more. The overall treatment course is approximately the same as for conventional radiation therapy with 2 Gy/f. Clinical experience indicates that tumor control is consistently lower in every stage of the disease when compared with continuous conventional fractionation radiation therapy.[4,5] The inferior results are probably due to excessive regeneration of the tumors during the rest period and the prolonged entire treatment course. Rapid split-course fractionation may show tumor control similar to that with conventional continuous radiation therapy with 2 Gy/f, but with more severe late sequelae, such as bone necrosis and severe fibrosis, as the result of large daily fraction sizes.

Hyperfractionation

Hyperfractionation is the use of multiple small fractions two or three times a day with 4 hours or more between fractions. The fraction size may be 1.15–1.2 Gy per treatment with two treatments per day. This is equivalent to 2 Gy/fraction/day, 5 days a week, and can be given continuously up to 65–70 Gy. The overall treatment time remains unchanged, for example, 6–8 weeks. The acute toxicity of such an approach is generally comparable to or slightly more than the conventional once-daily radiation therapy with 2 Gy/f. The total dose may be increased since the fraction size is decreased. The intent of hyperfractionation with smaller fraction sizes (less than 1.8–2 Gy/f) is to reduce late effects or, with an increased total dose, to achieve equivalent late effects but with better tumor control. Clinical experience with this approach indicates 10–15% better local control for lesions of the oropharynx, hypopharynx, and supraglottic larynx without increase of survival. For somewhat better local control, the total dose is escalated from 75.9 to 82.5 Gy.[6,7] On the other hand, the randomized trials of RTOG[8–10] did not show significant improvement of local control and survival when compared with conventional radiation therapy. The EORTC trial[11] results, however, indicate increased local control as well as a trend toward improved survival.

Acclerated Fractionation

Accelerated fractionation uses the conventional dose per fraction—that is, 2 Gy, 2–3 fractions/day—for a total dose of 60 Gy. The overall treatment time is markedly shortened. The basic intent is to minimize the potential tumor growth or repopulation without changing the late effects, since the total dose, number of fractions, and dose per fraction remain the same as the conventional program. One difficulty with accelerated fractionation is the severe toxicity to the acute-responding tissues (i.e., the mucous membranes), which may necessitate reduction of the total dose or early termination of the program because of poor tolerance. This may compromise local tumor control. The most common accelerated fractionation schedule includes a boost treatment to the primary lesion through a reduced "field-within-field" boost technique[12,13] with two or three daily fractions per week, along with the conventional program (1.8–2 Gy/day, 5 days/week). Thus the dose to the primary lesion may amount to a total of 70 Gy delivered in 6 weeks with somewhat less volume of mucosal toxicity.

Another accelerated approach is to deliver radiation therapy in three fractions of 1.4–1.5 Gy/f each per day (TID), continuously for 12 days (CHART).[14,15] The total dose is limited to 50.4–54 Gy due to the severe mucosal toxicity, and patients often require intensive nutritional support and, not infrequently, hospitalization. The CHART data thus far show some improvement in local control but not in survival over a 2-year period.

There are a few nonrandomized trials on accelerated fractionation, and the data show no significant improvement in local control or survival in patients with oropharyngeal carcinomas.[16–18]

Accelerated Hyperfractionation

Altered fractionation radiation therapy at the Massachusetts General Hospital (MGH) is a hybrid between accelerated and hyperfractionated programs.[19,20] The scheme consists of 15–20% dose reduction per fraction, twice a day (1.6 Gy/f BID), for a total dose of 67.2–70.4 Gy in 6 weeks. The procedure can shorten the total treatment course, despite the necessity for a midcourse break of 10–14 days due to severe mucosal toxicity. Generally, the entire program is fairly well tolerated and is still 1 week shorter than the conventional radiation program.

Nonrandomized trials at the MGH showed better local control and survival in patients with advanced carcinoma of the oropharynx and larynx after BID radiation therapy. The data after TID therapy with 1 Gy/f and the EORTC randomized trial, however, show no improvement in either local control or survival.[21]

The altered fractionation radiation therapy programs of considerable promise can be summarized as follows:

1. Hyperfractionated program (University of Florida) with 1.15–1.2 Gy/f BID continuously to 74.4–79.2 Gy in 6.5–7 weeks.
2. Concomitant boost program (M.D. Anderson Hospital) with 1.8–2 Gy/f QD and concomitant boost of 1.2–1.5 Gy/f for a total dose of 70 Gy in 6 weeks.
3. Accelerated hyperfractionated program (Massachusetts General Hospital) with 1.6 Gy/f BID for 67.2–70.4 Gy in 6 weeks with a midcourse break.
4. CHART program (Mount Vernon Hospital) with 1.4–1.5 Gy/f continuously for 50.4–54 Gy in 12 days.

These treatment schemes are depicted in Figure 4.1.

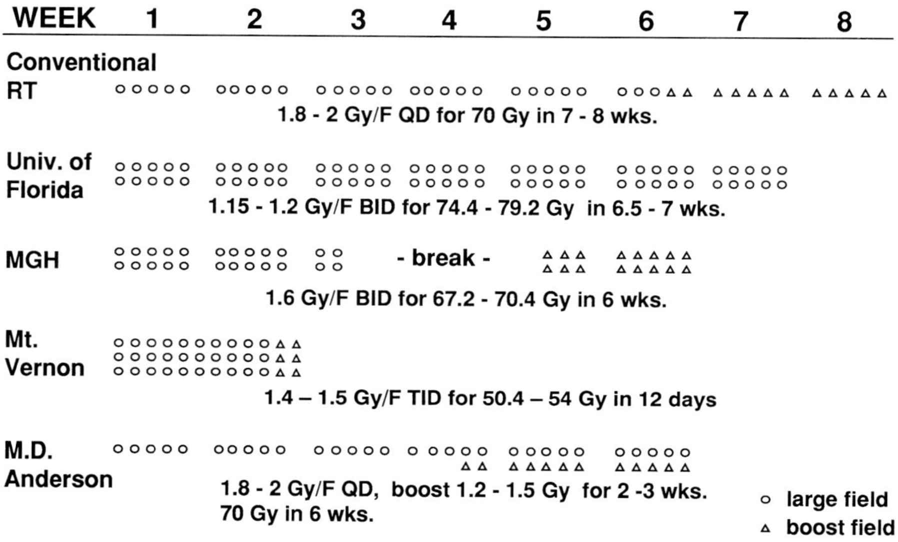

FIGURE 4.1   Diagram summarizing various forms of altered fractionation radiation therapy for head and neck carcinoma.

RADIOBIOLOGIC CONCEPTS OF ALTERED FRACTIONATION

The principle of altered fractionation radiation therapy for the treatment of human cancers is one of the strategies stemming from laboratory radiobiologic research. Studies of the results of dose–survival curves of cells, both normal and malignant, and acute- and late-responding tissues, of various radiobiologic characteristics of the cells of tumors and critical normal tissues, and of repair of sublethal damage for both normal and cancer cells after photon irradiation are relevant to the understanding and practice of altered fractionation radiation oncology. The biologic basis for various dose modification programs has been extensively discussed by Withers and co-workers.[22–25]

It has been observed that the repair of sublethal damage is almost complete in 4–6 hours. The shoulder of the survival curve is duplicated, although the degree of repair may be different in various biologic environments and tissues. The acute-responding oxygenated tissues, including skin, mucous membrane of the aerodigestive tract, and testes, have higher capacity of repair of sublethal damage than the chronically hypoxic cancerous cells and late-responding tissues, such as vasculoconnective tissue, spinal cord, lung, and kidney. For radiation treatment given in two or three fractions per day, the interval time between fractions should be 4–6 hours if complete repair is to be achieved. Shortening the interfraction time to 2–3 hours results in severe late complications[10] due to the significant increase of risk of damage to late-responding normal tissues.

Various biologic tissues respond differently to a change of dose per fraction. It was observed experimentally by Withers et al.[24,25] that the slopes of the dose–response curves for late-responding tissues are steeper or curvier than those for acute-responding tissues (Figure 4.2). The late-responding tissues are therefore dependent on the dose per fraction and not on overall treatment time, and they are much more sensitive to increased fraction size. With identical total dose and treatment time and large fractions, there is marked impairment of repair of sublethal damage to late-responding tissues, resulting in late complications (Figure 4.3). When using fraction sizes smaller than "standard" or conventional radiation therapy (<2 Gy/fraction), there is preferential sparing of the late-responding tissues relative to the acute-responding tissues. Thus the total dose required to produce a specified level of damage to or complications in late-responding tissues can be increased, perhaps with an increase in local tumor control.

Clinical and experimental studies indicate that both normal and malignant cells are capable of repopulating during and after radiation damage, although to varying degrees. Repopulation of squamous cell carcinomas tends to escalate after a lag period of 4–5 weeks after the initiation of radiation.[26,27] With total treatment time protracted beyond 40 days, repopulation of tumor cells is increased, followed by decreased tumor control from a given total dose. The increase of dose necessary to achieve an isoeffect is estimated to be about 0.6 Gy for each day after 40 days.[28] It is postulated that the best therapeutic strategy of altered fractionation radiation therapy is to deliver the maximum dose to the tumor as tolerated by late-responding tis-

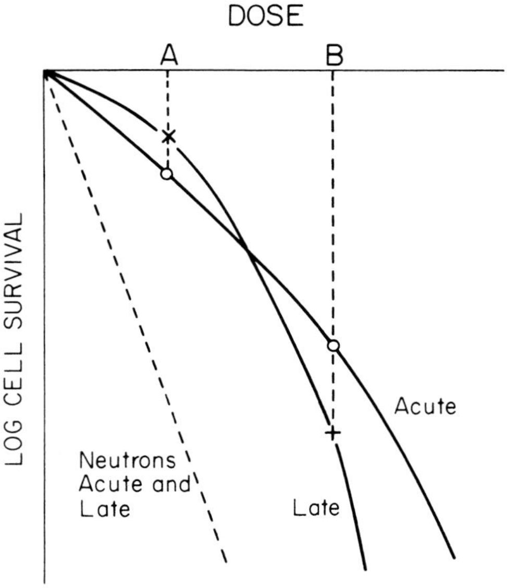

FIGURE 4.2 Diagram showing steeper slope for survival curve of late-responding target cells as compared to acute-responding cells. With decrease in x-ray dose per fraction, there is greater sparing of late effects and fewer late complications. (From Withers HR, Thames HD, Peters LJ: *Int J Radiat Oncol Biol Phys* 1982;8:2071–2076. Used with permission of authors.)

sues in the minimum total treatment time, consistent with limits of tolerance of the acute reactions.

The Dilemma of Altered Fractionation Radiation Therapy

Clinically, the extent of radiation toxicity on acute-responding tissues, such as the mucous membranes of the aerodigestive tract, is the determinant of the patient's tolerance and is related to fraction size, total daily, weekly, and overall doses, and overall treatment course. If the fraction size is large and the overall treatment course is shortened, there is severe acute toxicity, which may require reduction in total dose and may eventually lower the probability of tumor control.[29] Extremely rapid fractionation and high total dose often result in severe radiation complications.[30,31] There is an extremely delicate balance between fraction size, number of fractions per day, and overall total dose and treatment time in selecting the dose fractionation schedule. An attempt to simplify the interrelationship between changes of acute- and late-responding tissues versus fraction size and overall treatment time relative to toxicity, tolerance, tumor control probability, and complications is shown in Figure 4.4.

Which Altered Fractionation Program?

Various altered fractionation radiation therapy programs are available. It has not been established with certainty which fractionation schedule is best. The available data, however, indicate that conventional treatment is not indicated in all cases of

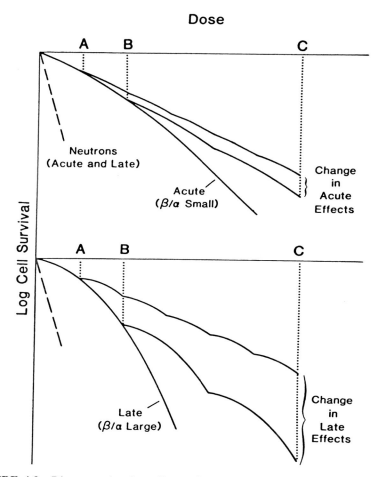

FIGURE 4.3   Diagrams showing effects of multifraction radiation in acute- and late-responding tissues. The late-responding tissues are more sensitive to a large change of fraction size. (From Withers HR, Thames HD, Peters LJ: Differences in fractionation response of acute and late responding tissues. In: Karcher KH, Kogeinik HD, Reinartz E, eds. *Progresses in radio-oncology 11*. New York: Raven Press, 1982;257–296. Used with permission.)

carcinoma of the head and neck, and altered fractionation radiation therapy can provide higher local control in selected cases. In order to determine the optimum fractionation scheme, altered fractionation radiation therapy programs are undergoing intensive investigation[32] and a prospective randomized trial conducted by RTOG is in progress. However, Withers and Horiot speculate that "both hyperfractionation alone and accelerated treatment hold promise for an improved therapeutic outcome; and accelerated hyperfractionation, by combining the advantages of both, may be even better."[23]

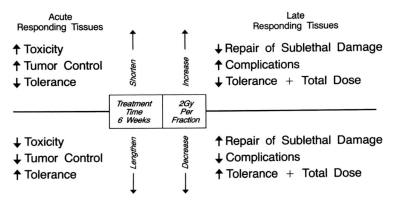

FIGURE 4.4   Effects of acute- and late-responding tissues related to treatment time and dose per fraction.

Massachusetts General Hospital BID Programs

The twice-daily (BID) program was initiated at the Massachusetts General Hospital in 1979 and consists of 1.6 Gy/f, two fractions per day, with a minimum of 4 hours between fractions, for 12 days, 5 days a week. All fields were treated per session with megavoltage radiation. After 38.4 Gy, patients were given a rest period of approximtely 10 days to 2 weeks. After the rest period or "break," the treatment was resumed with a shrinking field technique. Initially, one fraction of 1.8 Gy/f/day was given, up to 65–66 Gy. This is designated as the twice-daily/once-daily (BID/QD) regimen, which did not shorten the overall treatment time compared to the QD program. In August 1982, the twice-daily regimen was resumed after the break, using 1.6 Gy/f for 8 additional days, for a total dose of 67.4 Gy over 6 weeks. In some instances, an additional 1 or 2 days of twice-daily dosing was directed to the primary site through markedly reduced portals as a final boost, for a grand total of 70.4–72 Gy. This is designated the twice-daily/twice-daily (BID/BID) program, which can shorten the overall treatment course by about 7–10 days as compared to the QD scheme. The spinal cord dose was excluded after the first 38.4 Gy in 24 fractions of 1.6 Gy each. Figure 4.5 illustrates diagrammatically the course of treatment versus treatment time by QD, BID/QD, and BID/BID programs at the MGH.

As of 12/30/94, a total of 2500 patients with squamous cell carcinomas of the head and neck were treated with various accelerated hyperfractionated programs, and these formed the basis of data analyses in subsequent chapters of this text.

Acute and Late Effects After BID Radiation Therapy   Acute effects after twice-daily radiation therapy consist mostly of severe sore throat and development of patchy to confluent mucositis. The reactions vary in degree and extent in different anatomic sites and with portal size and irradiated volume and with the physical

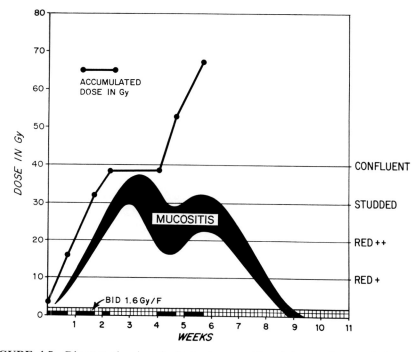

FIGURE 4.5   Diagram showing the biphasic mucositis of the oropharynx during twice-daily radiation therapy course versus dose and time. Extent of mucosal reaction shown on right of graph is divided into four categories.

condition of the patient. In general, the mucosal reaction follows a rather regular pattern. It occurs rapidly, reaching a peak of studded or confluent mucositis 2.5–3 weeks after commencement of therapy. It then decreases rapidly over the 10-day to 2-week therapy break. After twice-daily radiation therapy is resumed, mucositis is reactivated, but to a lesser extent, toward the completion of the course of radiation therapy. With the aid of topical analgesics, symptoms of mucosal reactions are generally well tolerated. Very few patients require hospitalization, nasogastric intubation, or feeding gastrostomy for severe dehydration during the course of irradiation.

Figure 4.6 relates the development and subsidence of biphasic radiation mucositis of the oropharynx and larynx related to radiation dose and time.

Arbitrary Interfraction Time for BID Program   In order to achieve a meaningful degree of repair of sublethal tissue damage, RTOG trial[10] indicated a minimum of 6 hours between fractions is required. At the MGH, however, all patients receive BID radiation therapy with an interfraction time of 4 hours or longer, and the late effects are insignificant. Normal tissues generally were in good condition and showed no undue skin or subcutaneous fibrosis at the irradiated site nor in-

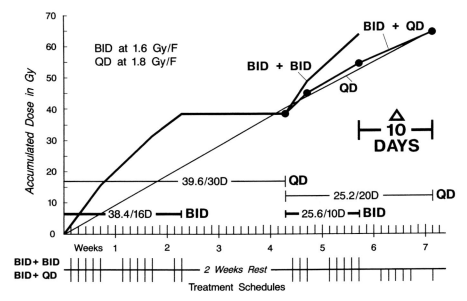

FIGURE 4.6 Comparison of accumulated doses before and after midcourse break between BID, BID/QD, and QD radiation therapy programs versus time (days idealized).

creased incidence of mucosal ulceration or osteoradionecrosis for an observation period as long as 15 years. No patient has developed radiation myelitis after the twice-daily program as outlined. The few patients who underwent salvage surgery to primary sites or neck dissection for nodal recurrence or persistent disease did not experience an unusually high incidence of postoperative complications when compared to the patients receiving conventional irradiation.[33]

MGH Experience and Results of Treatment

To assess the efficacy of the accelerated hyperfractionated radiation therapy program at the MGH, we evaluated the local control rates of patients treated with BID

TABLE 4.1 Five-Year Actuarial Local Control (LC) of T1–2 Carcinoma of the Oropharynx and Supraglottis: Comparison of Various Programs, 1970–1994

Program	LC	p Value
BID/QD vs. QD	100/77	NS
BID/BID vs. QD	80/77	NS
BID/BID vs. BID/QD	80/100	NS

TABLE 4.2   Five-Year Actuarial LC of T3 Carcinoma of the Oropharynx and Supraglottis: Comparison of Various Programs, 1970–1994

Program	LC	p Value
BID/QD vs. QD	63/45	0.05
BID/BID vs. QD	71/45	0.0001
BID/BID vs. BID/QD	71/63	0.04

programs from 1970 to 1994 and compared the results with those for patients having the same diseases and stages but treated with conventional once-daily (QD) radiation therapy. Standard life tables were obtained and the results were compared for statistical difference.

Evaluation of Accelerated Hyperfractionated Programs   A total of 545 patients with squamous cell carcinoma of the oropharynx and supraglottic larynx were treated by various programs and were available for analysis. There were 195 with T1–2 and 350 with T3 lesions: 236 were treated by QD program, 64 by BID/QD scheme, and 245 by BID/BID scheme. The 5-year actuarial local control rates for the T1–2 and T3 lesions after various programs are shown in Tables 4.1 and 4.2.

These findings, including previously published data,[34,35] indicate that sequential, nonrandomized trial of accelerated hyperfractionated BID programs yielded significant improvement of local control of advanced (T3) carcinoma of the oropharynx and supraglottis as compared to the historical control QD program at the MGH. The improvement is more marked in BID/BID than in BID/QD schemes; however, it is not significant (NS) for early T1–2 lesions.

Evaluation of Total Treatment Time and Doses of the Programs   Factors affecting local control of carcinomas of the oropharynx and larynx after accelerated

TABLE 4.3   Five-Year Actuarial Local Control of Oropharyngeal Carcinoma Related to Treatment Time: 1970–1994

Lesions	Days	n	LC (%)
T1–2	<45	107	88
	≥45	136	75
			$p = 0.007$
T3	<45	90	67
	≥45	88	44
			$p = 0.005$

TABLE 4.4   Five-Year Actuarial Local Control of Oropharyngeal Carcinoma Related to Total Dose: 1970–1994

Lesions	Dose	n	LC (%)
T1–2	≤ 67 Gy	149	79
	> 67 Gy	88	83
			$p = 0.05$
T3	≤ 67 Gy	113	45
	> 67 Gy	65	74
			$p = 0.003$

hyperfractionation programs related to the total treatment time and total treatment doses[36,37] are shown in the Tables 4.3 to 4.8.

The data indicate significant improvement in local control by shortening of the total treatment course, shortening of the treatment gap, and increased total doses in patients with advanced (T3–4) carcinoma treated by accelerated hyperfractionated radiation therapy. The treatment program with total treatment course completed in less than 45 days, with a treatment gap of less than 14 days or preferably 11 days, and a total dose of 70 Gy is considered to be optimum for maximal local control of advanced carcinoma of the oropharynx and larynx (T3) with minimum complications. The deleterious effects of prolonging treatment course[37] and gap are probably the results of repopulation of the tumors during the treatment gap.

DISCUSSIONS AND SUMMARY

1. The concept of altered fractionation is one of the major contributions from laboratory basic research that has changed the practice of radiation therapy of head and neck carcinomas.

TABLE 4.5   Five-Year Actuarial Local Control of Supraglottic Carcinoma Related to Treatment Time: 1970–1994

Lesions	Days	n	LC (%)
T1–2	≤ 45	83	93
	> 45	48	84
			$p = 0.1381$
T3–4	≤ 45	71	78
	> 45	44	56
			$p = 0.013$

TABLE 4.6 Five-Year Actuarial Local Control of Oropharyngeal Carcinoma Related to Treatment Dose: 1970–1994

Lesions	Dose	n	LC (%)
T1–2	>67 Gy	133	78
	≤67 Gy	188	73
			$p = 0.31$
T3	>67 Gy	105	73
	≤67	78	57
			$p = 0.05$
T4	>67 Gy	17	65
	≤67 Gy	41	37
			$p = 0.18$

2. In order to exploit the radiobiological phenomenon of repair of sublethal damage, a minimal interfraction interval of 4 hours or more is required.

3. The optimum fraction size (1.2 versus 1.6 Gy), number of daily fractions (two versus three or more per day), total dose (65–75 Gy or higher), and total treatment time (6 versus 8 weeks) have not been established scientifically. A randomized clinical trial is required.

4. The accelerated hyperfractionated BID program with 1.6 Gy/f resulted in higher local control of advanced T3 carcinomas of the head and neck as compared to the results obtained with the historical QD radiation therapy programs.

TABLE 4.7 Five-Year Actuarial Local Control of Glottic Carcinoma Related to Treatment Time: 1970–1994

Lesions	Days	n	LC (%)
T1	≤45	436	92
	>45	220	92
			$p = 0.67$
T2–2a	≤45	103	85
	>45	38	78
			$p = 0.319$
T2b–3	≤45	119	65
	>45	68	47
			$p = 0.015$

TABLE 4.8   Five-Year Actuarial Local Control of T3 Carcinoma of Oropharynx and Larynx Related to Treatment Gap[a]

Treatment Gap	n^b	LC
≤ 14 days	80/32	80%
> 14 days	82/27	58%

[a]Further subdivision of the gaps into <11 days ($n = 28$) and $11-13$ days ($n = 5$ showed local control rates of 87% and 74%, respectively, with $p = 0.0166$, with dose constraint within $65-70$ Gy.[36]

[b]$n =$ (total number of patients at risk)

5. Recent studies[36,37] indicate that increasing the total dose to $67.4-70.4$ Gy and shortening the overall treatment time to less than 45 days profoundly and favorably affect local control of T3 carcinomas of the oropharynx and larynx; this benefit was less marked for early T1–2 lesions following the BID radiation therapy program.

6. In view of recent radiobiological progress in understanding the radioresponses of the acute- and late-responding tissues, the selection of a treatment schedule and of an altered fractionation radiation therapy scheme for head and neck carcinoma is of the utmost importance for local control and treatment complications.

7. Currently, all patients with advanced squamous cell carcinomas of the head and neck are treated with accelerated hyperfractionated BID radiation therapy at the Massachusetts General Hospital.

REFERENCES

1. Greenberg M, Eisert DR, Cox JD: Initial evaluation of reduced fractionation in the irradiation of malignant epithelial tumors. *Am J Roentgen Radium Ther Nucl Med* 1976;126:268–278.

2. Byhardt RW, Greenberg M, Cox JD: Local control of squamous cell carcinoma of the oral cavity and oropharynx with 3 vs. 5 treatment fractions per week. *Int J Radiat Oncol Biol Phys* 1977;2:415–420.

3. Cox JD, Byhardt RW, Komaki R, et al: Reduced fractionation and the potential of hypoxic cell sensitizers in irradiation of malignant epithelial tumors. *Int J Radiat Oncol Biol Phys* 1980;6:37–40.

4. Parsons JT, Bova FJ, Million RR: A re-evaluation of split-course technique for squamous cell carcinoma of the head and neck. *Int J Radiat Oncol Biol Phys* 1980; 6:1645–1652.

5. Marcial VA, Hanley JA, Hendrickson F, et al: Split-course radiation therapy of carcinoma of the tongue: results of a prospective national collaborative clinical trial con-

ducted by the Radiation Therapy Oncology Group. *Int J Radiat Oncol Biol Phys* 1983;9:437–443.

6. Million RR, Parsons JT, Cassisi NJ: Twice-a-day radiation technique for squamous cell carcinoma of the head and neck. *Cancer* 1985;55:2096–2099.

7. Parsons JT, Mendenhall WM, Cassisi NJ, Isaacs JH, Million RR: Hyperfractionation for head and neck cancer. *Int J Radiat Oncol Biol Phys* 1988;14:649–658.

8. Marcial VA, Pajak TF, Chang C, Tupchong L, Stetz J: Hyperfractionated photon radiation therapy in the treatment of advanced squamous cell carcinoma of the oral cavity, pharynx, larynx and sinuses using radiotherapy as the only planned modality: preliminary report by the Radiation Therapy Oncology Group (RTOG). *Int J Radiat Oncol Biol Phys* 1987;13:41–47.

9. Cox JD, Pajak TF, Marcial VA, et al: Dose–response for local control with hyperfractionated radiation therapy in advanced carcinomas of the upper aerodigestive tracts: preliminary report of radiation therapy oncology group protocol 83-13. *Int J Radiat Oncol Biol Phys* 1990;18:515–521.

10. Cox JD, Pajak TF, Marcial VA, et al: Astro plenary: interfraction interval is a major determinant of late effects, with hyperfractionated radiation therapy of carcinomas of upper respiratory and digestive tracts: results from radiation therapy oncology group protocol 83-13. *Int J Radiat Oncol Biol Phys* 1991;20:1191–1195.

11. Horiot JC: The EORTC radiotherapy group experience: phase III trials in hyperfractionation (HF) and accelerated fractionation (AF) in head and neck cancers. *Int J Radiat Oncol Biol Phys* 1991;21(suppl 1):108(abstr).

12. Ang KK, Peters LJ: Concomitant boost radiotherapy in the treatment of head and neck cancers. *Semin Radiat Oncol* 1992;2:31–33.

13. Schmidt-Ullrich RK, Johnson CR, Wazer DE, et al: Accelerated superfractionated irradiation for advanced carcinoma of the head and neck: concomitant boost technique. *Int J Radiat Oncol Biol Phys* 1991;21:563–569.

14. Dische S, Saunders MI: Continuous hyperfractionated, accelerated radiotherapy (CHART): an interim report upon late morbidity. *Radiother Oncol* 1989;16:65–72.

15. Saunders MI, Dische S, Grosch EJ, et al: Experience with CHART. *Int J Radiat Oncol Biol Phys* 1991;21:871–878.

16. Olmi P, Cellai E, Chiavacci A, Fallai C: Accelerated fractionation in advanced head and neck cancer: results and analysis of late sequelae. *Radiother Oncol* 1990;17:199–207.

17. Peracchia G, Salti C: Radiotherapy with thrice-a-day fractionation in a short overall time: clinical experiences. *Int J Radiat Oncol Biol Phys* 1981;7:99–104.

18. Svoboda VHJ: Accelerated fractionation: the Portsmouth experience, 1972–1984. In: *International workshop on clinical implications of non-conventional fractionation with emphasis on multiple fractions a day (MDF).* Proceedings of Varian's Fourth European Clinac Users Meeting, Malta, 1984.

19. Wang CC, Blitzer PH, Suit HD: Twice-a-day radiation therapy for cancer of the head and neck. *Cancer* 1985;55:2100–2104.

20. Wang CC: Accelerated hyperfraction. In: Withers HR, Peters LJ, eds. *Innovations in radiation oncology.* Berlin: Springer-Verlag, 1987;239–243.

21. van der Schueren E, van den Bogaert W, Vanuytsel L, van Limbergen E: Radiotherapy by multiple fractions per day (MFD) in head and neck cancer: acute reactions of skin and mucosa. *Int J Radiat Oncol Biol Phys* 1990;19:301–311.

22. Withers HR: Biologic basis for altered fractionation schemes. *Cancer* 1985;55: 2086–2095.

23. Withers HR, Horiot J: Hyperfractionation. In: Withers HR, Peters LJ, eds. *Innovations in radiation oncology.* Berlin: Springer-Verlag, 1985;223.

24. Withers HR, Thames HD, Peters LJ: Differences in the fractionation response of acutely and late-responding tissues. In: Karcher KH, Kogelnik HD, Reinartz E, eds. *Progress in radio-oncology II.* New York: Raven Press, 1982;287–296.

25. Withers HR, Thames HD, Peters LJ: A new isoeffect curve for change in dose per fraction. *Radiother Oncol* 1983;1:187–191.

26. Trott KR, Kummermehr J: Rapid repopulation in radiotherapy: a debate on mechanism. Accelerated repopulation in tumors and normal tissues. *Radiother Oncol* 1991;22: 159–160.

27. Trott KR, Kummermehr J: What is known about tumor proliferation rates to choose between accelerated fractionation or hyperfractionation? *Radiother Oncol* 1985;3:1–9.

28. Maciejewski B, Preuss-Bayer G, Trott, K: Three influences of the number of fractions and overall treatment time on the local tumor control of cancer of the larynx. *Int J Radiat Oncol Biol Phys* 1983;9:321.

29. Wang CC: The enigma of accelerated hyperfractionated radiation therapy for head and neck cancer. *Int J Radiat Oncol Biol Phys* 1987;14:209–210.

30. Bourhis J, Fortin A, Dupiis O, et al: Very accelerated radiation therapy: preliminary results in locally unresectable head and neck carcinomas. *Int J Radiat Oncol Biol Phys* 1995;32:747–752.

31. Delaney GP, Fisher RJ, Smee RI, Hook C, Barton MB: Split-course accelerated therapy in head and neck cancer: an analysis of toxicity. *Int J Radiat Oncol Biol Phys* 1995;32: 763–768.

32. Fu KK, Clery M, Ang KK, Byhardt TW, Maor MH, Beitler JJ: Randomized phase I/II trial of two variants of accelerated fractionated radiotherapy regimens for advanced head and neck cancer: results of RTOG 88-09. *Int J Radiat Oncol Biol Phys* 1995;32: 589–599.

33. Metson R, Freehling D, Wang CC: Surgical complications following twice-a-day versus once-a-day radiation therapy. *Laryngoscope* 1988;98:30–34.

34. Wang CC: Does changing the pattern of fractionation affect local control of head and neck carcinomas? 1995 Franz Buschke Lecture, 15th Annual Current Approaches, UCSF.

35. Wang CC: Local control of oropharyngeal carcinoma after two accelerated hyperfractionation radiation therapy schemes. *Int J Radiat Oncol Biol Phys* 1988;14:1143–1146.

36. Wang CC, Efird JT: Does prolonged treatment course adversely affect local control of carcinoma of the larynx? *Int J Radiat Oncol Biol Phys* 1994;29:657–660.

37. Wang CC, Efird J, Nakfoor B, Martins P: Local control of T3 carcinomas after accelerated fractionation—a look at the "gap." *Int J Radiat Oncol Biol Phys* 1996;35:439–441.

CHAPTER 5

CANCER OF THE SKIN

The skin has two layers: an outer epidermis and an inner dermis. The former consists of stratified squamous epithelium, the external layer of which is keratinized. The dermis contains connective tissue and elastic fibers and the subcutaneous tissue further down. The sebaceous glands and other glands of the skin are in the dermis and the adjacent subcutaneous tissue. All skin components can give rise to malignant tumors.

Malignant tumors arising from the skin of the head and neck region include basal cell carcinoma (BCC), squamous cell carcinoma (SCC), lymphoma, malignant melanoma, malignant fibrohistiocytoma, angiosarcoma, and skin appendage carcinoma, among others. The adnexal tumors consist of sebaceous, meibomian, eccrine, and apocrine gland carcinomas. The common basal cell carcinomas, so-called rodent ulcers, appear typically as pearly firm elevations, with occasional central ulceration surrounded by minute capillaries, and are commonly found on the skin of the eyelids, nose, and nasolabial sulcus. BCC may manifest various forms, including superficial multicentric, nodular or noduloulcerative, pigmented, morphea or sclerosing, and adenoid cystic varieties. It is unreliable to differentiate between BCC and SCC on clinical grounds. It is therefore important that a tissue biopsy be obtained before any form of treatment is given.

Other uncommon tumors of the skin of the head and neck include mycosis fungoides, lymphomas, and leukemic infiltrates; these tumors involve multiple sites as a generalized process, and their local problems may require local radiation therapy.

The TNM staging system recommended by the American Joint Committee on Cancer[1] is as follows:

Tis   Carcinoma in situ
T1   Tumor 2 cm or less in greatest dimension

T2   Tumor more than 2 cm but not more than 5 cm in greatest dimension
T3   Tumor more than 5 cm in greatest dimension
T4   Tumor invades deep extradermal structures (i.e., cartilage, skeletal muscle, or bone)
Nx   Regional lymph nodes cannot be assessed
N0   No regional lymph node metastases
N1   Regional lymph node metastases

Squamous cell carcinomas of the skin of the head and neck region may involve the regional lymph nodes. For lesions of the midface, temporal area, nose, and lips, the metastases tend to occur in the preauricular, submandibular, and submental nodes. The incidence of metastases, however, is low, that is, about 5%.[2] Elective neck treatment either by neck dissection or radiation therapy for N0 neck is not indicated. For the clinically positive neck, radical neck dissection, with or without adjuvant radiation therapy, is warranted.

SELECTION OF THERAPY AND INDICATIONS

There are many ways to treat skin cancers. These include surgical excision, curettage, radiation therapy,[3-5] cryosurgery,[6] Mohs' micrographic surgery,[7] and topical 5-FU cream.[8] Although Mohs' procedure can be used for treatment of basal cell carcinoma of the skin, it is better reserved for the management of advanced lesions and/or recurrent tumors after curative surgery or radiation therapy. For early and moderately advanced lesions, surgery and irradiation remain the mainstays of curative procedures.

The selection of treatment modalities depends on the following 4C's:

CURE
COSMESIS
COST
CONVENIENCE

Surgery — The Treatment of Choice

1. Small lesions treated by excision expediently without sequential dysfunction or esthetic impairment.
2. Small lesions of the neck and scalp.
3. Lesions of the dorsum of the hand or arising from scar, thermal burns, and chronic radiation dermatitis.
4. Lesions arising in atrophic and aged skin, lupus vulgaris, and infected tumors in the pinna of the ear with chondritis.
5. Large, destructive lesions where extensive loss of soft tissue is evident and where plastic repair is necessary if cured by radiation therapy.

6. Extensive tumor infiltrating the underlying bone.
7. Skin appendage carcinomas and invasive melanomas.

Radiation Therapy — The Treatment of Choice

1. Carcinomas arising in the midline of the face, eyelids, nose, and lip, the so-called facial triangle (Figure 5.1).
2. Large, deeply infiltrative lesions of the skin of the face without bone involvement.
3. BCC and SCC arising in the skin of the auricle.
4. Lesions involving the commissure of the mouth.
5. Lesions arising in the preauricular or postauricular areas and nasolabial sulcus.

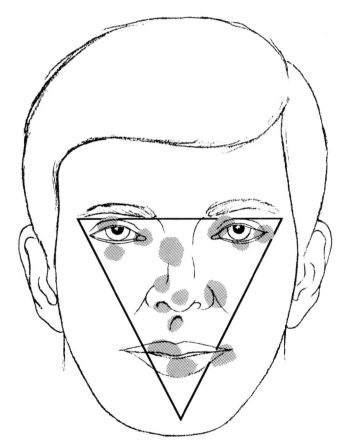

FIGURE 5.1 Diagram showing the so-called facial triangle, illustrating various sites of cancer of the skin most suitable for radiation therapy.

EVALUATION OF SKIN CANCERS

Before a radiotherapeutic procedure is considered, the size, thickness, and margins of the lesion must carefully be assessed. The margins are best evaluated in bright light with the aid of magnifying glasses. The lesion should be palpated gently. The surrounding hair follicles as well as skin texture and color should be compared between the normal skin and the lesion. The use of a Woods lamp (ultraviolet light) may help in differentiating between the tumor and the adjacent normal skin. Unfortunately, carcinoma and keratosis cannot be differentiated by a Woods lamp alone.

When the lesion is situated on the skin of the cheek and lip, bidigital palpation by gloved finger may be very informative as to the depth of infiltration of the lesion. When the lesion is fixed to adjacent bone, appropriate radiographs, including CT scans, should be obtained to evaluate the possibility of bone involvement.

RADIOTHERAPEUTIC MODALITIES AND ACCESSORIES

Most superficial cancers of the skin currently are treated by low-energy electrons, commonly 6–9 MeV. Low megavoltage photons (4–6 MV) or cobalt-60 radiations are used for the treatment of large and thick invasive tumors and/or regional lymph node metastases. BCC of the eyelid is best treated by low-energy x-rays, such as with the Phillips 50 kVp contact unit (Figure 5.2).

In addition to external beam therapy, brachytherapy can be employed. The afterloading interstitial implant procedure is preferred, using angiocath applicators and ^{192}Ir sources. For the past 4 years, a high dose rate (HDR) ^{192}Ir source has been available at the MGH; a large fraction, that is, 3–4 Gy/BID, is given as a boost fractionated for 2–3 days.

As a general rule, lesions on a curved surface are preferably treated by electrons while those on a flat surface are treated by brachytherapy alone or combined with electrons.

For radiation therapy of skin cancers, lead shields are used for proper exposure of the lesion and protection of the adjacent normal tissues. Table 5.1 shows the various thicknesses of lead needed to reduce the incident beams to 5% in low orthovoltage x-rays. Individually made lead cutouts, especially for the eye, nose, and gum shields, are used in the treatment of appropriate tumors (Figures 5.3 and 5.4). For electron beam therapy, 6–9 MeV beams are frequently used. The low-energy electrons have skin-sparing characteristics, and a thin layer of bolus must be added to the surface of the tumor to achieve D_{max} on the skin, as shown in Figure 5.5. An individual Cerrobend cutout with appropriate aperture is made to the shape of the lesion and placed under the window of the linear accelerator. These simple gadgets are extremely important for the treatment of skin cancers.

Radiation Therapy Dosages and Fraction Size

Any lesion thicker than 1.0 cm cannot be treated satisfactorily by 50 kV or 100 kV x-radiations. Such lesions are treated either by low-energy electrons or low-energy

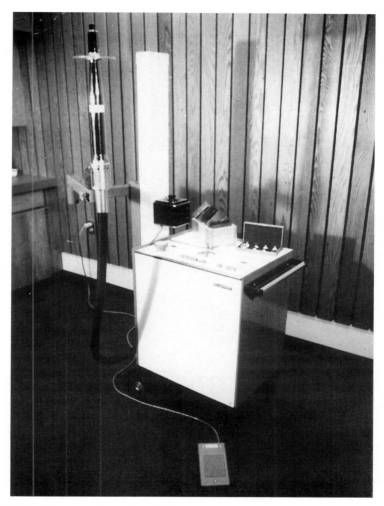

FIGURE 5.2   Photograph showing Phillips 50 kV contact machine for treatment of small carcinoma of the eyelid.

TABLE 5.1   Fractionation Radiation Therapy (RT) for Skin Cancer[a]

Lesion Size: 1.5–2.0 cm	
Fitzpatrick (Princess Margaret Hospital)[10]	35 Gy, 5 Gy/f, in 5 days
Moss (University of Oregon)[3]	45 Gy, 3–4 Gy/f, in 3–4 weeks
Wang (MGH)	45 Gy, 9 Gy/f, in 1 week
	45 Gy, 5 Gy/f, in 2 weeks
	52 Gy, 4 Gy/f, in 2.5 weeks

[a]No differences in dosage of RT for squamous and basal cell carcinomas.

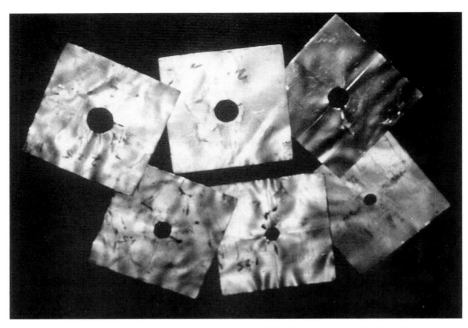

FIGURE 5.3 Special lead sheets and cutouts to tailor-fit the shape and size of the lesions for use with the 50 kV contact machine.

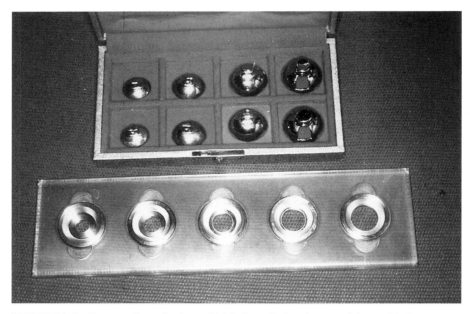

FIGURE 5.4 Top tray shows lead eye shields for radiation therapy of the eyelid. Bottom tray shows lead "nipple" cutouts suitable for treatment of cancer of the inner canthus of the eye.

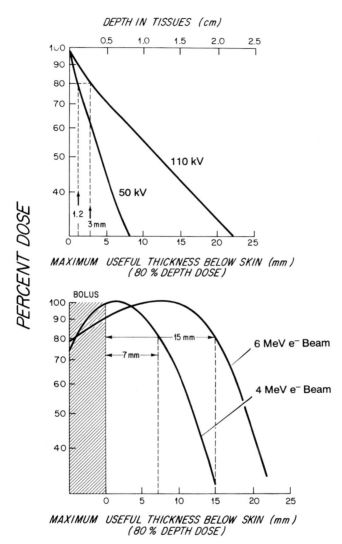

FIGURE 5.5 Comparison of percent depth dose data of radiations versus maximal therapeutic thickness of the lesions suitable for radiation therapy.

electrons in combination with an interstitial implant. For external beam x-ray therapy, various time–dose–fraction schemes[9] are available and have proved to be effective. The cosmetic results are related to the fraction size and total dose. Fractionation radiation therapies are presented for lesions 1.5–2.0 cm in diameter and for lesions 5–6 cm in diameter in Tables 5.1 and 5.2.

One notes that the treatment schemes are extremely variable, depending on the availability of treatment machine time, patient population (i.e., young or old, male or female), likelihood of patient's long-term survival, and so on. Our program of radiation therapy for skin cancer at the MGH has been used for the past 35 years and has proved to be highly effective with acceptable cosmetic results. The program is as follows:

1. For small lesions of 0.5–1 cm in size, a single treatment of 24 Gy is curative. It is rarely used but may be given to debilitated, aged patients who have difficulty attending daily radiation therapy sessions on an out-patient basis.

2. For lesions 1.5–2.5 cm in size, 45 Gy in five fractions or 45 Gy in nine fractions is commonly used, depending on the patient's skin, age, and ability to attend daily therapy sessions.

TABLE 5.2   Fractionation RT for Skin Cancer[a]

Lesion Size: 1.5–2.0	
Princess Margaret Hospital	7 Gy × 5 (113)[b]
University of Oregon	3 Gy × 15 (92)
University of Florida	3 Gy × 15 (92) or 4 Gy × 10 (96)
University of Arizona	7 Gy × 5 (113) or 5 Gy × 8 (108)
University of Alabama	9 Gy × 5 (167)
Christie	10 Gy × 3 (123) or 20 Gy × 1
MGH	9 Gy × 5 (167) or 5 Gy × 9 (123)
	4 Gy × 13 (125)
	20–23 Gy × 1 (rarely used)

Lesion Size: 5.0–6.0 cm	
PMH	3 Gy × 20 or 4 Gy × 10
	3 Gy × 15 plus implant
University of Oregon	3 Gy × 20
University of Florida	1.8 Gy × 35
University of Arizona	3 Gy × 20
University of Alabama	3 Gy × 10 plus implant 35 Gy
Christie	35 Gy plus implant
	Implant to 60 Gy alone
MGH	4 Gy × 13 or 3 Gy × 20
	3 Gy × 10 plus implant

[a]Data were surveyed by Kyle Colvett, M.D., 1994 (resident at MGH).
[b]Numbers in parentheses are TDF values.

3. For a somewhat larger lesion, or more desirable cosmesis, a prolonged course of treatment is prescribed, that is, 52 Gy divided into 13 daily fractions.

4. Large tumors are treated with 60 Gy in 25 fractions.

5. For large lesions suitable for combined external beam and interstitial implants, generally a total dose between 65 and 70 Gy is planned, that is, 30 Gy in 10 daily fractions by x-rays or electrons plus 30–35 Gy by implant.

6. Experience has shown that a TDF value of 120–130 as shown in Figure 5.6 is required for permanent local control of most small- to medium-sized carcinomas of the skin of the head and neck. For a larger and thicker lesion, a higher dose is required.

Technical Pointers

1. Patient should lie comfortably on the treatment couch and be immobilized.

2. Protect the underlying radiosensitive structures, such as the cornea and lens of the eye, mandible, teeth, gum, and nasal septum, with waxed lead shields. For sites that cannot be protected by intervening lead shields, select appropriate energies of x-rays, electrons, or implant or combination of various therapeutic modalities.

3. Due to the surface-sparing effects of low-energy electrons, add a bolus over the tumor when a 6–9 MeV electron beam is employed. (See Figure 5.5.)

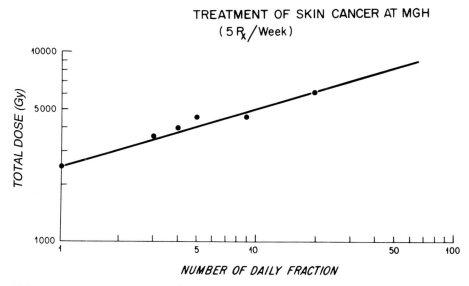

FIGURE 5.6 Isobioeffect curve for treatment of small to medium-sized cancers of the skin at the Massachusetts General Hospital. TDF values range between 125 and 135.

TABLE 5.3   6 MeV Electron Beam with 0.5 cm Bolus[a]

	Depth in Patient	Depth Dose (%)
Surface does	0.0 cm	84
Maximum	0.5 cm	100
0.5 cm bolus plus	1.0 cm	80
0.5 cm bolus plus	2.0 cm	40

[a]Varian 2100 C data.

4. For extensive lesions involving bone and muscle, consider surgery first with adjuvant postoperative radiation therapy.
5. Use the same dose and treatment scheme for squamous cell carcinoma and basal cell carcinoma.
6. Always evaluate the lesion at 2 weeks after treatment for skin reactions and radiation coverage. If the irradiated lesion and the adjacent tissue do not show brisk erythema to the point of moist desquamation, give an additional 9–10 Gy on top of the previously prescribed dose through a smaller field.
7. The lesion should heal in 4–6 weeks, leaving a smooth pliable scar. Any nodularity or ulceration in 6 months should be investigated by biopsy for recurrence.

The data in Tables 5.3 and 5.4 are related to the 6–9 MeV electron dose distribution at depth, for daily clinical management of skin carcinoma.

RADIOTHERAPEUTIC RESULTS

Carcinoma of the skin is highly curable by radiation therapy with local control rates of 90% or better. When basal cell carcinoma involves bone, the local control rate is poor but the patient may live with the disease for many years and therefore a relentless surgical approach could be rewarding. Metastatic squamous cell carcinoma of the skin to the regional nodes has a poor prognosis with a 3-year NED (no evidence of disease) rate of approximately 30%.

Table 5.5 shows the results of treatment of skin as reported in the literature.

TABLE 5.4   9 MeV Electron Beam with 1.0 cm Bolus[a]

	Depth in Patient	Depth Dose (%)
Surface does	0.0 cm	90
Maximum	0.6 cm	100
1.0 cm bolus plus	1.0 cm	82
1.0 cm bolus plus	2.0 cm	55

[a]Varian 2100 C data.

TABLE 5.5 Local Control After Treatment of Skin Cancer

Regato[11]
  594/654 patients—93% by RT
Lauritzen et al.[12]
  2802/2900 patients—96.5% by Surgery or RT
Freeman and Duncan[13]
  2235/2288 patients—98% by Surgery or RT
Sweat gland (well differentiated)—5 year survival, 70%[11]
Merkel cell carcinoma—50%[11]

SPECIFIC SITES OF RADIOTHERAPEUTIC INTEREST

Carcinoma of the Eyelid

For all practical purposes, basal cell carcinomas of the eyelid are considered to be cancers of the skin and they are treated as such.[10,14,15] When the lesion involves the inner canthus, surgical removal would mean either plastic repair or damage to the lacrimal duct. Radiation therapy can often achieve both good functional and cosmetic results and control of the disease comparable to that produced by a surgical procedure and therefore is preferred. Tumors of the canthi tend to involve the bony orbit rather early, especially at the inner canthus. When this occurs, control by radiation therapy is uncommon—about 25%—and therefore orbital exenteration may be required in order to save the patient's life. Postoperative radiation therapy may be considered as an adjuvant procedure.

Because of the superficial nature of most early cancer of the eyelid and the necessity for avoiding irradiation of the underlying radiosensitive structures of the eye, radiation therapy must be highly individualized. Radiations of low penetration are highly desirable, such as 4–6 MeV electrons or 50 kV x-rays using Phillips contact machine (the only kilovoltage machine used for clinical radiation therapy at the MGH at the present time).

The doses used for treatment of carcinoma of the eyelids are similar to radiation therapy for carcinoma of the skin: that is, for small lesions, 45 Gy in 5 daily fractions; for moderately advanced lesions, 45 Gy in 2 weeks; and for large lesions, 4 Gy per fraction for 13 days.

Technical Pointers

1. Because of the smaller portal to be used and the radiosensitive structures of the eye, the daily setup of treatment should be handled by the attending radiation oncologist.
2. Use inner waxed lead eye shields or beam-blocking devices to protect the cornea and lens.
3. The eye is anesthetized with topical anesthetic (0.5% paracaine hydrochloride).

The eyeshield is rinsed with saline solution or tap water after it is cleaned by alcohol. (The residue of the alcohol is irritating to the conjunctiva.)

4. Individual cutouts with at least 0.5 cm visible normal margins are used.

5. Bandage the anesthetized eye for about 30 minutes after each irradiation to prevent foreign bodies gaining access to the eye.

Squamous cell carcinoma of the eyelid is an uncommon disease and its management is identical to that for basal cell carcinoma in terms of extent of coverage and radiation dose and fractionation. Metastases from carcinoma of the eyelids occur in about 10% and carry a grave prognosis. The parotid lymph nodes are the most common site of involvement. The management of such metastases is a combination of surgical resection and radiation therapy.

Sebaceous gland carcinoma of the eyelid is rare, with high incidence of regional lymph node and distant metastases (i.e., approximately 25%).[16] For a small lesion, radiation therapy is the treatment of choice with good local control and satisfactory cosmesis.[16] The large infiltrative tumors associated with orbital invasion are better managed by surgical resection with adjuvant postoperative radiation therapy. Owing to their high propensity for lymph node metastases, elective ipsilateral parotid and neck irradiation with 45–50 Gy in 4 weeks appears worthwhile.

The results of radiation therapy for carcionoma of the eyelid are shown in Table 5.6.

Carcinoma of the Skin Overlying the Nasal Cartilage and the Nasolabial Sulcus

Carcinomas arising from the bridge and tip of the nose and nasal alae present a difficult problem for radiation dosimetry.[4,5] The so-called saddle lesion, covering both nasal alae, would be better treated by a combination of low-energy electrons and interstitial implant. The nasal cartilage has a high radiation tolerance, and radiochondritis following a therapeutic dose of radiotherapy has not been encountered in our practice and is a mythical misconception in the literature.

Carcinoma arising from the nasolabial sulcus tends to burrow beneath the skin and into the premaxillary fossa and adipose tissue and the true tumor extension often escapes accurate detection. The treatment of choice for these lesions is a combination of external beam therapy and interstitial implant.

Technical Pointers

1. Use 6–9 MeV electrons along with a 0.5 cm bolus over the lesion, and treat 1–1.5 cm below the skin surface.

TABLE 5.6   Local Control of Carcinoma of the Eyelid

Regato[14] — 108/117, 95%
Wildermuth and Evans[15] — 67/71, 93%
Fitzpatrick et al.[10] — 1106/1166, 95%
Wang — 290/300, 97%

2. A lead shield should be inserted into the nostrils to protect the nasal floor and septum.
3. Protect the underlying gum posterior to the upper lip with a lead shield.
4. Due to the slope of both nasal alae with increase of distance from the electron target, the peripheral dose is constricted toward the center, with a decrease of depth dose in the periphery. Use a wider portal, considerably more than in photon therapy.
5. The dose and treatment scheme is the same as for skin cancer in general.
6. For combined electron beam and brachytherapy, give 30 Gy in 2 weeks and 35 Gy in 3 days, respectively.

Carcinoma of the Skin of the Auricle of the Ear

When the lesion is infected and deeply ulcerative, exposing the cartilage, surgical excision is preferred. For early, superficial lesions arising from the pinna or concha of the ear, radiation therapy alone may be used with good local control and cosmetic results. Because of the irregular curvature of the surface of the auricle of the ear, x-ray therapy for this disease often produces "hot spots" and "cold spots" in the irradiated field, which may result in radiochondritis or local recurrence. The treatment of choice for these lesions is low-energy electrons; the incidence of radiochondritis is much lessened.

Technical Pointers

1. Protect the middle ear by inserting a lead cylinder (in the shape of the auditory canal, a so-called ear plug).
2. Protect the mastoid sinus by placing a waxed lead shield behind the auricle.
3. Protect the concha of the ear, if not involved with disease, by a small lead shield.
4. Use 6–9 MeV electrons to treat the entire thickness of the ear.
5. Place a 0.5 cm bolus over the lesion for maximal dose on the skin.
6. Dose schedule is the same as radiation therapy for skin cancer in general.

The treatment results are shown in Table 5.7.

TABLE 5.7   Local Control of Carcinoma of the Skin Over the Nose and Ear

Regato[11]
53/56, 95%
Fitzpatrick[17]
Nose: 285/320, 89%
Ear: 672/743, 90%

Carcinoma of the Skin Overlying Preauricular or Postauricular Sites

Carcinomas arising from these sites should not be treated by external beam alone, since the radiation dose to the temporomandibular joint (TMJ) or temporal bone may result in complications such as TMJ ankylosis or temporal bone necrosis. These lesions can be managed satisfactorily by a combination of low-energy electron beam and interstitial implant.

Technical Pointers

1. Use 6–9 MeV electrons and treat 1–1.5 cm below the surface.
2. Use varying thicknesses of bolus to determine the depth dose desired.
3. For moderate-sized lesions, plan 30 Gy of electrons in 2 weeks to be followed by a 30–35 Gy interstitial implant.
4. For the preauricular implant, insert sources horizontally [i.e., anteroposterior (AP) direction]. For postauricular lesions, insert sources vertically; the auricle is then sutured and folded forward over the preauricular area.
5. Be certain the auriculomastoid sulcus is adequately covered.

MISCELLANEOUS SKIN TUMORS OF RADIOTHERAPEUTIC INTEREST

Skin Appendage Carcinomas

Carcinomas of sebaceous glands, eccrine sweat glands, and apocrine glands may occur in the head and neck region.[18,19] Sebaceous gland carcinoma occurs most frequently on the eyelids as a malignant lesion of the meibomian gland. Widespread aggressive metastatic disease is often seen with eyelid lesions. Carcinoma of eccrine sweat glands and apocrine glands are locally invasive and tend not to metastasize. Treatment of these malignant appendage tumors is mostly by radical resection. The role of radiation therapy is not well recognized. Our experience, however, indicates that these lesions respond to high-dose (i.e., 70–75 Gy) irradiation well with good local control. If the lesions remain localized, yet unresectable, a trial course of radiation therapy is worthwhile.[16]

Merkel Cell Tumor

Merkel cell tumors are small cell neuroendocrine undifferentiated neoplasms of the skin, which occur on sun-exposed areas, especially on the face and arms in elderly men and women, and not infrequently run a fulminating clinical course with regional and distant metastases.[20–23] This type of tumor is quite radiosensitive and responds to a modest dose of radiation therapy. Generally, a dose of 45–50 Gy in 3–4 weeks is sufficient for local control. Due to the propensity to distant metastases, the eventual outcome for patients is extremely poor. Chemotherapy has been used but its efficacy remains primarily palliative.[21] (See Case Illustrations.)

Keratoacanthoma[24,25]

Keratoacanthoma is a benign lesion and histologically similar to well differentiated carcinoma; it can grow to 1–2 cm in a few weeks.[24,25] This type of lesion is often umbilicated and covered with a central keratin plug. The diagnosis can often be made on clinical grounds. Although biologically it may undergo spontaneous resolution, leaving a depressed scar, those lesions occurring on the eyelid, nose, and lip may cause significant loss of soft tissue, with resultant facial and functional deformity, and therefore require radiation therapy for local control.

A dose of 25 Gy in 1 week or its equivalent is sufficient for most lesions. If the tumor fails to show good regression in 2 weeks with such doses, an additional higher radiation dose (i.e., 60–65 Gy) should be given as if it were a genuine squamous cell carcinoma. (See Case Illustrations.)

Lentigo Maligna

Circumscribed precancerous melanosis or melanotic freckle of Hutchinson is a noninvasive melanotic lesion occurring primarily on the faces of elderly persons. It is usually a flat, tan lesion with irregular borders and areas of lighter pigmentation. Treatment of choice is surgical excision. In areas of cosmetic and functional importance, such as the eyelid, pinna of the ear, and bridge and ala of the nose, radiation therapy is employed in lieu of surgery and can achieve satisfactory local control.[26] Doses similar to those for the treatment of carcinoma of the skin are recommended—that is, 45 Gy in nine daily fractions or its equivalent. (See Case Illustrations.)

Kaposi's Sarcoma

Kaposi's sarcoma is a multicentric, incurable lesion. The tumors are extremely radiosensitive, and for the small, symptomatic lesion a single dose of 10 or 15 Gy in three fractions should produce lasting regression. Kaposi's sarcoma associated with acquired immunodeficiency syndrome (AIDS) can also be irradiated with good local control. A dose of 25–30 Gy in 1 week or its biological equivalent should suffice. Unfortunately, the survival of the AIDS patient is short in terms of months.

CASE ILLUSTRATIONS

To illustrate the salient features of the different kinds of skin cancer and their treatment techniques and results, a series of cases are presented in Figures 5.7 through 5.14.

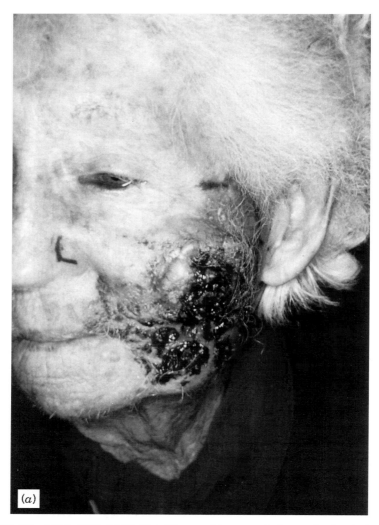

(a)

FIGURE 5.7   M.M. #244-96-69. This 87-year-old woman had an enlarging lesion on the left cheek and biopsy revealed well-differentiated squamous cell carcinoma. There was no regional adenopathy. Radiation therapy was given using a combination of 12 and 15 MeV electrons for 30 Gy and lateral wedge pair cobalt-60 x-rays for 40 Gy in 45 days. The total TDF value was 136. (a) Pretreatment photograph.

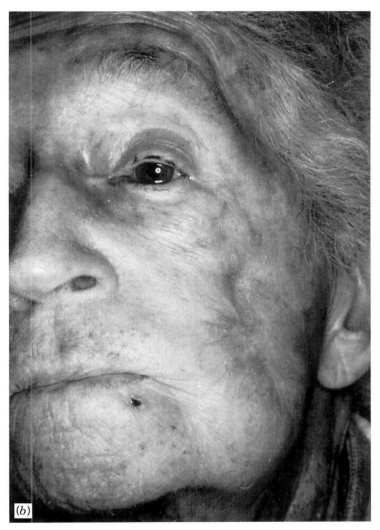

FIGURE 5.7   (b) Postradiation therapy photograph 1 year after treatment.

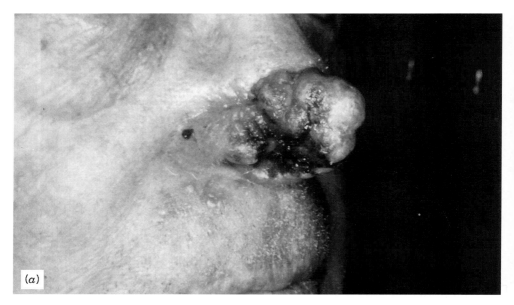

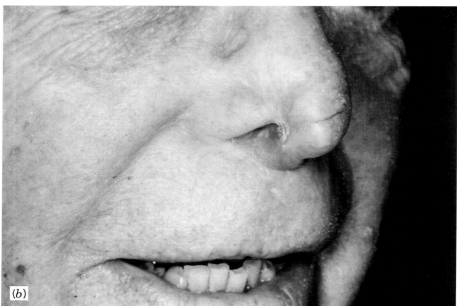

FIGURE 5.8 J.R. #234-31-01. This 83-year-old man had a recurrent basal cell carcinoma on the right nasal ala, previously treated by excision and skin graft. The recurrent lesion was treated with 12 MeV electrons for 30 Gy in 10 daily fractions, followed by interstitial implant of 30 Gy in 60 hours. The patient was NED. (a) Pretreatment photograph. (b) Postradiation therapy photograph $2\frac{1}{2}$ years after implant.

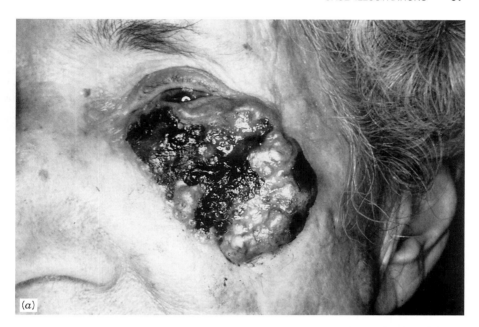

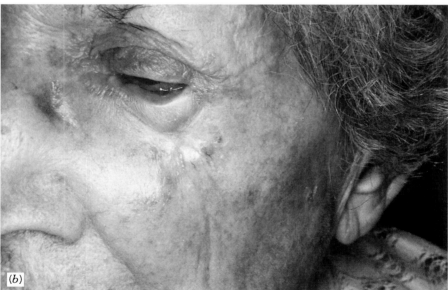

FIGURE 5.9   E.C. #238-88-54. This 83-year-old woman presented with a large mobile and exophytic basal cell carcinoma of the left malar region involving the lower eyelid. Radiation therapy consisted of 45 Gy using 9 MeV electrons with 0.5 cm bolus in nine daily fractions. Three weeks later, an additional 10 Gy in a single treatment was given using a 6 MeV electron beam. The eye was protected. (a) Pretreatment photograph. (b) Postradiation therapy photograph $1\frac{1}{2}$ years later. TDF = 145.8.

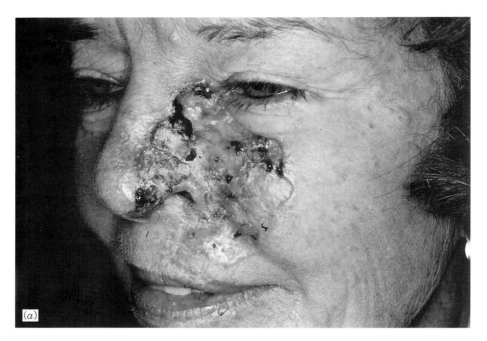

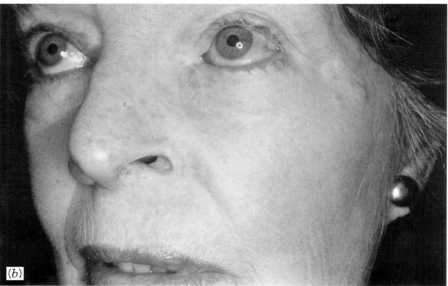

FIGURE 5.10   P.P. #2735009. This 63-year-old woman noticed a scaly, eczematoid squamous cell carcinoma on the left side of her face and nose for 5 years. The lesion was freely mobile from the underlying structures and measured 7×7 cm.[2] No parotid or cervical adenopathy was evident. The lesion was treated with 64 Gy in 25 fractions over 35 elapsed days with good response and she was NED 5 years after radiation therapy. (a) Pretreatment photograph. (b) Postradiation photograph showing excellent response with good cosmesis.

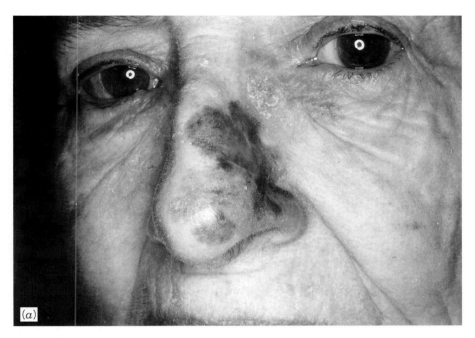

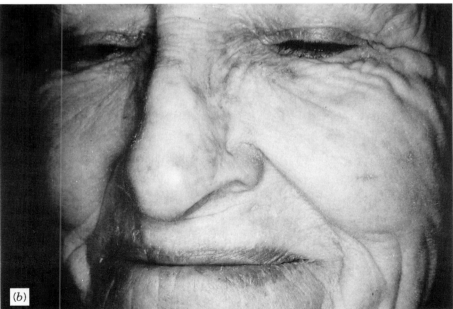

FIGURE 5.11 A.C. #166-82-95. This 81-year-old woman had lentigo maligna on the left side of the nose for 10 years. The lesion was treated using 6 MeV electrons, 5 Gy per fraction per day for 45 Gy in 13 elapsed days. Three weeks later, due to lack of severe reaction, an additional 10 Gy was given in a single fraction. She was last seen 2 years after radiation therapy and the pigmented lesion had completely disappeared with good skin and subcutaneous tissue in evidence. (a) Pretreatment photograph. (b) Postradiation therapy photograph.

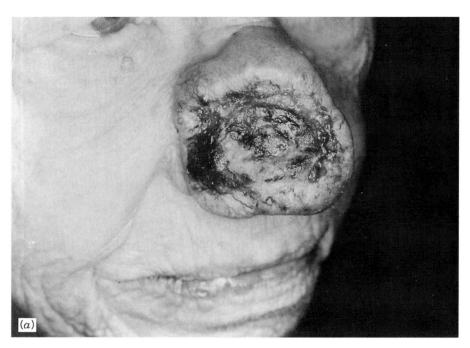

(a)

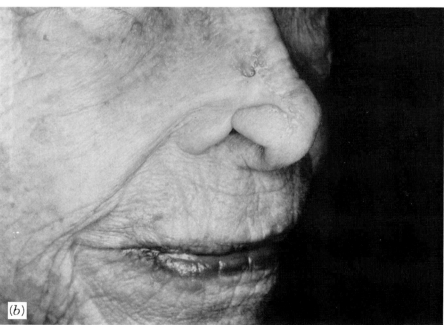

(b)

FIGURE 5.12 E.J. This 93-year-old woman noted a rapidly enlarging mass on her nose for 3 months. Biopsy showed squamous cell carcinoma. The clinical course was that of kerato-acanthoma. The lesion was treated for 32 Gy in 10 days with 4 Gy per fraction of 12 MeV electrons. The tumor completely vanished, leaving a relatively normal looking nose. (a) Pre-treatment photograph. (b) Postradiation therapy photograph.

100

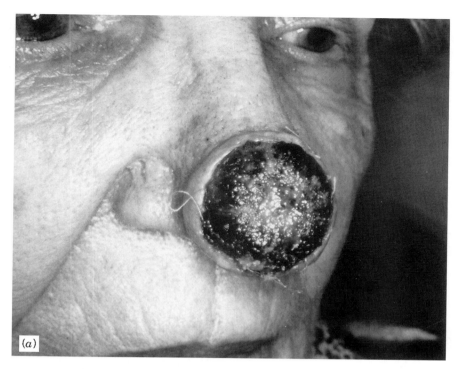

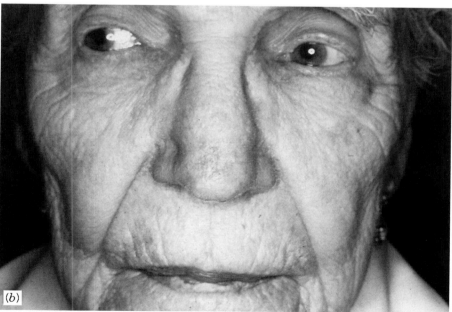

FIGURE 5.13 B.D. #199-52-70. This 85-year-old woman presented with rapidly enlarging keratoacanthoma on the tip of the nose of 6 weeks' duration. Radiation therapy of 12 Gy, 4 Gy per fraction, using a 280 kV machine was given. Five weeks later, due to persistence of disease, an additional 5 Gy was given. When last seen the patient was NED $3\frac{1}{2}$ years after radiation therapy. (a) Pretreatment photograph. (b) Postradiation therapy photograph.

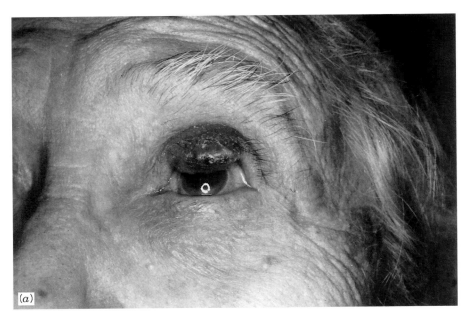

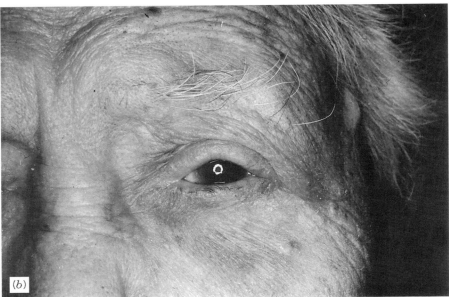

FIGURE 5.14 This 98-year-old woman had a small lump in the left upper eyelid for 6 months. Incisional biopsy revealed a Merkel cell tumor. Physical examination indicated a 1.5 cm × 2.5 cm × 1.0 cm nodule in the left upper eyelid with a 2.0 cm metastatic left preauricular lymph node. The eyelid lesion was treated with a small field, with the eye protected, to 51 Gy over 16 days, and the left parotid node was treated with a separate field to 60 Gy over 29 days, using a combination of electrons and ^{60}Co radiation. Treatments were given with the twice-daily program with 2 Gy per fraction. There was complete disappearance of both lesions after the treatment. Later, the patient developed fulminating cervical and supraclavicular metastatic lesions and received chemotherapy for palliation. (a) Pretreatment photograph. (b) Post-treatment photograph.

SUMMARY

Cancers of the skin of the head and neck are very common. Basal cell carcinoma and squamous cell carcinoma are the common histologic types and in the early stage are curable in about 90–95% of patients. The selection of various therapy methods is highly important in cancer management and depends on the availability and skill of the specialists, the location and size of the lesion, the cosmetic and functional results anticipated after the treatment, the cost and effects, and the convenience to the patient. Many small accessible basal cell carcinomas of the face can be treated expediently by excisional biopsy, electrodesiccation, and curettage. The large and superficial lesions arising in difficult sites, for which surgery may result in significant cosmetic mutilation, are best dealt with by radiation therapy. Surgical excision may be used for large, deeply infiltrative lesions with bone involvement in accessible location. The Mohs procedure is a time-consuming, laboratory-taxing, and tissue-destroying procedure and is generally reserved for treatment of recurrent carcinoma.

The use of radiation therapy for Merkel cell tumor, keratoacanthoma, lentigo maligna, and Kaposi's sarcoma has gradually been recognized and in selected cases may be rewarding.

Radiation therapy for carcinoma of the skin requires careful planning and techniques with various energies of photons and electrons intermixed with brachytherapy and calls for greater professional skills, ingenuity, and individuality. Proper selection of quality and quantity of radiations and fraction size, with careful protection of adjacent and underlying structures, can result in extremely high cure rates and excellent cosmesis without complications. This requires personal interest and enthusiasm on the part of the radiation oncologist.

REFERENCES

1. American Joint Committee on Cancer. *Manual for staging of cancer*, 4th ed. Philadelphia: Lippincott, 1992.
2. McGavran MH: Skin tumors. In: Ackerman LV, Rosai J, eds. *Surgical pathology*. 5th ed. St Louis: CV Mosby, 1974.
3. Moss WT, Bran WN, Battifora H: Metastasis of squamous cell carcinoma of the skin by region and frequency of surgical control of metastasis. In: Moss WR, Brand WN, Battifora AH, eds. *Radiation oncology*, 5th ed. St Louis: CV Mosby, 1979.
4. del Regato JA, Vuksanovic M: Radiotherapy of carcinomas of the skin overlying the cartilages of the nose and ear. *Radiology* 1962;79:203–208.

5. Parker RG, Wildermuth O: Radiation therapy of lesions overlying cartilage. *Cancer* 1962;15:57–65.

6. Zacarian S, ed: *Cryosurgical advances in dermatology and tumors of head and neck. Dermatology.* Springfield, IL: Charles C Thomas, 1977.

7. Mohs FE: Chemosurgery: microscopically controlled surgery for skin cancer—past, present and future. *J Dermatol Surg Oncol* 1978;4:41–54.

8. Klein E, Helen F, Milgram H, et al: Tumors of the skin, effects of local use of cytostatic agents. *Skin* 1962;1:89.

9. Strandquist M: Time–dose relationship. *Acta Radiol* 1977;55(suppl):1.

10. Fitzpatrick PJ, Jamieson DM, Thompson GA, et al: Tumors of the eyelids and their treatment by radiotherapy. *Radiology* 1972;104:661–665.

11. del Regato JA: *Ackerman & del Regato's cancer-diagnosis, treatment and prognosis,* 6th ed. St Louis: CV Mosby 1985;203–206.

12. Lauritzen RE, Johnson RE, Spratt JS Jr: Pattern of recurrences in basal cell carcinoma. *Surgery* 1965;57:813–816.

13. Freeman RG, Duncan WC: Recurrent skin cancer. *Arch Dermatol* 1973;107:395–399.

14. del Regato JA: Roentgen therapy of carcinoma of the eyelids. *Radiology* 1949; 52:564–573.

15. Wildermuth O, Evans JC: The special problem of cancer of the eyelid. *Cancer* 1956; 9:837–841.

16. Pardo F, Wang CC, Albert D, et al: Sebaceous carcinoma of the ocular adnexae: a role of radiotherapy. *Int J Radiat Oncol Biol Phys* 1988;15:167.

17. Fitzpatrick PJ: Radiation therapy of tumors of the skin of the head and neck. In: Thawley SE, Panje WR, Batsakis JG, Lindberg RO, eds. *Comprehensive management of head and neck tumors.* Philadelphia: Saunders, 1987;1208–1220.

18. Miller WL: Sweat gland carcinoma: a clinicopathologic problem. *Am J Clin Pathol* 1967;47:767–780.

19. Wertkin MG, Bauer JJ: Sweat gland carcinoma: current concepts of surgical management. *Arch Surg* 1976;111:884–885.

20. Sibley RK, Dehner LP, Rosai J: Primary neuroendocrine (Merkel cell?) carcinoma of the skin. *Am J Surg Pathol* 1985;9:95–108.

21. George TK, Santagnese A, Bennett JM: Chemotherapy for metastatic Merkel cell carcinoma. *Cancer* 1985;56:1034–1038.

22. Goepfert H, Remmler D, Silva E, Wheeler B: Merkel cell carcinoma (endocrine carcinoma of the skin) of the head and neck. *Arch Otolaryngol* 1984;110:707–712.

23. Warner TF, Uno H, Hafez GR, et al: Merkel cells and Merkel cell tumors: ultrastructure, immunocytochemistry and review of the literature. *Cancer* 1983;52:238–245.

24. Finley AG: Keratoacanthoma. *Aust J Dermatol* 1954;2:144.

25. Shimm D, Duttenhaver J, Doucette J, et al: Radiation therapy of keratoacanthomas. *Int J Radiat Oncol Biol Phys* 1983;9:759–761.

26. Harwood AR: Conventional radiotherapy in the treatment of lentigo maligna and lentigo melanoma. *J Am Acad Dermatolol* 1982;6:310–316.

27. O'Brien PH, Brasfield RD: Kaposi's sarcoma. *Cancer* 1966;19:1497–1502.

28. Holecek MJ, Harwood AR: Radiotherapy of Kaposi's sarcoma. *Cancer* 1978;41:1733–1738.

CHAPTER 6

CANCER OF THE ORAL CAVITY

GENERAL COMMENTS

Squamous cell carcinomas arising from the various anatomic sites of the oral cavity shown in Figures 6.1a and b are relatively common malignancies of the head and neck. The TNM Staging System for Oral Cancer as recommended by the American Joint Committee in 1992 is as follows[1]:

T1   Tumor 2 cm or less in greatest dimension
T2   Tumor more than 2 cm but not more than 4 cm in greatest dimension
T3   Tumor more than 4 cm in greatest dimension
T4   Tumor invades adjacent structures, for example, through cortical bone into deep (extrinsic) muscle of tongue, maxillary sinus, or skin

Pathologically, the majority of cancers of the oral cavity are squamous cell carcinomas. As a general rule, when the location of the lesion is further away from the lips toward the oropharynx or closer to the midline of the oral cavity, the tumor tends to be less differentiated and associated with a higher incidence of lymph node metastases. Thus the lip and buccal mucosa carcinomas have a much lower incidence of lymphatic spread than do the lesions of the tongue and oropharynx; that is, lesions of the tonsils and hard palate have much less chance of developing regional metastases than do soft palate carcinomas. Since squamous cell carcinoma represents dysplastic mucosal membrane, there is almost always some degree of mucosal change associated with the tumor. The lesion shows some bleeding, often after detailed examination and scraping with tongue depressors. Early mucosal lesions may

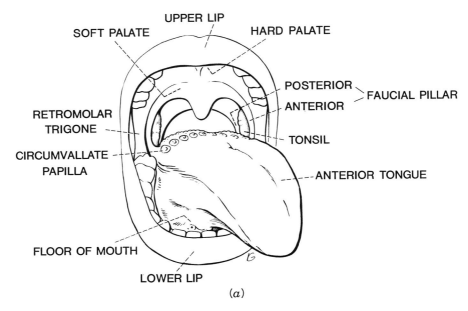

(a)

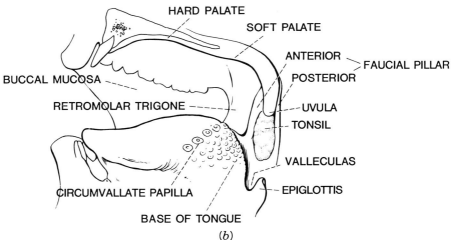

(b)

FIGURE 6.1   Diagrams showing various anatomic sites of the oral cavity: (a) anterior view and (b) lateral view.

appear as only superficial granularity or an indurated nodule or as a shallow ulceration that may have minimal subjective symptoms. Advanced tumors often extend deeply into the underlying muscles or bone causing fixation of the organ and resulting in difficulty in speech and deglutition. Metastases commonly occur to the ipsilateral submandibular, subdigastric, superior, and midjugular nodes although cross metastases to the contralateral neck may also occur with lesions across the midline of the oral cavity or lesions arising from the tip of the tongue or anterior floor of the mouth. The incidence of cervical lymph node metastases varies with different tumor sites, and for early lesions, T1, ranges from 10% to 20%; for the intermediate lesions, T2, the range is 25% to 30%; and for advanced lesions, T3 and T4, 50% to 70%.[2] Distant metastases below the clavicle are uncommon, with an incidence of approximately 10–15%, and are related to the extent of the primary tumor and the status of the cervical nodes. For the Stage I lesion the incidence is 6%; for Stage II, 20%; and for the advanced stages the rates increase to 30–40%.[3,4] The majority of patients who die with distant metastases also have evidence of recurrent disease above the clavicle and these metastases occur late in the course of the disease.

Multiple primary tumors may occur synchronously or metachronously in the upper aerodigestive tract. Patients with a single tumor, which was cured either by surgery or radiation therapy, have a significant risk (approximately five- to sixfold) of developing a second tumor in the head and neck area.[5] Patients with Stage III and Stage IV head and neck carcinoma who are cured by aggressive combined therapies have a 6% per annum risk of developing a second tumor.[6] Radiation therapy modalities for treatment of carcinoma of the oral cavity consist of external beam low megavoltage radiations, that is, cobalt-60 units or 4–6 MV x-rays from linear accelerators, electron beam, interstitial implant with iridium-192, and intraoral cone (IOC) using kilovoltage radiations or electrons. Frequently, one or more of these modalities are employed to achieve maximum tumor control and minimal complications.

For the lesions with high propensity for nodal metastases, radiation therapy includes the primary lesion as well as the first echelon of lymph nodes as a comprehensive treatment program. Because of the limited tolerance of the mandible,[7] treatment of oral cancer entirely by external beam generally produces lower local tumor control and higher complications than the treatment with mixed modalities, and therefore interstitial implant and/or intraoral cone (IOC) radiations are required to boost the primary site as a part of the integrated radiotherapeutic procedure.

Interstitial implant has been a standby procedure for treatment of oral cancers for the past few decades[8] and is used to irradiate the residual nidus after the lesion is shrunken by external radiation therapy. The implant should not be carried out without prior external irradiation because of the probability of implantation of the unirradiated tumor cells along the needle tracts during implantation. Due to the invasive nature and the associated complications, interstitial implant is limited primarily for lesions lateral to the mandibular arch, such as the lip and buccal mucosal carcinoma. Since 1975 at the MGH, its use for carcinoma of the tongue and floor of the mouth has been superseded by IOC radiation therapy.

Intraoral cone therapy is used for most of the early lesions lying within the mandibular arch of the oral cavity. These commonly include the oral tongue, floor of the mouth, and occasionally the retromolar trigone and palate. For lesions with well defined margins, which are encompassable by the cone, IOC radiation therapy may be given at the very outset of the therapy program as an initial boost to the primary lesion to be followed by comprehensive external beam radiation therapy. On the other hand, if the lesions are poorly defined, it is advisable to proceed with external beam therapy first for approximately 20 Gy in 2 weeks, employing large portals to better define the margins of the lesion by the development of tumoritis. This initial "mouth bath" is found to be highly important for the management of carcinoma of the oral cavity. After the margins of the tumor are well defined, they should be photographed and tattooed for permanent recording of the lesion. In general, daily IOC radiation therapy is not well tolerated after a high dose of comprehensive external radiation therapy, that is, 45–50 Gy, because of severe symptomatic radiation mucositis, and the lesion is often poorly localized from tumor regression if not initially tattooed.

If the lesions are not suitable for boost by IOC or interstitial implant, external radiation therapy through the reduced portal technique, either opposing lateral portals or ipsilateral wedge pair approach or ipsilateral electrons, should be given to bring the total dose to a level of 70–72 Gy. Submental electron boost, sparing the mandible, may supplement external beam radiation therapy. If none of the radiation therapy boost techniques is possible, limited surgical excision of residual disease in the form of nidusectomy should be considered. Thus, nidusectomy could be considered a surgical boost procedure.

Results of radiation therapy for carcinoma of the oral cavity are generally related to the size of the primary lesion (T stage) and the presence or absence of metastatic nodes (N stage) or the level of the nodal involvement.[9] In early lesions, T1, the local control rates approach 75–80% and for intermediate lesions, T2, 50–60%. For advanced carcinomas, T3 and T4, local control rates range from 20% to 30%. For lesions without node involvement, the cure rates range from 50% to 70%, while the presence of metastatic nodes reduces rates by one-half to one-third.

The location of the metastatic nodes greatly influences the patient's survival. The classification of the Memorial Sloan-Kettering Cancer Center assigns five levels of nodal distribution in the cervical region as follows[9]:

Level I	Submandibular and submental nodes
Level II	Upper third deep jugular nodes
Level III	Middle third jugular nodes
Level IV	Lower third jugular nodes
Level V	Posterior triangle nodes

In general, patients presenting with metastases in Levels I and II will have higher survival rates than patients with involvement of Level IV and V nodes.

From the standpoint of anatomic origin and management, carcinoma of the oral cavity can be subdivided as follows: lip, oral tongue, floor of the mouth, retromolar trigone and anterior tonsillar pillar, buccal mucosa, gingiva, soft palate, and hard palate. A detailed discussion of each of these lesions is presented in the following sections.

REFERENCES

1. American Joint Committee on Cancer: *Manual for staging of cancer*, 4th edition Philadelphia: J. B. Lippincott 1992.

2. Lindberg R: Distribution of cervical lymph node metastases from squamous cell carcinoma of the upper respiratory and digestive tracts. *Cancer* 1972;29:1446.

3. Kotwall C, Sako K, Razack MS, et al: Metastatic patterns in squamous cell cancer of the head and neck. *Am J Surg* 1987;154:439.

4. Merino OR, Lindberg RD, Fletcher GH: An analysis of distant metastases from squamous cell carcinoma of the upper respiratory and digestive tracts. *Cancer* 1977;40:145.

5. Shikhani AH, Metanoski GM, Jones MM et al: Multiple primary malignancies in head and neck cancer. *Arch Otolaryngol Head Neck Surg* 1986;112:1172.

6. Vikram B, Strong EW, Shah JP, Spiro RH: Second malignant neoplasms in patients successfully treated with multimodality treatment with advanced head and neck cancer. *Head Neck Surg* 1984;6:734.

7. Wang CC, Doppke KP, Biggs PJ: Intra-oral cone radiation therapy for selected carcinomas of the oral cavity. *Int J Radiat Oncol Biol Phys* 1983;9:1185–1189.

8. Pierquin B, Chassagne D, Baillet F, et al: The placement of implantation in tongue and floor of mouth cancer. *JAMA* 1971;215:961.

9. Shaj JP, Cendon RA, Farr HW, Strong EW: Carcinoma of the oral cavity: factors affecting treatment failure at the primary site and neck. *Am J Surg* 1976;132:504.

A. CARCINOMA OF THE LIP

Cancer of the lip is a relatively common tumor of the head and neck. In 1995 statistics approximately 3600 new cases will be diagnosed annually.[1] Squamous cell carcinoma of the lip behaves differently from other cancers of the oral cavity and is somewhat similar to carcinoma of the skin. These lesions occur mostly after the fifth decade of life and are rare in the black race but are commonly seen in patients with outdoor occupations having heavy exposure to sunshine. Pipe smokers have a high incidence of lip cancer as do persons whose lower lips protrude forward, resulting in direct exposure to the sun. Basal cell carcinoma does not occur in the lip per se but may originate in the skin with secondary involvement of the lip. Other malignancies include salivary gland tumors, melanoma, and malignant fibrous xanthoma.

Approximately 90% of squamous cell carcinomas occur in the lower lip, 90% are in males, and 90% are well differentiated carcinomas less than 1 cm in size. Approximately 5% of lip cancers occur in the upper lip, frequently near the midline. Tumors involving the commissure and adjacent lip are infrequent, approximately 1–2%.[2] The incidence in both sexes is roughly equal for upper lip cancer.

Lip cancers may be associated with chronic immunosuppressed status in patients with kidney and/or liver transplants.

The American Joint Committee (AJC) staging for lip cancer as published in 1992 is identical to that for cancer of the oral cavity and is as follows[3]:

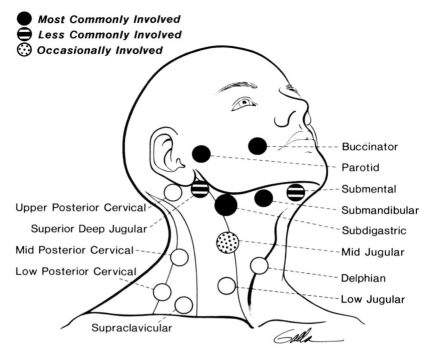

● *Most Commonly Involved*
⊜ *Less Commonly Involved*
⊙ *Occasionally Involved*

FIGURE 6A.1 Lymph node involvement from carcinoma of the upper lip.

T1	Tumor 2 cm or less in greatest dimension
T2	Tumor more than 2 cm but not more than 4 cm in greatest dimension
T3	Tumor more than 4 cm in greatest dimension
T4	Tumor invades adjacent structures (e.g., through cortical bone, tongue, skin of neck)

The lymphatic network of the upper lip is more extensive than that of the lower lip and drains to the preauricular and infraparotid, buccinator, submandibular, and then to the superior jugular nodes, shown in Figure 6A.1. The lymphatics of the lower lip drain to the submental and submandibular nodes and to the subdigastric nodes as shown in Figure 6A.2. The lymphatic vessels in the lower lip near the midline cross from one side to the other (Figure 6A.3). This fact is of great importance in therapeutic considerations involving the spread of lower lip cancer. The lymphatic crossing in the upper lip is unlikely, however.

The incidence of lymph node metastases in lower lip carcinoma averages less than 10% but is closely related to (1) cellular differentiation of the tumor, (2) location of the primary, and (3) size of the primary lesion. Cross et al.[4] showed that the incidence for Grade I lesions is 7%, for Grade II it's 23%, and for Grade III it's 35%. Wurman et al.[5] reported that T1 lesions (2 cm) had an incidence of 5% and for T2 (2–4 cm) and T3 lesions (4 cm) the rates increased to 52% and 73%, respectively. Recurrent lip cancers, after definitive therapies, are likewise associated with a high incidence of metastases. Lund et al.[6] reported that metastases occurred more frequently for those lesions recurring after prior treatment as compared to untreated lesions, that is, 23% versus 3%. The differences were more marked for those advanced lesions (T2—20% versus 2% and T3—46% versus 16%, respectively).

Contrary to lower lip cancers, lesions arising from the upper lip have a slightly higher incidence of lymph node metastases. For the commissural lesions, the incidence of metastases is approximately 20% at diagnosis.[2] With the exception of a midline location, upper lip carcinomas tend to metastasize to the ipsilateral lymph nodes. The lower lip lesions near the midline have a higher incidence of contralateral metastases. Even when metastases develop, the disease is known to occur in an orderly fashion and rarely skips the first echelon of nodes to the inferior jugular nodes. Distant metastases are extremely rare, approximately 10–15%,[7,8] especially for patients with uncontrolled primary lesions.

The motor function of the lips is enervated by the facial nerve and the sensory function of the upper and lower lips is supplied by the second and third division of the trigeminal nerve, respectively. Thus the major portion of the skin and upper lip is enervated by the infraorbital nerve and the lip commissure and lower lip by the mental nerve. Knowledge of the neurological distribution of various nerve innerva-

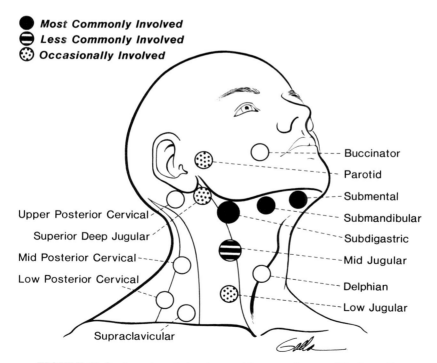

FIGURE 6A.2 Lymph node involvement from carcinoma of the lower lip.

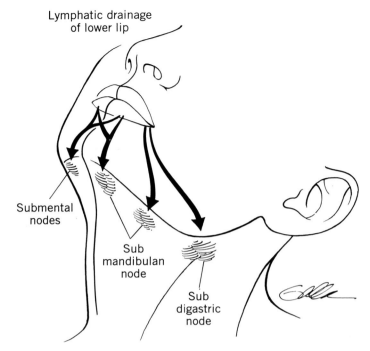

FIGURE 6A.3 Cross-lymphatics in lower lip.

tion is important as perineural spread of carcinoma of the lip may occur, resulting in numbness of the upper and lower lip, although this pattern of metastases is rare.[9,10]

SELECTION OF THERAPY

Since radiation therapy or surgery has yielded equally high cure rates for small limited cancers—that is, 3-year NED rates of 90%—the selection of treatment modality must depend on the cosmetic result following the procedure.

Surgery Is Preferred for the Following Conditions:

1. A small carcinoma of the lip, which can be dealt with expediently and successfully by V-shaped excision if the procedure will not result in cosmetic and functional deformity.
2. Extensive cancers that involve the mandible.
3. Cancer associated with significant loss of soft tissue, which requires major reconstruction after the lesion is controlled by radiation therapy.

4. Advanced tumors with nodal metastases.

5. Radiation failures.

Radiation Therapy Is Preferred for the Following Conditions:

1. Superficial lip cancers involving more than one-third of the entire lip.

2. Tumors involving the commissure and upper and lower lips.

3. Recurrent tumors after prior surgical excision.

4. Patients who refuse surgery.

Although radical neck dissection with adjuvant radiation therapy is clearly necessary for metastatic nodes, that is, N1 and N2 disease, prophylactic or elective neck dissection or irradiation for N0 neck in patients with lip cancer is not indicated. The arguments are as follows: (1) low grade lesions of the lower lip rarely metastasize to the lymph nodes and less than 10% of the lesions with N0 neck at the time of diagnosis will subsequently develop nodal metastases during the entire course of the disease[5,11]; (2) therapeutic neck dissection has favorable results as a prophylactic neck dissection with occult nodes[12]; and (3) a small group of patients developing metastases can still be cured[13] and yet a majority of the patients (90%) are spared unnecessary elective neck dissection or irradiation.

RADIOTHERAPEUTIC MANAGEMENT

As a rule, therapy is directed to the primary lesion if there are no palpable nodes or if the primary lesion is well differentiated. For superficial, small tumors, T1, radiation therapy consists of low megavoltage electron beams or interstitial implant. Generally, a dose of 45–50 Gy with 3–4 Gy per fraction external photon or electron therapy in 3–4 weeks should suffice. Due to the high sensitivity of the lip mucosa, radiation mucositis is generally rather severe but well tolerated. For large tumors, T2 and T3, involving more than one-half of the lip, or tumors extending below the buccogingival sulcus, making shielding of the underlying mandible impossible, a combination of 30 Gy in 2 weeks by external photons or electrons and 35 Gy in 3–4 days by interstitial implant offers the best local control and cosmesis. Osteoradionecrosis of the underlying mandible is a distinct possibility if high-dose external beam therapy is given to the entire thickness of the lip, including a large segment of the mandible. This must be avoided. For far advanced tumors with metastatic nodes or recurrent tumors after previous surgical procedures, 4 MV photons or cobalt-60 radiations are used to include the primary tumor and the first echelon of lymph nodes. In such circumstances, it is important to boost the primary site to a total dose of 60 Gy in 5 weeks and later consider a localized boost to the primary site by an interstitial implant for an additional 10–12 Gy. If the primary disease is controlled, any residual nodes in the neck are dealt with by neck dissection.

INTERSTITIAL IMPLANT FOR CARCINOMA OF THE LIP

Small carcinomas (T1) of the lip may be entirely and expediently dealt with by external beam therapy alone and therefore are not usually considered for interstitial implant. For the large, bulky T2 lesions, external radiation therapy is given first for shrinkage of the exophytic component, to be followed by boost radiations via interstitial implant. Ordinarily, a single plane implant at the mid-thickness of the lip is planned with the needles being inserted vertically from the chin percutaneously toward the midplane of the lip. In order to deliver a maximal dose to the lesion on the surface of the lip, a rubber tube of 1 cm in diameter is sutured to the surface of the lip, acting as a bumper to receive the radioactive isotope, as shown in Figure 6A.4. This is in the form of extended implant similar to the dosimetric benefit of a crossing needle. For the extensive growth involving the lip commissure, the lateral portion of the upper and lower lips are sutured together and a plane of needles is placed vertically midway between the skin and mucosa, covering both upper and lower lips as well as the commissure and its adjacent buccal mucosa. In most patients, lip implant is usually done under local anesthesia. An afterloading angio-cath $-$ ^{192}Ir technique is highly satisfactory for lip implantation.

Technical Pointers

1. A lead or Cerrobend cutout is made for the individual lesion with a minimum of 1 cm margin of normal tissue.
2. Insert a waxed lead shield between the lip and alveolar ridge (Figure 6A.5).

AFTER LOADING ANGIOCATH IMPLANT for CANCER of LIP

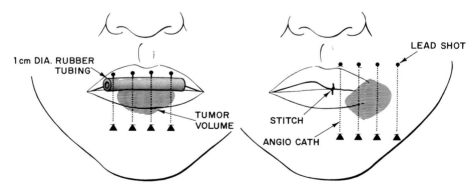

FIGURE 6A.4   Left diagram shows interstitial implant with a rubber tubing sutured on the lip to serve as a "bumper" to receive isotope as an "overextending" implant. This acts as a crossing needle. Right diagram shows stitching of the upper and lower lips during interstitial implant for carcinoma of the lip involving the lip commission.

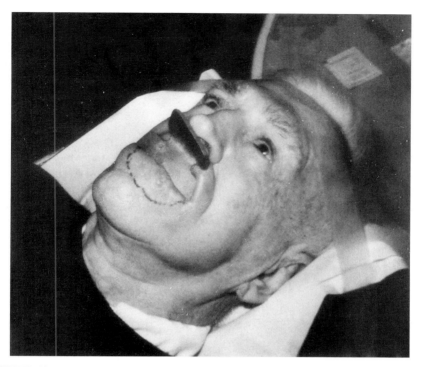

FIGURE 6A.5   Photograph showing lead shield inserted between lip and gum during radiation therapy.

3. For electron beam therapy select 9 MeV with a 0.5 cm bolus over the lesion.
4. For interstitial implant, insert the needles percutaneously midway between the skin and mucosa (0.5 cm from the implanted plane).
5. Use rubber tubing for extending the implant in lieu of a crossing needle.
6. A boost dose of 30 Gy in 3–4 days should be delivered in addition to the 30–35 Gy external photons or electrons.

RADIOTHERAPEUTIC RESULTS

Local control and the cosmetic and functional results for cancer of the lip depend on the size and location of the primary tumor and the status of the lymph nodes. For small lip cancers (T1 and T2), local control by radiation therapy or surgery is extremely good, ranging between 80% and 90%.[7,12,14,15] For larger lesions, T3 and T4, the rates are lower, being in the neighborhood of 60% to 40%, respectively. As a rule, very few recurrences occur after 3 years. del Regato and Sala[13] reported a series of 498 patients with cancer of the lower lip. The rates of local control were extremely satisfactory after either surgery or radiation therapy. Of 306 patients with lesions less than 2 cm in size treated by surgery, the control rate was 98% (299/306) and for patients with lesions ranging from 2 to 12 cm in diameter, mostly treated by radiation therapy, the local control rate was 91% (174/192). Dick et al.[14] reported local control rates of 98% (282/287) after radiation therapy. Similar results were reported by Petrovich et al.,[11] indicating a recurrence rate of 11% after appropriate therapy. Similar good results were reported by Cerezo et al.[16]

Survival is much better for tumors of the lower lip than for the upper lip and commissural lesions. Recurrent carcinomas of the lip after previous radiation therapy may be salvaged by surgery with good local control and survival. On the other hand, recurrences after previous definitive surgery tend to be massive with higher incidence of nodal metastases and poor survival, and the results of salvage by radiation therapy are usually poor. Metastatic cervical disease can be managed successfully by surgery in approximately 50% of cases. Modlin[8] reported 52% (13/25) and del Regato and Sala[13] recorded 56% (30/54). For lesions associated with fixed nodes, the rates were one-half of those with mobile nodes, approximately 25%.

The prognosis for carcinoma of the upper lip is relatively less favorable. Jorgensen et al.[7] reported an 84.5% survival, which was reduced to 56% in patients with nodal metastases.

MGH EXPERIENCE

Although carcinoma of the lip is a common cancer of the oral cavity, the number of patients referred for radiation therapy is very small because most lesions are traditionally treated by surgery. From 1960 through 1994, a total of 125 patients received radiation therapy, 118 patients with previously untreated carcinoma of the lip and 7 patients with gross postoperative recurrence. Of the former group, 105 lesions occurred in the lower lip, 6 in the upper lip, and 7 in the lip commissure. The male to female ratio was 10:1 for the lower lip lesions. The treatment results are shown in Table 6A.1.

TABLE 6A.1   Three-Year Local Control (LC) of Squamous Cell Carcinoma of the Lip After Radiation Therapy: MGH Experience

Area of Lip	LC	Total
LOWER LIP		
T1–2N0	88/92 (96%)	
T3N0	13/15 (87%)	101/107 (94%)
T1–3N1–3	1/7 (14%)	
UPPER LIP	1/3 (33%)	
T1–2N0	3/7 (43%)	
T1–3N1–3	0/2 (0%)	4/10 (40%)

Of 92 patients with T1–2 carcinoma of the lower lip, 88 or 96% were cured by radiation therapy alone for 3 or more years. For patients with T3 lesions, 13 or 87% were NED. There were 8 radiation failures, 2 of whom were salvaged by surgery, thus yielding an overall local control rate of 96%. Ninety-four percent presented without node involvement at the time of diagnosis, and, of these, 94% were locally NED for 3 or more years after radiation therapy, while in 7 patients with N1–N3 disease, only one was NED. Of 10 patients with upper lip carcinoma without nodes, 4 were NED. Two patients had neck metastases; one survived 3 years. Of 107 patients with lower lip carcinoma and N0 neck at initial diagnosis surviving after radiation therapy for 3 or more years, only 4 or 4% subsequently developed nodal metastases and were salvaged by surgery.

CASE ILLUSTRATIONS

To illustrate the examples of radiation therapy for carcinoma of the lip with the techniques and results a series of cases are presented in Figure 6A.6 through 6A.8.

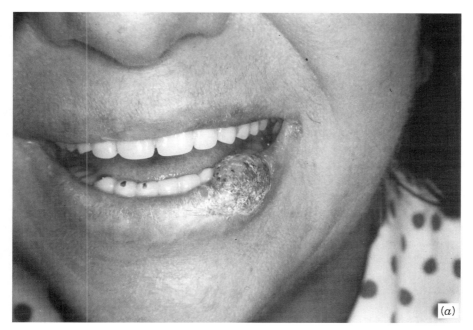

FIGURE 6A.6 B.F., a 57-year-old woman, had squamous cell carcinoma of the left lower lip for 6 months. No nodes are present and she was in Stage T2N0. Radiation therapy totaled 45 Gy in 2 weeks. The gum and teeth were protected. (a) Preradiation therapy photograph. (b) Postradiation photograph 8 years later.

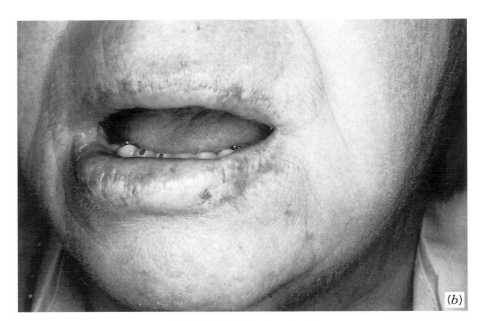

FIGURE 6A.6 *Continued*

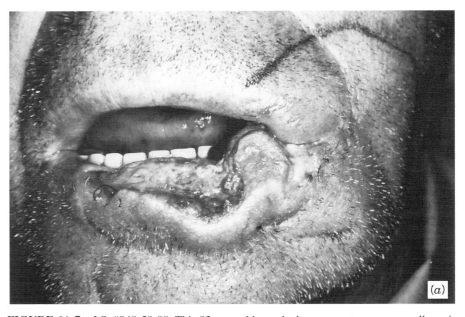

FIGURE 6A.7 J.S. #048-59-98. This 82-year-old man had a recurrent squamous cell carcinoma of the left lower lip, treated by excision of half of lower lip with nasolabial fold flap reconstruction with massive recurrence 3 years after surgery. No cervical adenopathy. Radiation therapy was given with 30 Gy in 10 fractions in 15 days, followed by interstitial implant for 40 Gy in 100 hours. An additional 21 Gy in 7 daily fractions was given after implant. He was NED 5 years posttreatment. (a) Preradiation therapy photograph. (b) Photograph showing interstitial implant. (c) Postradiation therapy photograph.

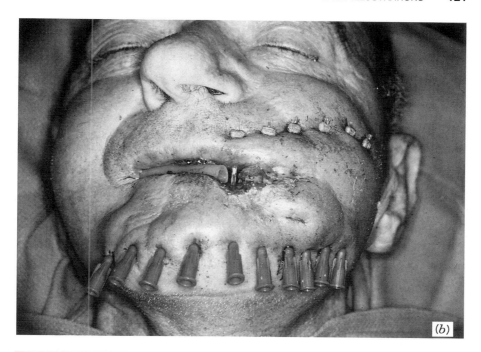

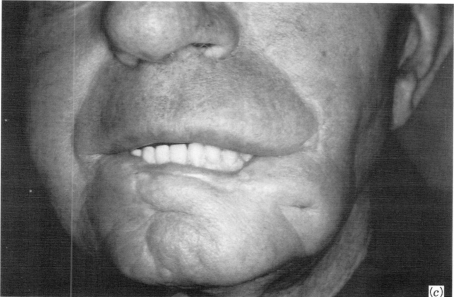

FIGURE 6A.7   *Continued*

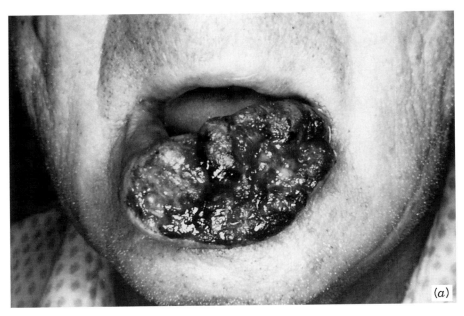

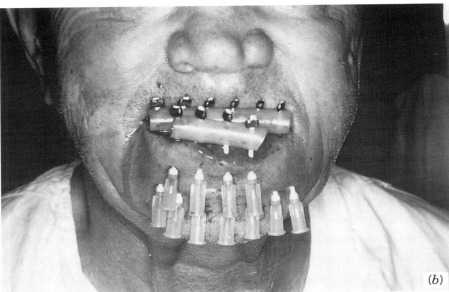

FIGURE 6A.8 F.N. #248-24-42. This 72-year-old man had progressively enlarging tumor in the lower lip. He smoked 3 to 4 cigars regularly. Biopsy showed squamous cell carcinoma, T3N0. Tumor did not involve the buccogingival sulcus and was freely mobile, and without cervical node involvement. Radiation therapy was given to the primary lesion for 45 Gy in 23 days in 15 fractions, using 12 MeV electrons followed by angiocath afterloading 192 Ir interstitial implant for 30 Gy in 40 hours. An additional 10 Gy in 5 fractions was given after implant. He was seen 7 years after radiation therapy and was NED. During this interval he had a right upper neck dissection for one metastatic node in the submandibular triangle with good recovery. (a) Preradiation therapy photograph of the lesion. (b) Photograph showing interstitial implant with rubber tubing to create "bumper" effect. (c) Postradiation therapy photograph.

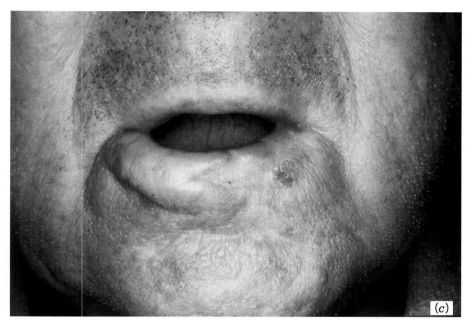

FIGURE 6A.8   *Continued*

SUMMARY

Squamous cell carcinoma of the lip is a highly curable malignancy. Both surgery and radiation therapy produce similarly high cure rates. For the larger tumors involving more than one-third of the lip and lip commissure, radiation therapy produces better cosmetic and functional results. Radiation therapy failures can still be salvaged by surgery with high success but the reverse is seldom true. Treatment must be tailored to the cell grade and location of the lesions, as well as the presence or absence of metastatic nodes. The substance of the lip generally can tolerate a very high dose of radiation therapy thus resulting in favorable "therapeutic ratio" and, therefore, localized tumor can be expected to be highly curable by radiation therapy. The mandible should be spared from high dose of radiations if osteoradionecrosis is to be avoided. This can be achieved by using a combined low megavoltage electron beam and interstitial implant. Careful treatment planning for this disease is rewarding.

REFERENCES

1. *CA-A Cancer Journal for Clinician*: Cancer Statistic. January/February 1995;45:1.
2. MacKay EN, Sellers AH: A statistical review of carcinoma of the lip. *Can Med Assoc J* 1964;90:670.

3. *Manual for staging of cancer*, 4th ed.American Joint Committee on Cancer, 1992.

4. Cross JE, Guralnick E, Daland EM: Carcinoma of the lip: a review of 563 case records of carcinoma of the lip at Pondville Hospital. *Surg Gynecol Obstet* 1948;87:153.

5. Wurman LH, Adams GL, Meyerhoff WL: Carcinoma of the lip. *Am J Surg* 1975; 130:470.

6. Lund C, Sogaard H, Elbrond O, et al: Epidermoid carcinoma of the lip. Histologic grading in the clinical evaluation. *Acta Radiol Ther Phys Biol* 1975;14:465–474.

7. Jorgensen K, Elbron O, Anderson AP: Carcinoma of the lip: a series of 869 cases. *Acta Radiol* 1973;12:177–190.

8. Modlin J: Neck dissections in cancer of the lower lip. *Surgery* 1950;28:404–412.

9. Byers RM, O'Brien J, Waxler J: The therapeutic and prognostic implications of nerve invasion in cancer of the lower lip. *Int J Radiat Oncol Biol Phys* 1978;4:215–217.

10. Schmidseder R, Dick H: Spread of epidermoid carcinoma of the lip along the inferior alveolar nerve. *Oral Surg Oral Med Oral Pathol* 1977;43:517.

11. Petrovich Z, Kuisk H, Tobochnik N, et al: Carcinoma of the lip. *Arch Otolaryngol* 1979;105:187–191.

12. Wilson JSP, Kemble JVH: Cancer of the lip at brisk. *Br J Oral Surg* 1972;9:186.

13. del Regato JA, Sala JM: The treatment of carcinoma of the lip. *Radiology* 1959;73:839.

14. Dick D: Clinical and cosmetic results in squamous cancer of the lip treated by 140 kV radiation therapy. *Clin Radiol* 1962;13:304–312.

15. Lampe I: The place of radiation therapy in the treatment of carcinoma of the lower lip. *Plast Reconstr Surg* 1959;24:34.

16. Cerezo L, Liu FF, Tsang R, Payne X: Squamous cell carcinoma of the lip: analysis of the Princess Margaret Hospital experience. *Radio Oncol* 29:142–147, 1993.

B. CARCINOMA OF THE ORAL TONGUE

The oral tongue is a muscular organ composed of the paired styloglossus, hyoglossus, genioglossus, and palatoglossus muscles and is covered by a mucous membrane with stratified squamous epithelium. The circumvallate papillae, which anatomically belong to the base of the tongue, are situated posteriorly in a V configuration and separate the base of the tongue from the oral tongue. The tongue is divided into the tip, dorsum, lateral borders, and undersurface. Approximately 90% of carcinomas occur in the lateral border, 8% in the dorsum, and 2% in the tip. The oral tongue is a more common site for cancers than the base of the tongue by a ratio of 3:1. The blood supply is the lingual artery, which is a branch of the external carotid artery. One lingual artery may be sacrificed without danger of necrosis, but if both lingual arteries are ligated there is an increased risk of loss of the tongue and almost certainly the base of the tongue as well. The sensory nerve serving the anterior tongue is the lingual nerve (V) while the taste buds are innervated by the chorda tympani (VII). The hypoglossal nerve (XII) is the motor nerve and supplies all of the intrinsic and extrinsic muscles except the palatoglossus, which is innervated by the vagus nerve (X).

Squamous cell carcinoma of the oral tongue is a common type of oral cancer, and in the early stage these lesions are often asymptomatic and pain is surprisingly uncommon. Patients complain of irritation or chancre but rarely seek immediate medical attention. The tumor frequently invades the underlying muscles and tends to spread along the muscle plane, with poorly defined borders. Lumps in the neck, bleeding, dysphagia, odynophagia, otalgia, and fixation of the tongue with resultant slurring of speech are late symptoms and signs indicating advanced disease. Since carcinoma of the tongue may infiltrate the tongue root, base of the tongue, and floor of the mouth submucosally, evaluation of the extent of the tumor calls for careful inspection and digital palpation for tumor induration adjacent to the visible tumor. Inability to protrude the tongue fully indicates the presence of deep muscular invasion and advanced disease.

The lymphatic network of the oral tongue is quite complex. In general, the lymphatic vessels of the anterior tongue drain to the jugulo-omohyoid nodes with or without involvement of the submental nodes (Figure 6B.1). In the mid and pos-

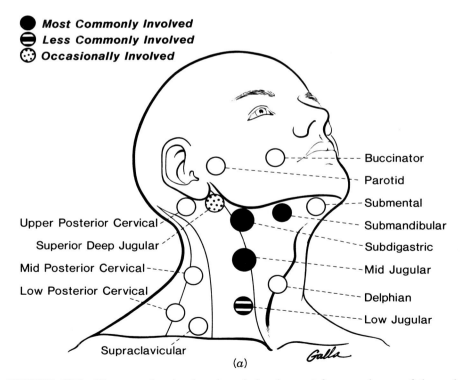

FIGURE 6B.1 Diagrams showing lymph node involvement from carcinoma of the oral tongue: (a) anterior portion of the tongue and (b) posterior portion of the oral tongue.

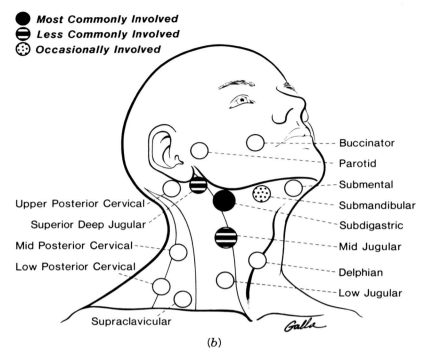

● Most Commonly Involved
⊜ Less Commonly Involved
⦂ Occasionally Involved

Buccinator

Parotid

Submental

Upper Posterior Cervical

Superior Deep Jugular

Mid Posterior Cervical

Low Posterior Cervical

Submandibular

Subdigastric

Mid Jugular

Delphian

Low Jugular

Supraclavicular

Galla

(b)

FIGURE 6B.1   *Continued*

terior oral tongue, the lymphatics drain to the submandibular and subdigastric nodes. The lymphatics of the posterior oral tongue drain to the upper jugular and subdigastric lymph nodes (Figure 6B.1). There are many bilateral crossings in the midline of the dorsum and tip of the tongue, and therefore contralateral metastases are not uncommon. As in the lower lip area, this crossover of the lymphatics is of prime therapeutic significance in considering the spread of cancers of the tongue.

The tongue is endowed with a rich supply of lymphatics, and squamous cell carcinomas arising form this anatomic site tend to have metastasized to the lymph nodes when the disease is initially diagnosed. The incidence is extremely high. For T1N0, T2N0, and T3N0 lesions, the rates of occult metastases are 20%, 30%, and 40–70%, respectively, and of these, 15–20% have bilateral involvement.

SELECTION OF THERAPY

The management of carcinoma of the oral tongue is controversial, depending on the size, location, and growth pattern of the primary lesions as well as the lymph node status in the neck.

Small T1 and T2 Lesions

Although both surgery and radiation therapy are effective in controlling small cancers,[1] it is not unreasonable to consider transoral surgical resection for small, well-defined lesions (T1) involving the tip and anterolateral border of the tongue.[2-4] Such lesions can be cured by resection expediently without resultant functional morbidity. This is particularly true in older and feeble patients, who apparently can tolerate oral surgery much better than they do a prolonged course of curative radiation therapy.

Radiation therapy is preferred for small, ill-defined posterior oral tongue lesions that are inaccessible for surgical excision through the oral route. The large, superficial, exophytic T1 and T2 lesions without a great deal of muscle involvement are most amenable to treatment with radiation therapy, with high control rates and excellent cosmetic results. For the moderately advanced, medium-sized tumors (T2) with involvement of the adjacent floor of the mouth, surgical treatment would have to include partial glossectomy, partial mandibulectomy, and radical neck dissection; therefore comprehensive radiation therapy to the primary site and neck lymph nodes is preferred, and surgery is reserved for salvage of residual or recurrent disease.

Advanced T3 and T4 Lesions

Advanced (T3 and T4) disease with deep muscular invasion, often associated with cervical lymph node metastasis, is unlikely to be curable by radiation therapy or surgery alone and therefore is best managed by a planned combination of surgery and radiation therapy.

Importance of Management of Neck Lymph Nodes

With the exception of small, exophytic, mucosal tumors, treatment of carcinoma of the tongue must include treatment of primary lesions and the regional cervical lymph nodes because of the high incidence of occult metastases, even in patients with N0 necks. Therefore, in patients with infiltrative T1N0 and T2N0 lesions treated by excision alone via the oral route, the neck must be considered at risk for occult metastases, with an incidence of 30–40%.[5,6] The neck should be examined carefully and regularly or irradiated selectively to prevent lymph node recurrence.[7-11] Elective or so-called prophylactic functional upper neck dissection, however, has been used as a sampling procedure,[12] but the beneficial effects are questionable. For the N1 and N2 neck, a combination of therapeutic neck dissection and radiation therapy is the procedure of choice after the primary lesion is controlled.[13-15]

RADIOTHERAPEUTIC DECISION-MAKING AND MANAGEMENT

After definitive radiation therapy is decided on, the selection of radiation therapy modalities is governed by the following factors:

1. Size of the primary lesion (T stage) and lymph node status (N stage).
2. Location of the primary lesion (i.e., anterior versus posterior).
3. Presence or absence of dentition.
4. Medical condition of the patient.
5. Local experience and personal preference.

In general, the smaller the primary lesion and the more anteriorly situated the lesion, the more suitable for interstitial implant[16–19] or IOC radiation therapy.[20,21] Patients who cannot undergo surgery because of intolerance of general anesthesia are rarely candidates for interstitial implant even with local anesthesia.

Comprehensive radiation therapy to the primary site and first echelon lymph nodes is essential for the treatment of carcinoma of the oral tongue and is carried out with a dose of 50–55 Gy over 5–6 weeks. Treatment of the primary lesion is enhanced with either interstitial implant or by IOC electron beam therapy boost, bringing the total dose to approximately 70–72 Gy in about 6 weeks. Such an approach can deliver a very high dose to the primary tumor in the tongue, yet avoids excessive irradiation to the mandible. For advanced (T3 and T4) disease, interstitial implantation or IOC is ineffective, and therefore external beam therapy through multiple portals is used for a total dose of 72 Gy. Since the mandible can not tolerate such a high dose by opposing lateral portals, the primary lesions must be boosted by brachytherapy or a submental approach or limited resection (nidusectomy). The concept is to use nidusectomy to remove any residual disease as a surgical boost in lieu of radiation boost.

Technical Pointers

A. *For External Beam Therapy*
   1. Patient is to lie supine and be immobilized with a face mask. Neck nodes should be lead wired. Use a bite block to depress the tongue.
   2. Tattoo the anterior and posterior margins of the lesion, with a least 1 cm of normal tissue, for daily setup for IOC.
   3. Gold grains are inserted at the tattoos for external beam localization.
   4. External beam portals include the primary tumor and submandibular and subdigastric lymph nodes. The superior border lies 1.5 cm superior to the dorsum of the tongue; the inferior border is at the thyroid notch or below the vallecula and posterior to the posterior bodies of the cervical vertebrae (Figure 6B.2).
   5. Parotid glands may be spared if the lesion is anteriorly situated.
   6. Give 45–50 Gy through opposing lateral portals. With 21–24 Gy IOC, the total dose adds up to approximately 70–75 Gy. An additional dose of 15 Gy with electrons should be given for N1–2 residual nodes, if no RND is planned.

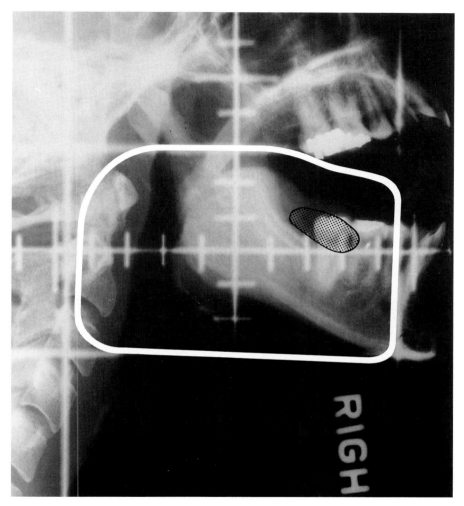

FIGURE 6B.2   Simulation film showing placement of portal in lateral projection for T1N0 carcinoma of the oral tongue.

B. *For IOC Boost*

1. Patient should lie supine, comfortably. Select appropriate cone size and shape.
2. Lesion is stained with toluidine blue dye.
3. The tip of the tongue is held by the patient's fingers or by a clamp for stabilization.
4. Insert the cone toward the lesion, sparing the mandible.

5. Deliver a boost dose of 21–24 Gy with 2.5–3 Gy per fraction, followed by comprehensive external radiation therapy.

6. Depending on the thickness of the lesion, use 9 or 12 MeV electrons with a 5 mm bolus over the lesion.

C. For Interstitial Implant

1. Follow the Patterson–Parker dosimetry rule. For a single plane, place the full-strength sources inside the tumor. For a double plane implant, place the half-strength sources in each plane to sandwich the tumor. For volume implant, place two-thirds to one-half of half-strength sources outside the tumor and the remainder inside the lesion.

2. Use an afterloading technique, angiocath–^{192}Ir, precutaneous trans-submental route.

3. Suture the tip of the tongue to the floor of the mouth or fix it by angiocaths.

4. For a 1-cm lesion in the lateral border of the tongue, use a single plane. For a 1.5-cm lesion, place the medial plane in the tongue medial to the lesion and the outer plane in the gutter of the floor of the mouth, held in place by a rubber tubing.

5. In lieu of crossing sources, use a rubber tubing over the dorsum of the tongue for over implant instead. With a high dose rate (HDR) apparatus, computerize to add intensity at the top of the crossing plane.

6. Lesions larger than 4 cm are not suitable for brachytherapy and are best treated by combined surgery and external beam radiation therapy.

7. To protect the mandible, place a dental roll in the floor of the mouth to separate the sources from the mandible.

RADIOTHERAPEUTIC RESULTS

Results of radiation therapy for carcinoma of the oral tongue are related to the size of the primary lesion and the presence or absence of metastatic lymph nodes and are comparable to those achieved with surgery.

Small mucosal tumors can be treated successfully with either radiation therapy or surgical excision, with similar results. The reported series indicate a 5-year survival rate of approximately 80% for T1 lesions and 50% for T2 lesions.[16] Local control for advanced T3 and T4 lesions was poor with either surgery or radiation therapy, with 5-year survival rates of approximately 25% and 30%, respectively.[25] Survival rates are considerably better, by approximately a factor of 2, in patients without affected lymph nodes than in those with affected lymph nodes.

Extensive lymph node disease (N2 or N3 neck) is rarely salvageable by either radiation therapy or surgery and currently is managed with combined modalities, including chemotherapy. The chemotherapeutic response is usually measured in terms of weeks or months. Chemotherapy given before surgery does not appear to increase the morbidity of subsequent therapies but may exaggerate the acute mucosal reaction during radiation therapy.

MGH EXPERIENCE

From 1970 through 1994, a total of 292 patients with carcinoma of the oral tongue were treated definitively with curative radiation therapy. The 5-year actuarial local control (LC) rate for the entire group of patients after radiation therapy alone was 60%, and disease-specific survival (DSS) rate was 66% (Table 6B.1). For T1 and T2 lesions, the corresponding LC rates were 86% and 64%, and DSS rates were 96% and 67%, respectively. Large tumors (T3–4) generally responded poorly to radiation therapy, with a local control rate of 33% and a disease-specific survival rate of 42%. The disease in the neck indicated very poor local control and survival. Those patients with N1 disease had only one-half of the local control and survival of those without node involvement. Those patients with extensive neck disease (N2–3) had approximately 15% local control and survival, as shown in Table 6B.1.

For early lesions without nodal disease, Stage I (T1N0) and Stage II (T2N0), the local control rates were 85% and 69%, and disease-specific survival rates were 95% and 72%, respectively, as shown in Table 6B.2.

TABLE 6B.1   Five-Year Actuarial LC and DSS Rates After Radiation Therapy

Lesions	n	LC (%)	DSS (%)
T1	62	86	96
T2	139	64	67
T3	63	42	55
T4	28	9	9
T3–4	91	33	42
Total	292	60	66
N0	222	67	77
N1	36	39	36
N2–3	13	13	16
Nx	21		
		$p = 0.0001$	$p = 0.0001$

TABLE 6B.2   Five-Year Actuarial LC and DSS Rates After Various Boost Techniques for Oral Carcinoma: 1970–1994

	n	LC (%)	DSS (%)
T1N0			
IOC	44	90	97
Brachytherapy	10	70	100
External beam	4	66	50
		$p = 0.33$	$p = 0.07$
T2N0			
IOC	79	81	85
Brachytherapy	21	38	42
External beam	19	52	62
		$p = 0.0001$	$p = 0.0001$

Boost Techniques: 1970–1994

From 1970 to 1994, various boost techniques were used for the treatment of oral tongue carcinoma consisting of external irradiation only, interstitial implant, or IOC. Table 6B.3 shows the 5-year actuarial local control rates for Stage I (T1N0) and Stage II (T2N0) lesions after various treatment boost modalities.

The IOC boost techniques resulted in the highest 5-year actuarial local control when compared to brachytherapy and external beam only boosts, that is, 80–90%, 40–70%, and 50–65%, respectively. The differences were significant with $p = 0.0001$, as shown in Table 6B.3.

The radiation complications following various boost techniques were minimum, as shown in Table 6B.4. Of 177 patients with T1N0 and T2N0 lesions, only 6 patients or 3% experienced significant radiation complications. This low incidence is probably due to the use of IOC boost programs, comprising approximately 70% of the group.

Metastatic disease in the neck from carcinoma of the oral tongue presents a difficult management problem. The incidence of neck failure in patients with early lesions is high. For the T1N0 and T2N0 lesions, 4 of 31 patients (13%) and 30 of 64 patients (47%), respectively, developed metastatic lymph nodes when the neck re-

TABLE 6B.3   Five-Year Actuarial LC Rates for T1N0 and T2N0 Lesions After Radiation Therapy

	n	LC (%)	DSS (%)
Stage 1	58	85	95
Stage 2	119	69	72
		$p = 0.005$	$p = 0.0004$

TABLE 6B.4   Incidence of Complications After Boost Techniques Versus Stage

	n	# Ulcer	# Osteoradionecrosis
T1N0			
IOC	44	1	0
Brachytherapy	10	1	0
External beam	4	0	0
T2N0			
IOC	79	0	1
Brachytherapy	21	1	1
External beam	19	1	0

ceived partial or no elective radiation therapy prior to 1978 at the MGH, as shown in Table 6B.5.

Salvage surgery was performed in patients who failed curative radiation therapy. For the 55 patients undergoing postradiation surgery to the primary sites, the salvage rates for T1 and T2 were 86% and 66% (Table 6B.6). The salvage rate for T3 was low, being 46%. Patients with large tumors (T4) and extensive lymph node disease (N2 to N3) were rarely salvageable with surgery. Including the results of salvage surgery, the ultimate local control rates after radiation therapy of oral tongue carcinoma for T1–3 were 97%, 74%, and 60%, respectively.

A planned combination of surgery and radiation therapy was carried out in 27 patients with T3–4 disease. Radiation therapy was given either preoperatively with 45 Gy or postoperatively with 55–60 Gy. For the entire group of 27 patients, the 5-year actuarial local control and disease-specific survival rates were 82% and 72%, respectively, as shown in Table 6B.7.

Results of Twice-Daily Radiation Therapy for Carcinoma of Oral Tongue

From 1979 through 1994, 159 patients received twice-daily radiation therapy; the results are shown in Table 6B.8. Twenty-five patients had T1 disease; the 5-year actuarial local control rate was 91%. For 85 patients with T2 disease, the LC rate was

TABLE 6B.5   Incidence of Nodal Recurrence from Occult Metastasis in Patients with T1N0 and T2N0 Lesions (No Elective Neck Irradiation): 1960–1980

Lesions	n	# patients w/RND	#D/N dz/DWD[a]	Total
T1N0	31	1	3/6 — 33%	4/31 — 13%
T2N0	64	23	7/30 — 23%	30/64 — 47%
Total	95	24	10/36 — 28%	30/95 — 36%

[a]Number of patients who died of the disease; number of patients who died of disease in the neck alone.

TABLE 6B.6 Five-Year Actuarial Rates Following Salvage Surgery for Radiation Failures for Carcinoma of the Oral Tongue: 1970–1994

Lesions	n	Surgical Salvage	Ultimate LC
T1	62	82%	97%
T2	139	79%	74%
T3	63	24%	60%
T4	28	0%	0%

82%. The corresponding rate for T3–4 lesions was 46%. When these rates were compared with results of 133 patients receiving once-daily radiation therapy from 1970 to 1994, the difference was statistically significant for the T2 and T3 lesions ($p = 0.0001$), respectively, but not for T1 lesions. The DSS data comparing BID and QD programs are also shown in Table 6B.8.

SUMMARY

Squamous cell carcinoma of the oral tongue is a common cancer of the head and neck. Its therapeutic management is extremely complex. The small, mucosal tumors can be treated successfully with either radiation therapy or surgical excision with equally good results. Once the tumors become large or extend to the underlying muscle, the incidence of metastatic lymph nodes is high. For T1N0 and T2N0 lesions, if the neck is not treated though clinically normal, approximately one-fourth to one-third of patients will develop lymph node disease during the course of the disease. When the disease becomes advanced (T3 and T4), the incidence of occult and overt neck disease ranges from 50% to 70%.

Except for small, mucosal lesions, radiation therapy therefore must consist of comprehensive external beam radiation to the primary site and the first echelon lymph nodes with approximately 50–60 Gy, with local boost to the primary lesion either via interstitial implant or IOC to a total tumor dose of approximately 70–75 Gy in 6 weeks. Occasionally, in lieu of radiation boost, limited surgical excision of the residual disease or nidusectomy at the primary site is effective.

When the primary lesion is treated only by simple excision, the neck must be considered at risk for relapse due to occult metastases and should be closely ob-

TABLE 6B.7 Five-Year Actuarial LC and DSS Rates for T3–4 After Combined Surgery and Radiation Therapy: 1970–1994

Lesions	n	LC (%)	DSS (%)
T3–4	27	82	72

TABLE 6B.8 Five-Year Actuarial LC and DSS Rates for Carcinoma of the Oral Tongue: BID Versus QD

	n	LC (%)	DSS (%)
T1			
BID	25	91	100
QD	37	82	93
		$p = 0.040$	$p = 0.24$
T2			
BID	85	82	84
QD	54	43	45
		$p = 0.0001$	$p = 0.0001$
T3–4			
BID	49	46	52
QD	42	21	33
		$p = 0.001$	$p = 0.02$

served. Other options are to perform a functional neck dissection for sampling purposes or postoperative radiation therapy to the neck electively.

The program of combined IOC boost and comprehensive external beam radiation therapy has resulted in approximately 80–90% local control of T1N0 and T2N0 carcinoma of the oral tongue, and at the MGH it is the procedure of choice.

Extensive tumors (large T3 and T4 lesions with or without N2 or N3 neck) are rarely curable with radiation therapy. At present, a combination of surgery and radiation therapy, either preoperative or postoperative, is preferred. Accelerated hyperfractionation radiation therapy has resulted in some improvement of local control, particularly for the T2–3 lesions.

The role of chemotherapy for these advanced tumors is disappointing, and the duration of response is usually measured in terms of weeks or months. Its use before radiation therapy or surgery does not appear to increase the patient's chance of survival.

REFERENCES

1. Saxena VS: Cancer of the tongue: local control of the primary. *Cancer* 1970;26: 788–794.

2. Ange DW, Lindberg RD, Guillamondegui OM: Management of squamous cell carcinoma of the oral tongue and floor of mouth after excisional biopsy. *Radiology* 1975; 116:143–146.

3. Spiro RH, Strong EW: Epidermoid carcinoma of the mobile tongue, treatment by partial glossectomy alone. *Am J Surg* 1971;122:707–710.

4. Spiro RH, Strong EW: Surgical treatment of cancer of the tongue. *Surg Clin North Am* 1974;4:759–765.

5. Johnson JT, Leipzig B, Cummings CW: Management of T1 carcinoma of the anterior aspect of the tongue. *Arch Otolaryngol* 1980;106:249–251.

6. Odell EW, Jani P, Sherriff M, Ahluwalia SM, Hibbert J, Levison DA, Morgan PR: The prognostic value of individual histologic grading parameters in small lingual squamous cell carcinomas. The importance of the pattern of invasion. *Cancer* 1994;74:789–794.

7. Million RR: Elective neck irradiation for TxN0 squamous cell carcinoma of the oral tongue and floor of mouth. *Cancer* 1971;34:149–155.

8. Bagshaw MA, Thompson RW: Elective irradiation of the neck in patients with primary carcinoma of the head and neck. *JAMA* 1971;217:456–458.

9. Benak S, Buschke F, Galante M: Treatment of carcinoma of the oral cavity. *Radiology* 1970;96:137–143.

10. Biller HF, Ogura JH, Davis WH, et al: Planned preoperative irradiation for carcinoma of the larynx and laryngopharynx treated by total and partial laryngectomy. *Laryngoscope* 1969;79:1387–1395.

11. Leborgne F, Leborgne JH, Barlocci L, Ortega B: Elective neck irradiation in the treatment of cancer of the oral tongue. *Int J Radiat Oncol Biol Phys* 1987;13:1149–1153.

12. Strong EW: Carcinoma of the tongue. *Otolaryngol Clin North Am* 1979;12:107–114.

13. Hanks GE, Bagshaw MA, Kaplan HS: The management of cervical lymph node metastases by megavoltage radiotherapy. *AJR Am J Roentgenol* 1969;105:74–82.

14. Jesse RH, Lindberg RD: The efficacy of combining radiation therapy with a surgical procedure in patients with cervical metastasis from squamous cancer of the oropharynx and hypopharynx. *Cancer* 1975;35:1163–1166.

15. Lindberg R, Jesse RH: Treatment of cervical lymph node metastasis from primary lesions of the oropharynx, supraglottic larynx and hypopharynx. *AJR Am J Roentgenol* 1968;102:132–137.

16. Botstein C, Silver C, Ariaratnam L: Treatment of carcinoma of the oral tongue by radium needle implantation. *Am J Surg* 1976;132:523.

17. Decroix Y, Ghossein N: Experience of the Curie Institute in the treatment of cancer of the mobile tongue. *Cancer* 1981;47:496–502.

18. Horiuchi J, Okuyama T, Shibuya H, Takeda M: Results of brachytherapy for cancer of the tongue with special emphasis on local prognosis. *Int J Radiat Oncol Biol Phys* 1982;8:829–835.

19. Fu KK, Chan EK, Phillips TL, et al: Time, dose and volume factors in interstitial radium implants of carcinoma of the oral tongue. *Radiology* 1976;119:209–213.

20. Griffin TW, Gerdes AJ, Simko TG, et al: Per oral irradiation for limited carcinoma of the oral cavity. *Int J Radiat Oncol Biol Phys* 1977;2:333–335.

21. Wang CC: Radiotherapeutic management and results of T1N0, T2N0 carcinoma of the oral tongue: evaluation of boost technique. *Int J Radiat Oncol Biol Phys* 1989;17:287–291.

C. CARCINOMA OF THE FLOOR OF THE MOUTH

The floor of the mouth is a crescent-shaped area between the lower gingiva and the undersurface of the tongue. It extends from the anterior inner aspect of the lower gingiva laterally to the insertion of the anterior tonsillar pillar into the tongue. Anteriorly, it is divided in half by the lingual frenulum. The floor of the mouth is covered by a mucous membrane with stratified squamous epithelium. Laterally, the sublingual glands are separated by the midline genioglossus and the geniohyoid muscles. The genial tubercles are bony protuberances that occur at the point of insertion of these two muscle groups on the symphysis. The floor of the mouth contains several muscles, including the mylohyoid, hyoglossus, and diagastric muscles.

Anatomically, there is a gap between the mylohyoid and hyoglossus muscles, through which the superficial portion of submaxillary gland is continuous via the gap with the deep portion of the gland. The submaxillary duct (Wharton's duct), which is about 5 cm long, and the hypoglossal nerve (12th cranial) also pass through the gap to enter the sublingual space and the former terminates in the sublingual papilla. This gap is a weak portion of the floor of the mouth, which is vulnerable for carcinoma to gain easy access into the submandibular and sublingual areas, presenting as a soft tissue mass, mimicking an enlarged lymph node or large submaxillary gland.

The lingual nerve, a branch of the submaxillary nerve, provides sensation to the floor of the mouth. The arterial supply comes from the lingual artery, a branch of the external carotid.

Carcinoma of the floor of the mouth is often located in the anterior portion of the floor adjacent to Wharton's duct orifice and frequently spreads along the directional course of the submaxillary duct. The early lesions are seldom symptomatic and commonly diagnosed by a dentist during ordinary dental work. In extensive lesions, the tumor may extend deeply into the muscle, the adjacent tongue and alveolar ridge, and onto the submandibular triangle. The far-advanced lesions may invade the neighboring mandible.

The lymphatic network of the floor of the mouth drains to the submental nodes anteriorly and submandibular nodes posteriorly, then to the subdigastric and deep jugular nodes as shown in Figure 6C.1. In contrast to the oral tongue, the incidence of lymph node metastases is low for the T1 lesions, that is, less than 10%. For the extensive tumors such as T3 and T4, however, the incidence of lymph node metastases is high, ranging from 50% to 75%, respectively, and of these 20% are bilateral.[1-3]

Evaluation of the extent of carcinoma of the floor of the mouth includes careful inspection to ascertain whether the lesion extends to the undersurface of the tongue or adjacent gingiva. The presence of normal mucosa between the lesion and the gingiva without fixation almost precludes significant bone involvement. Bimanual palpation with the gloved finger is essential to define the tumor mass, nodal disease in the submandibular triangle, and/or enlargement of the submaxillary gland. As in the groin, there are palpable nodes in the submandibular area in a normal, healthy individual. These normal nodes tend to be small and freely mobile, ranging in diameter from 1 to 1.5 cm, and should not be interpreted as metastatic nodes in patients with carcinoma of the floor of the mouth. At times, their differentiation may be extremely difficult without a biopsy or careful observation as to their changing character during or after radiation therapy. When the lesion is adherent to the gingiva, it is important that radiographic examination be obtained, including Panorex and CT scans or intraoral dental films directly over the lesion. Although the AJC staging

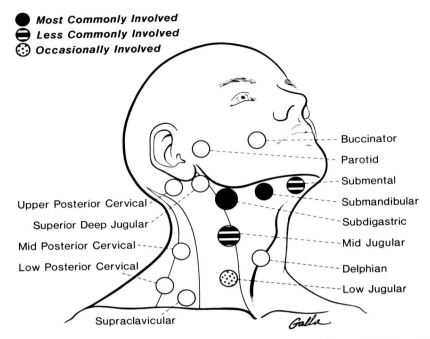

- ● **Most Commonly Involved**
- ⊜ **Less Commonly Involved**
- ⊙ **Occasionally Involved**

Buccinator
Parotid
Submental
Submandibular
Subdigastric
Mid Jugular
Delphian
Low Jugular

Upper Posterior Cervical
Superior Deep Jugular
Mid Posterior Cervical
Low Posterior Cervical

Supraclavicular

FIGURE 6C.1 Diagram showing lymph node involvement in carcinoma of the floor of the mouth.

system for oral carcinoma is strictly by tumor size, the presence or absence of tumor adherence to the gingiva certainly would influence the choice of therapeutic modality and the incidence of radiation therapy complications and subsequent treatment outcome.

SELECTION OF THERAPY

When the tumor is small or limited to the mucosa, it is highly curable by radiation therapy[4-6] alone with excellent cosmesis, and therefore radiation therapy is the treatment modality of choice. For the moderately advanced lesion, T2 or early exophytic T3, a trial course of radiation therapy may be given first, with surgery being reserved for salvage of residual disease. For the infiltrative lesion with fixation or tethering to the adjacent mandible, though the surface size is still small and/or categorized as T1, surgical excision with a rim of the mandible[7] (i.e., marginal mandibulectomy) may be considered, as shown in Figure 6C.2, followed by postoperative radiation therapy. For large, extensive, infiltrative lesions, T3 and T4, with marked involvement of adjacent muscle of the tongue and mandible, a planned combination of radical resection and postoperative radiation therapy is the procedure of choice.

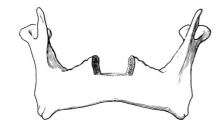

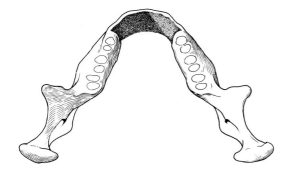

FIGURE 6C.2. Diagram showing concept of partial mandibulectomy or rim resection for treatment of carcinoma of the floor of the mouth.

RADIOTHERAPEUTIC MANAGEMENT

Radiation therapy for early lesions, T1 and T2, consists of external beam therapy with interplay of IOC. For small, well defined lesions, IOC may be given at the very outset. For poorly defined lesions, large field radiation therapy in the form of a "mouth bath" with 20 Gy in 2 weeks is delivered for better delineation of the tumor margins by the development of tumoritis, and this is followed by IOC radiation therapy for approximately 21 Gy in 7–10 daily fractions. Additional external radiation therapy is given to bring the total dose to the primary site up to 68–70 Gy in 6 weeks or its biological equivalent. In patients with small oral aperture and full dentition, localized boost by submental electrons with 18 MeV electrons may be given to the primary site or by reduced external beam therapy with anterior and lateral wedge pair for 20 Gy in 2 weeks after 45 Gy opposed lateral portal treatment is achieved.

Another option for localized boost to the primary site is by interstitial implant. It is to be noted that interstitial implant for carcinoma of the floor of the mouth carries significant risk of localized soft tissue ulceration and osteoradionecrosis of the mandible and is not recommended for lesions adherent to or involving the gingiva.

Because of the low incidence of occult metastases in the superficial T1N0 and early T2N0 lesions, elective neck irradiation or neck dissection is not indicated.

Technical Pointers

A. External Radiation Therapy

1. Insert gold seeds 1 cm anterior and posterior to the margins of the lesion. Neck nodes are wired by lead.
2. Patient should lie supine and be immobilized with a face mask.
3. A bite block is used to depress the tongue and floor of the mouth. Make a Cerrobend cutout to include the submental, submandibular, and subdigastric nodes and to spare the parotid glands.
4. The superior border of the portal is 1.5 cm over the dorsum of the tongue, the inferior border is at the thyroid notch, the anterior border is at the mental symphysis, and the posterior border is at the vertebral bodies shown in Figure 6C.3.
5. For advanced T2–3N2–3 lesions, bilateral lower anterior neck (LAN) elective irradiation is used.
6. The upper lip is excluded from the radiation portal and the lower lip is pushed forward outside the field by using a dental roll if the lesion is close to the lower buccogingival sulcus.

B. IOC Boost Procedure

1. Patient is to lie supine. Select the appropriate cone size and shape.
2. Make a personalized mold to displace the tongue backward and expose the FOM. Stain the lesion with toluidine blue dye for better visualization.
3. Insert the cone directly over the lesion. Add a 5 mm bolus over the lesion and deliver 21 Gy with 2.5–3 Gy per fraction 9 MeV electrons.
4. An alternative option is to boost the FOM lesion with the IOC apparatus through a submental route, using 18 MeV electrons with 2 Gy per fraction for 15 Gy, carefully sparing the mandible, to be followed by comprehensive external beam therapy for 50 Gy.

C. Interstitial Implant

1. This procedure carries a high risk of ulceration or osteoradionecrosis of the mandible.
2. Use an afterload technique through a submental percutaneous route.
3. The tip of the tongue is transfixed to the floor and the Ir source is placed through the dorsum of the tongue. There is no need for crossing sources.
4. Most lesions in the anterior floor of the mouth call for a small volume implant.

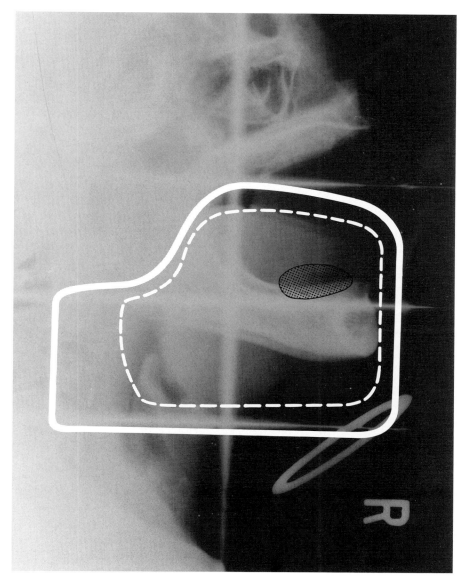

FIGURE 6C.3   Simulation film showing Cerrobend cutout to shield parotid glands when treating carcinoma of the anterior floor of the mouth.

RADIOTHERAPEUTIC RESULTS

The results of treatment by radiation therapy are comparable to those achieved with radical surgery. The early mucosal lesions, T1 and T2, are controlled satisfactorily by a combination of external radiation therapy intermixed with intraoral cone electron beam therapy or interstitial implant, with local control rates of approximately 80% and 60%, respectively.[6,8,9] Extensive infiltrative lesions, T3 and T4, with involvement of the gum and the mandible or deeply infiltrative into the adjacent musculature, often with cervical lymph node metastases, are rarely controlled by radiation therapy alone with local control rates of approximately 20–30%.[4,10,11] The tolerance of the mandible to radiation is low and prevents the use of external beam therapy alone. Likewise, the use of brachytherapy has resulted in an extremely high incidence of osteoradionecrosis of the mandible.[10] Therapeutic neck dissection for nodal metastases does not jeopardize survival as compared to elective neck dissection for N0 neck.[12] Unfortunately, carcinoma of the floor of the mouth is frequently associated with multiple primaries in the upper aerodigestive tract, ranging from 25% to 33% after successful treatment of the previous tumors. This certainly accounts for the poor results of overall survival of the patients.[13]

MGH EXPERIENCE

From 1970 through 1994, 309 patients with carcinoma of the floor of the mouth were treated by radiation therapy. Of these, 111 patients were treated with accelerated (BID) radiation therapy.

The incidence of nodal metastases at the time of diagnosis for early lesions is remarkably low, being 10% for T1 and 18% for T2 lesions. When the lesions become large and extensive, invading adjacent musculature and bone, the incidence is high, averaging approximately 70%.

TABLE 6C.1   Five-Year Actuarial LC and DSS Rates After Radiation Therapy for Floor of Mouth Carcinomas: 1970–1994

Lesions	n	LC (%)	DSS (%)	Ultimate LC (%)
T1	92	90	95	95
T2	159	71	75	81
T1–2	251	79	82	
T3	31	29	23	29
T4	27	26	36	30
T3–4	58	28	27	
Total	309	69	72	
N0	261	74	77	
N1	27	53	52	
N2–3	21	25	20	
		$p = 0.0001$	$p = 0.0001$	

**TABLE 6C.2   Five-Year Actuarial LC and
DSS Rates Related to Stages After Radiation
Therapy: 1970–1994**

Stages	n	LC (%)	DSS (%)
Stage 1	88	92	97
Stage 2	134	71	76
		$p = 0.0005$	$p = 0.0001$

Table 6C.1 shows the 5-year actuarial local control and disease-specific survival rates following radiation therapy. Of the entire group of 309 patients, the local control (LC) and disease-specific survival (DSS) rates were 69% and 72%, respectively. For the T1 and T2 lesions, the corresponding rates were 79% and 82%, respectively. For extensive disease, T3 and T4, the local control rates was 28% and the DSS rate 27%.

The local control and disease-specific survival according to the stages of the disease are shown in Table 6C.2.

Salvage surgery was carried out on patients who failed after radiation therapy. On 69 patients who underwent such a procedure, 17 or 25% were NED. Thus, including patients successfully rescued by salvage surgery, the ultimate local control rates for T1 and T2 lesions were 95% and 83%, shown in Table 6C.3.

Unfortunately, not all patients who failed radiation therapy could undergo salvage surgery. In patients with T4 disease, only 15% achieved local control, and none of 31 patients with T3 lesions were successfully salvaged by surgery.

Radiotherapeutic boost techniques for the treatment of carcinoma of the floor of the mouth consist of external beam only, intraoral cone (IOC), or interstitial implant. Table 6C.4 shows the 5-year actuarial local control rates of T1N0 and T2N0 lesions after various boost techniques from 1970 through 1994.

Of the T1N0 group, 17 patients were treated by an interstitial implant boost technique, 27 patients by IOC, and 39 patients by external beam boost only. The 5-year actuarial local control rates were 93%, 91%, and 94%, respectively, with $p = 0.88$. For the T2N0 group, 23 patients received interstitial implant boost, 36 patients were treated with IOC, and 71 patients by external beam boost. The corresponding rates were 72%, 79%, and 69%, respectively, with $p = 0.75$, as shown in Table 6C.4.

TABLE 6C.3   Local Control, Surgical Salvage, and Ultimate LC: 1970–1994

Lesions	n	LC (%)	Surgical Salvage (%)	Ultimate LC (%)
T1	92	90	22	95
T2	159	75	30	83
T3	31	32	0	32
T4	27	26	15	37

TABLE 6C.4   Five-Year Actuarial LC and DSS Related to Various Boost Techniques of Radiation Therapy: 1970–1994

	n	%LC	%DSS
T1N0			
External boost	39	94	97
IOC	27	91	100
Brachytherapy	17	93	100
		p = 0.88	p = 0.84
T2N0			
External boost	71	69	71
IOC	36	79	91
Brachytherapy	23	72	70
		p = 0.75	p = 0.14

The incidence of radiation complications in terms of soft tissue ulceration and osteoradionecrosis was high with the interstitial implant. As shown in Table 6C.5, of 40 patients receiving interstitial implant alone, 10 or 25% developed major radiation complications (i.e., soft tissue ulceration and/or osteoradionecrosis), as contrasted to external radiation therapy only and IOC after which only 5% (6/110) and 5% (3/63), respectively, developed complications. The difference was significant with $p = 0.0016$.

TABLE 6C.5   Incidence of Radiation Complications After Various Boost Techniques Related to Stages

	n	Ulceration	Osteoradionecrosis	Total
T1N0				
External boost	39	3	0	3/39, 8%
IOC	27	0	0	0/27, 0%
Brachytherapy	17	5	0	5/17, 29%
Total	83	10%	0%	
T2N0				
External boost	71	3	0	3/71, 4%
IOC	36	2	3	5/36, 14%
Brachytherapy	23	3	2	5/23, 22%
Total	130	6%	4%	
Combined T1–2	Total			
External boost	5%			
IOC	5%			
Brachytherapy	25%			

TABLE 6C.6   Incidence of Nodal Recurrence in Patients in Whom No Significant Elective Neck Radiation Therapy Was Given: 1970–1994

Lesions	n	# Patients w/RND	# Patients d/N dz[a]	Total Neck Failures
T1N0	90	1	2/4	3/90 — 3%
T2N0	135	10	8/29	18/135 — 13%

[a]Number of all patients who died of cancer; number of patients who died of neck disease alone.

Management of Neck Nodes in Early Carcinoma of the Floor of the Mouth

For small lesions without node involvement, T1N0 and superficial T2N0, the treatment toward the primary site is quite adequate. Most patients in the series received partial or no irradiation to the neck, yet the incidence of neck recurrence is remarkably low.

From 1970 to 1994, in a group of 90 patients with T1N0 and 135 patients with T2N0, as shown in Table 6C.6, one in T1 and 10 in T2 developed nodal recurrence treated by radical neck dissection and the majority succumbed to the disease. Including the neck failures alone in patients who succumbed to the disease, two in T1N0 and eight in T2N0, the total incidence of nodal disease in the neck was 3% (3/90 and 13% (18/135) for T1N0 and T2N0, respectively. Therefore elective neck treatment in patients with T1N0 or early T2N0 floor of the mouth carcinomas, either by radiation therapy or surgery, is not indicated. Patients with clinical nodal disease should be managed aggressively. The present data show that the survival of patients with nodes involvement is half that of patients without nodal disease.

Results of Combined Radiation Therapy and Surgery

Of 33 patients with T3–4 lesions who underwent planned combined radiation therapy and surgery, the 5-year actuarial local control and disease-specific survival rates were 80% and 62%, respectively, as shown in Table 6C.7.

TABLE 6C.7   Five-Year Actuarial LC and DSS Rates for T3–4 Cancer of Oral Cavity After Combined Surgery and Radiation Therapy: 1970–1994

Stages	n	LC (%)	DSS (%)
T3–4	33	80	62

**TABLE 6C.8   Five-Year Actuarial LC and DSS Rates
After BID Versus QD Radiation Therapy: 1970–1994**

	n	LC (%)	DSS (%)
T1			
BID	23	94	93
QD	69	89	95
		$p = 0.43$	$p = 0.84$
T2			
BID	61	77	87
QD	98	69	70
		$p = 0.2$	$p = 0.02$
T3–4			
BID	27	40	38
QD	31	18	18
		$p = 0.17$	$p = 0.06$

RESULTS OF BID RADIATION THERAPY

From 1979 through 1994, 111 patients with carcinoma of the floor of the mouth received BID radiation therapy. The results of treatment as compared to QD radiation therapy are shown in Table 6C.8.

The 5-year actuarial local control rates for T1, T2, and T3–4 were 94%, 81%, and 62%, respectively. The corresponding rates for QD radiation therapy were 89%, 77%, and 68%

SUMMARY

Carcinoma of the floor of the mouth is a readily recognizable cancer and can be diagnosed early. It is quite dissimilar to carcinoma of the oral tongue from the standpoints of pattern of spread and incidence of nodal metastases, as well as radiation tolerance of its adjacent tissues. Early lesions tend to develop nodal metastases much less often than oral tongue carcinoma and the T1N0 and T2N0 lesions can be treated successfully by radiation therapy alone with satisfactory cosmetic and functional results. Advanced disease, T3 and T4 with nodes involvement, is better treated by combined radiation therapy and surgery. In certain large, exophytic tumors, a trial course of radiation therapy is justified with salvage surgery being reserved for failures.

External beam therapy to the primary site is a major portion of the radiation treatment, to be boosted by reduced portals or by IOC if feasible. Interstitial implant has been found to be associated with a high incidence of soft tissue ulceration or osteoradionecrosis. AT the present time, if the primary site cannot be boosted by IOC, electron beam radiation therapy through submental approach has been used with good results.

Squamous cell carcinoma of the floor of the mouth carries a high incidence of multiple carcinomas arising from the upper air and food passages, approximately one in four. Therefore patients with this disease must be followed regularly for life in order to detect any subsequent malignancies and offer appropriate therapy.

REFERENCES

1. Ballard BR, Suess GR, Pickren JW, et al: Squamous cell carcinoma of the floor of the mouth. *Oral Surg Oral Med Oral Pathol* 1978;45:568–579.
2. Kolson H, Spiro RH, Roswit B, et al: Epidermoid carcinoma of the floor of the mouth. *Arch Otolaryngol* 1971;93:280–283.
3. Wang CC, Doppke KP, Biggs PJ: Intra-oral cone radiation therapy for selected carcinomas of the oral cavity. *Int J Radiat Oncol Biol Phys* 1983;9:1185–1189.
4. Pierquin B, Chassagne D, Baillet F, et al: The place of implantation in tongue and floor of mouth cancer. *JAMA* 1971;215:961–963.
5. Campos JL, Lampe I, Fayos JV: Radiotherapy of carcinoma of the floor of the mouth. *Radiology* 1971;99:677–682.
6. Harrold CC: Management of cancer of the floor of the mouth. *Am J Surg* 1971;122:487–493.
7. Guillamondegui OM, Jesse RH: Surgical treatment of advanced carcinoma of the floor of the mouth. *AJR Am J Roentgenol* 1976;126:1256–1259.
8. Fu KK, Lichter A, Galante M: Carcinoma of the floor of the mouth: an analysis of treatment results and the sites and causes of failures. *Int J Radiat Oncol Biol Phys* 1976;1:829–837.
9. Fayos JV, Lampe I: Treatment of squamous cell carcinoma of the oral cavity. *Am J Surg* 1972;124:493–500.
10. Marks JE, Lee F, Smith PG, et al: Floor of the mouth cancer: patient selection and treatment results. *Laryngoscope* 1983;93:475–480.
11. Million RR, Cassisi NJ: Oral cavity. In: Million RR, Cassisi NJ, eds. *Management of head and neck cancer*. Philadelphia: Lippincott 1984.
12. Correa JN, Bosch A, Marcial V: Carcinoma of the floor of the mouth: review of clinical factors and results of treatment. *AJR Am J Roentgenol* 1967;94:302–312.
13. Fitzpatrick PJ, Tepper BS: Carcinoma of the floor of mouth. *J Assoc Can Radiol* 1982;33:148–153.

D. CARCINOMA OF THE RETROMOLAR TRIGONE AND ANTERIOR PILLAR

The retromolar trigone (RMT) is a triangular area that covers the anterior aspect of the ascending ramus of the mandible, posterior to and between the upper and lower third molars. The mucous membranes of this site blend medially with the anterior tonsillar pillar and laterally with the buccal mucosa and are intimately attached to the ascending ramus of the mandible and pterygomandibular ligament or raphe.

Bone involvement by the tumor rarely occurs. The lesions spread primarily antero-laterally to involve the posterior gingival ridge, buccal mucosa, and floor of the mouth, posteriorly to the adjacent tonsillar fossa and base of tongue, and medially to the soft and hard palates. This area is innervated by the lingual nerve and there-fore is anatomically within the oral cavity. Most of these tumors are moderately to well differentiated carcinomas. Advanced lesions may spread to the gingival ridge with bond destruction and to the pterygoid fossa, resulting in trismus. Therefore ra-diographic imaging studies including Panorex, CT scans, or MR scans are often in-dicated to evaluate the extent of mandibular and pterygoid involvement.

Thus squamous cell carcinomas arising from the retromolar trigone and anterior faucial pillar are generally considered under one heading.

The lymphatic drainage of the retromolar trigone is to the submandibular, subdi-gastric, and superior jugular nodes, commonly ipsilateral. Involvement of sub-mandibular and posterior cervical nodes is most unusual.[1] For the early lesions, the incidence of nodal metastases is low. For T1 and T2 lesions, the incidence is 10% and 20%, respectively. However, for the advanced lesions, T3 and T4, the incidence is high, ranging from 45% to 60% and of these 10% are bilateral. When the soft palate or base of the tongue is extensively involved, the superior deep jugular and contralateral subdigastric nodes are at risk of involvement, as shown in Figure 6D.1.

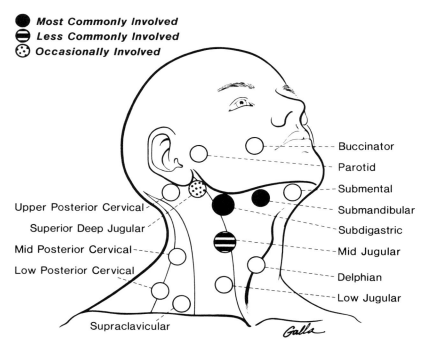

FIGURE 6D.1   Lymph node involvement in carcinoma of the retromolar trigone and ante-rior pillar.

SELECTION OF THERAPY

Treatment of this disease can be by either by radical surgery or radiation therapy. Primary surgery in the form of partial mandibulectomy with or without partial glossectomy and palatectomy generally is attended by marked facial deformity and impairment of swallowing mechanism and often results in a high incidence of marginal recurrence. Therefore, for superficial T1, T2, and T3 lesions, radiation therapy is considered the treatment of choice, with surgery being reserved for salvage. Extensive and deeply infiltrative T3 and T4 disease, if operable, should be considered for primary radical surgery and reconstructive procedure to be followed by postoperative radiation therapy.

Due to intimate adherence of the mucous membrane to the medial angle of the jaw, external radiation therapy with high dose for RMT tumors may result in radiation complications including soft tissue ulceration and/or osteoradionecrosis, reportedly in the range of 20–30%.[2] Proper selection of patients for high-dose radiation therapy may reduce radiation complications.

RADIOTHERAPEUTIC MANAGEMENT

The early lesions, T1N0 and T2N0, without involvement of the base of the tongue or soft palate are treated initially by opposing lateral portals for approximately 20 Gy, followed by ipsilateral and AP wedge pair technique for 45–50 Gy, as shown in Figure 6D.2; thus the contralateral parotid gland is spared the full dose. Small,

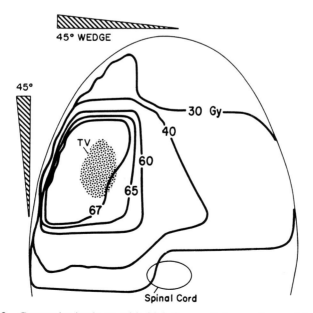

FIGURE 6D.2 Composite isodoses with 20.8 Gy parallel opposing portals (mouth bath) and 48.8 Gy AP and lateral wedge pair.

well defined, superficial tumors may be dealt with effectively by a combination of ipsilateral oblique wedge pair and IOC boost technique in cooperative patients, as shown in Figure 6D.3.

For large T3 and some T4 lesions, particularly associated with marked involvement of the base of the tongue, therapy consists of a postoperative external beam for 60 Gy through opposed lateral portals with equal loading, shrinking field technique covering the primary site and the submandibular, subdigastric, and superior deep jugular nodes (Figure 6D.4). For N1, N2, and N3 and/or extensive T2, T3, and T4 lesions, elective neck irradiation with 45–50 Gy to the lower neck is given, to be followed by neck dissection if residual nodes are present.

Technical Pointers

1. Patient is to lie supine and be immobilized by a face mask. Neck nodes are lead wired.
2. For poorly defined lesions, the initial 20 Gy dose is given through large right

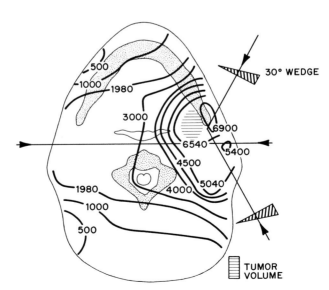

FIGURE 6D.3 Composite isodoses of IOC with 15 Gy, parallel opposing lateral (19.8 Gy) and ipsilateral oblique wedge pair for early carcinoma of the RMT, and AP for a total dose of 65 Gy.

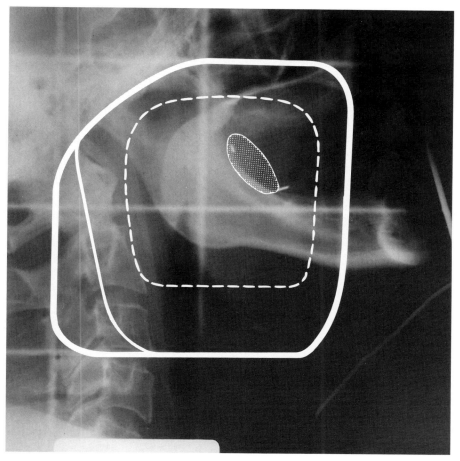

FIGURE 6D.4 Simulation film showing placement of portal and shrinking field for extensive RMT carcinoma with neck node involvement. Anterior and posterior borders of lesion are marked with gold seeds.

and left lateral portals with 1.8 Gy/f as a mouth bath for evaluation of the tumor margins by the development of tumoritis.

3. After tumor extent is determined, its borders are tattooed.

4. Use a wedge pair technique, that is AP and lateral 90° angle, for an additional 45 Gy. Further reduce the portals to bring the total dose to 68–70 Gy for T1–2 lesions and to 72 Gy for advanced tumors.

5. Another option is to use the IOC boost procedure after an initial 20 Gy for a localized lesion or appositional electron beam or wedge pair of reduced portals through different angle, that is, AP and lateral or ipsilateral oblique wedge pair.

6. For lateralized lesions, minimize irradiation to the contralateral parotid gland to decrease the severity of xerostomia.

RADIOTHERAPEUTIC RESULTS

For small tumors, T1 and T2 lesions, the local control rates by radiation therapy alone are high, ranging from 70% to 80%[3] with excellent cosmesis. The radiotherapeutic results for advanced tumors are poor, with local control rates ranging from 30% to 40%[4]; the control rates may be improved by a combination of surgical resection and postoperative radiation therapy.

MGH EXPERIENCE

From 1970 through 1994, a total of 246 patients with carcinoma of the retromolar trigone and anterior pillar were treated by radiation therapy. Of these, 120 patients received once-daily radiation therapy and 126 patients were treated by BID irradiation. Only two patients with T3−4 lesions had planned combined surgery and radiation therapy.

The 5-year actuarial local control (LC) and disease-specific survival (DSS) rates following radiation therapy are shown in Table 6D.1. Of the entire group of 246 patients, the LC and DSS rates were 58% and 62% after radiation therapy alone. For the T1, T2, and T3−4 lesions, the rates were 86%, 68%, and 36%, respectively. Those patients without node involvement (N0) had a local control rate of 63%. The presence of nodal disease, N1, reduced the rate to 46%, and N2−3, 41%.

For early lesions, Stages I and II, the results of radiation are extremely satisfactory, as shown in Table 6D.2.

TABLE 6D.1   Five-Year Actuarial LC and DSS Rates

Lesions	n	LC (%)	DSS (%)
T1	34	86	86
T2	117	68	70
		$p = 0.03$	$p = 0.11$
T3−4	95	36	45
T3	66	35	44
T4	29	88	46
		$p = 0.46$	$p = 0.34$
Total	246	58	62
N0	188	63	68
N1	34	45	69
N2−3	24	38	26
		$p = 0.03$	$p = 0.0001$

TABLE 6D.2   Results of BID and QD Radiation for Stages I and II

Stages	n	LC (%)	DSS (%)
Stage 1	31	89	87
Stage 2	95	70	74
		$p = 0.05$	$p = 0.12$

Thirty-eight patients who failed radiation therapy underwent salvage surgical procedures, and, of these, 21 or 55% were NED. There were 100% for T1 ($n = 2$), 43% for T2 ($n = 14$), 56% for T3 ($n = 18$), and 75% for T4 ($n = 4$). Thus the local control rates, including successful surgical salvage, were 94%, 75%, 55%, and 55% for T1, T2, T3, and T4 lesions, respectively.

Radiation complications following radiation therapy alone were relatively insignificant. Of 99 patients who were NED after radiation therapy alone, only 6 or 6% experienced radiation ulcer, which healed after conservative measures. Twelve patients or 12% developed osteoradionecrosis of the mandible, requiring sequestrectomy or partial mandibulectomy.

Since most of the squamous cell carcinomas are well differentiated, the incidence of occult metastases is low. Of the 31 patients with T1N0 surviving after radiation therapy at 3 years, none had RND and only 2 or 6% had neck failure and succumbed to the disease only in the neck in spite of most patients having only partial neck radiation therapy. Of 95 patients with T2N0 disease, 11 patients failed in the neck, and of these 4 of 9 were rescued by RND and 2 patients died of disease only in the neck. The incidence of occult neck disease in patients with T2N0 lesions was 11/95 or 12%.

Study of the pattern of radiation failures indicates that most treatment failures were due to uncontrolled primary lesions with or without neck disease. Therefore, in 188 patients with N0 neck, 17 or 9% underwent elective neck irradiation or neck dissection for metastatic neck disease; of these, 8 or 50% died with disease. Of 34 patients with N1 disease, 9 or 26% had RND. Of these, 4 or 44% succumbed to disease. For the N2–3 disease, only one had an RND but failed to survive. The remainder were inoperable and died with uncontrolled malignancy. It seems that neck dissection did not appear to add additional advantages in terms of patient survival.

RESULTS OF BID AND QD RADIATION THERAPY

From 1979 through 1994, 102 patients with squamous cell carcinoma of the retromolar trigone and anterior tonsillar pillar received BID radiation therapy. Of these, 13 had T1 disease and 49 had T2 disease and the 5-year actuarial local control rates were 92% and 71%, respectively. For T3–4 lesions, the corresponding rate was 54%, as shown in Table 6D.3A. The QD results are shown in Table 6D.3B.

In comparison to the QD radiation therapy from 1970 through 1978, there was a

TABLE 6D.3A   Five-Year Actuarial LC and DSS Rates After BID Radiation Therapy: 1979–1994

Lesions	n	LC (%)	DSS (%)
T1	13	92	76
T2	49	71	80
T3–4	40	54	50

TABLE 6D.3B   Five-Year Actuarial LC and DSS Rates After QD Radiation Therapy: 1970–1978

Lesions	n	LC (%)	DSS (%)
T1	21	83	92
T2	68	65	66
T3–4	55	24	41

significant increase of local control in T3–4 lesions in favor of BID radiation therapy ($p = 0.0002$), as shown in Table 6D.4.

TABLE 6D.4   Comparison of BID and QD Radiation Therapy Results

Lesions	LC	DSS
T1	$p = 0.56$	$p = 0.13$
T2	$p = 0.41$	$p = 0.09$
T3–4	$p = 0.0002$	$p = 0.1$

SUMMARY

Squamous cell carcinoma of the retromolar trigone is a relatively common cancer of the oral cavity. It must not be confused with carcinoma of the faucial tonsil[4] or posterior gingival ridge cancers, due to their differences in the pattern of spread, therapeutic management, and treatment results, although their locations may be quite similar. Most of these tumors are moderate to well differentiated. Approximately one-fifth of the patients with this disease present with homolateral lymph node metastases when the diagnosis is initially made. Early lesions are highly curable by radiation therapy alone with local control rates of 86% and 68% for T1 and T2 lesions, respectively. The large, infiltrative lesions, T3 and T4 with or without node involvement, are best treated by planned combination of composite resection with plastic closure and postoperative radiation therapy. For the past 15 years, most inoperable T3 and T4 lesions are managed by the BID program with some improvement in local control rates and patient survival.

Primary radical surgery is attended by significant facial deformity and impairment of speech and swallowing function and often results in a high incidence of marginal recurrence, and therefore is not considered to be the treatment of choice for the early lesions but may be reserved for the extensive carcinoma. Metastatic disease in the neck in patients with early lesions is low; elective neck treatment for T1N0 and T2N0 lesions, either surgical or radiotherapeutic, is seldom warranted.

REFERENCES

1. Byers RM, Anderson B, Schwartz EA, et al: Treatment of squamous carcinoma of the retromolar trigone. *Am J Clin Oncol* 1984;7:647–652.

2. Larson DL, Linberg, Lane E, et al: Major complications of radiotherapy in cancer of the oral cavity. *Am J Surg* 1983;146:531–536.

3. Lo K, Fletcher GH, Byers RM, et al: Results of irradiation in the squamous cell carcinomas of the anterior faucial pillar–retromolar trigone. *Int J Radiat Oncol Biol Phys* 1987;13:969–974.

4. Wang CC: Management and prognosis of squamous cell carcinoma of the tonsillar region. *Radiology* 1972;104:667–671.

E. CARCINOMA OF THE BUCCAL MUCOSA

Anatomically, the buccal mucosa is composed of the inner lining of the cheeks and lips, extending superiorly and inferiorly to the buccogingival junction and terminating posteriorly at the junction with the mucous membrane overlying the retromolar trigone and anterior tonsillar pillar. The mucosa is fixed to the underlying buccinator muscle, which is covered on the outside by the skin of the face. The motor and sensory functions are innervated by cranial nerves VII and V, respectively.

Squamous cell carcinoma is relatively uncommon and comprises approximately 5% of the oral carcinomas or 1% of the head and neck cancers. It occurs commonly in patients of old age and rarely before age 40. There is a higher incidence in persons with tobacco-chewing habit.[1,2] These tumors in their early stages are rarely symptomatic. Large tumors or advanced lesions are associated with pain, ulceration, infection, and trismus, which may indicate unresectability. Most of the tumors are relatively well differentiated and frequently associated with areas of leukoplakia. The common sites for buccal mucosa tumors are the mid- and posterior portion of the cheek along the "bite line." Because the mucous membrane is closely attached to the underlying muscle, early invasion of the buccinator muscle by the ulcerative infiltrative lesions is likely to occur. The tumors may also spread lateroposteriorly to the deep lobe of the parotid gland, to the pterygoid fossa, and superiorly and inferiorly to the adjacent alveolar ridge, to the commissure of the lip, and, in advanced stages, may perforate the skin of the cheek. The papillary, verrucous, and exophytic mucosal growths are usually well differentiated with low incidence of lymph node metastases, that is 10–20% for T1 and T2 lesions. Infiltrative, advanced tumors, often associated with muscle invasion, have a high propensity to lymph node metastases—as high as 50–60%.[3,4] The lymph nodes commonly involved include the submandibular, subdigastric, and deep superior jugular, and occasionally the submental and parotid nodes (Figure 6E.1).

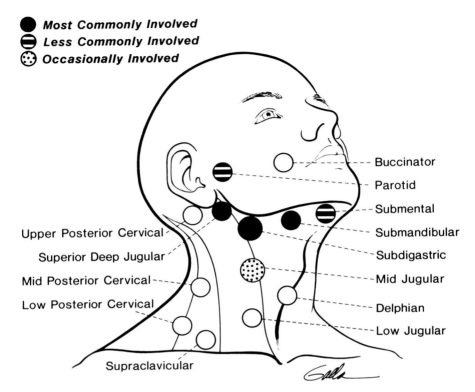

● *Most Commonly Involved*
⊜ *Less Commonly Involved*
⊙ *Occasionally Involved*

Buccinator
Parotid
Submental
Submandibular
Subdigastric
Mid Jugular
Delphian
Low Jugular

Upper Posterior Cervical
Superior Deep Jugular
Mid Posterior Cervical
Low Posterior Cervical
Supraclavicular

FIGURE 6E.1   Diagram showing lymph node involvement in carcinoma of the buccal mucosa.

SELECTION OF THERAPY

For small, superficial T1 lesions with well defined margins, primary simple per oral surgical excision is effective. The procedure not only provides expedient ridding of the malignancy but also eradicates any adjacent leukoplakia. For intermediate lesions, T2, radiation therapy may result in a high cure rate with good functional and cosmetic results and therefore is preferred, while surgery is reserved for salvage. For advanced tumors, T3 and T4 with deep muscular invasion and involvement of the buccogingival sulci and the adjacent mandible, the cure rates following radiation therapy are poor. Therefore en bloc excision of the primary lesion and its regional lymph node metastases followed by flap closure[1,2] and postoperative radiation therapy is the treatment of choice. The management of verrucous carcinoma of the buccal mucosa is often controversial. The concept of potential malignant degeneration after radiation therapy as reported in the literature[5,6] is debatable. It is true that such well differentiated lesions are difficult to control with homeopathic doses of radiation therapy and the recurrences may be more aggressive and hard to manage. Also, some cases of so-called verrucous carcinoma, diagnosed by small biopsy, undergoing malignant changes after radiation therapy are in fact due to sampling error, because the entire specimen is not available for pathologic examination prior to radiation therapy. A few patients with a diagnosis of verrucous carcinoma were treated by radiation therapy at the MGH and were NED for 10 or more years without malignant degeneration.

RADIOTHERAPEUTIC MANAGEMENT

Evaluation of the tumors for radiation therapy should include careful digital palpation of the cheek to ascertain the depth of invasion, extent of mucosal spread, and mobility of the lesions. Involvement of the retromolar trigone or buccogingiva should additionally be evaluated by Panorex and CT scans to rule out the possibility of bone involvement of the mandible. Any tumor extension to the gingiva or retromolar trigone probably precludes the use of interstitial implant as a major treatment modality because of its insufficient coverage and attendant risk of osteoradionecrosis of the mandible. Therefore external beam therapy should be heavily relied on as the major contributor of radiations.

The early lesions, T1 and most of T2, without node involvement are managed by combined external photons and boost techniques using electron beam or interstitial implant or intraoral cone therapy. For moderately advanced lesions with or without node involvement radiotherapeutic management of the disease must include treatment of the primary lesion and the first echelon lymph nodes mostly by an external beam technique through ipsilateral and anterior wedge pair field, as shown in Figure 6E.2, for a basic tumor dose of approximately 50 Gy in 6 weeks followed by electron beam, interstitial implant or IOC boost radiation therapy, sparing the mandible, for an additional 20 Gy (Figure 6E.2). The composite isodoses are shown in Figure 6E.3. The tissues of the buccal cheek can tolerate a high dose of radiation therapy without significant radiation sequelae. For early lesions with well differentiated histology, elective neck radiation therapy is seldom indicated.

Technical Pointers

1. Patient is to lie supine and be immobilized.
2. Margins of the lesion in the cheek are marked by gold grains in four directions, at least 0.5 cm for localization.
3. Use lateral and AP wedge pair portals for about 50 Gy, to be followed by implant or electron beam boost for 20–25 Gy.
4. For interstitial implant, insert "needles" percutaneously along the base of the lesion, rather than intraorally. Use a single vertical plane.
5. Use a dental roll to push the implant away from the jaw, thus reducing the dose to the mandible and the risk of osteoradionecrosis.
6. When using an electron beam, be aware of the constriction of isodoses at depth, which may be much narrower than the entrance portal. Protect the

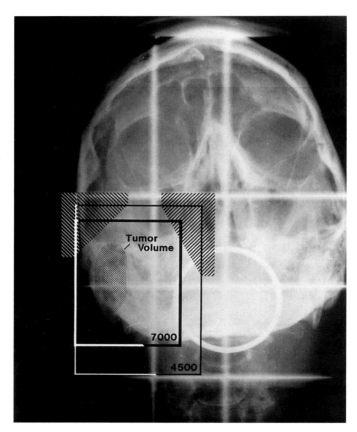

FIGURE 6E.2 Simulation films showing placement of radiation therapy portals for 45 Gy followed by appositional electron boost to 65 Gy or interstitial implant for T2N0 carcinoma of the buccal mucosa in (a) Anteroposterior (AP).

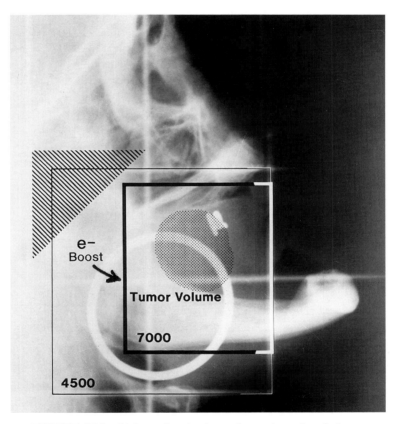

FIGURE 6E.2   (b) Lateral projection, using wedge pair techniques.

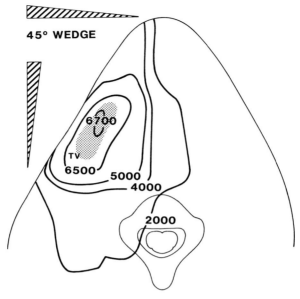

FIGURE 6E.3 Composite isodose consisting of 55 Gy AP and lateral wedge pair (BID program), followed by IOC 9 MeV electron boost with 12 Gy in four daily fractions. Patient is NED without complications.

mandible by inserting a piece of waxed lead shield between the gum and the cheek during irradiation.

7. To avoid a full dose to the mandible, use mixed beams, that is, external photon and lateral wedge pair and interstitial implant and/or electrons.

8. Total dose to the mandible should be limited to 60 Gy.

RADIOTHERAPEUTIC RESULTS

Results of treatment of carcinoma of the buccal mucosa are rather sparse. The published results from Memorial Sloan-Kettering Cancer Center indicate a 5-year survival rates of 42%. For small and intermediate lesions, Stages 1–2, the rates were 77% and 65%, respectively, and for Stages 3–4 the salvage rates were 27% and 18%, respectively.[7] The local control rates following radiation therapy ranged from one-half to two-thirds, depending on the stage of the primary lesions as well as the presence or absence of nodal metastases.[8–10] Large advanced tumors are rarely curable, with survival rates approximately one in five. Fixed cervical nodes generally had very poor outcome with local control rates of less than 10%. The most significant prognostic factor is tumor thickness. For lesions less than 6 mm, the prognosis is excellent regardless of the tumor size.[11] Neck failures occurred in less than 10% of the patients treated and elective neck radiation therapy is not indicated.

Fletcher[12] reported 97 patients with T1−4 lesions treated by radiation therapy. For T1 and T2 lesions, the local control rate was 79% (31/39) and for T3 and T4 lesions the rate was 66% (37/56). Ash[13] reported 5-year absolute survival of 35% in 374 patients, with most treated by radiation therapy. The local control rate for early lesions was 54% (T1N0) and for advanced lesions (T3) 30%; only 5% of patients with T4 were salvaged. Lampe[9] reported on 50 patients with buccal mucosa carcinoma and the 5-year NED survival was 50% after radiation therapy. These results were comparable to those achievable by surgery.[1,3,14,15]

MGH EXPERIENCE

At the MGH, most early and superficial carcinomas of the buccal mucosa were traditionally treated by surgical excision. The cases referred for radiation therapy therefore were patients with relatively large and advanced lesions. From 1970 through 1994, a total of 33 patients were treated by radiation therapy. The 5-year actuarial local control and disease-specific survival rates for T1−2 lesions were 68% and 77%, respectively. For T3 and T4 lesions, the local control rate was 30% with no disease-specific survivors, as shown in Table 6E.1.

The patterns of radiation therapy failure were analyzed.The majority of radiation therapy failures were due to uncontrolled disease at the primary site and, of these, more than two-thirds or 70% had nodal disease as well. Failure to control nodal metastases in the neck only accounted for three patients or 11%. Only one patient died of distant metastases without disease above the clavicles. Surgical salvage procedures were performed on six patients with T2 and T3 disease and all were NED after surgery. Thus, including surgical salvage patients, the overall 3-year NED rate of the entire group of patients was 55% (33/60).

TABLE 6E.1   Five-Year Actuarial LC and DSS Rates After Radiation Therapy: 1970−1994

Lesions	n	LC (%)	DSS (%)
T1	5	66	75
T2	22	60	78
T1–2	27	68	77
T3−4	6	30	0
Total	33	55	69

SUMMARY

Squamous cell carcinoma of the buccal mucosa is a relatively uncommon cancer. The small T1 lesion with well-defined borders can be managed successfully by simple excision or localized radiation therapy either by external radiation therapy, interstitial implant or IOC, or by a combination of these modalities. For the moderately advanced carcinomas, T2, comprehensive high-dose external radiation therapy encompassing the primary lesion and nodal drainage areas is advised. This is to be followed by radiation boost to the primary site either by intraoral cone (IOC), or interstitial implant, or electron beam to bring the total dose to 75–80 Gy in a 8 weeks. Care must be exercised to limit radiation dose to the mandible to 65–70 Gy in 7 weeks to avoid osteoradionecrosis. The residual nodes in the neck after partial or whole neck irradiation are treated by neck dissection. Extensive T3 and T4 infiltrative disease with or without node involvement is rarely curable by radiation therapy alone and, if operable, these lesions are currently managed by combined therapies, that is, adjuvant chemotherapy, radiation therapy, and surgery.

Radiation failures were primarily due to inability to control the primary lesions with disease in the neck. Failure by distant metastases alone accounted for 1 in 10 patients after irradiation.

REFERENCES

1. O'Brien JH, Catlin D: Cancer of the cheek (mucosa). *Cancer* 1965;18:1392–1398.

2. Conley J, Sadoyama JA: Squamous cell cancer of the buccal mucosa. *Arch Otolaryngol* 1973;94:330–333.

3. Modlin J, Johnson RE: The surgical treatment of cancer of the buccal mucosa and lower gingiva. *AJR Am J Roentgenol* 1955;73:620–627.

4. Skolnik EM, Campbell JM, Meyers RM: Carcinoma of the buccal mucosa and retromolar area. *Otolaryngol Clin North AM* 1972;5:327–331.

5. Fonts EA, Greenlaw RH, Rush BF, et al: Verrucous squamous cell carcinoma of the oral cavity. *Cancer* 1969;23:152–160.

6. Kraus FT, Perez-Mesa C: Verrucous carcinoma: clinical and pathologic study of 105 cases involving oral cavity, larynx and gingiva. *Cancer* 1966;19:26–38.

7. Bloom ND, Siro RH: Carcinoma of the cheek mucosa: a retrospective analysis. *Am J Surg* 1980;140:556–559.

8. MacComb WS, Fletcher GH: *Cancer of the head and neck.* Baltimore: Williams & Wilkins, 1967;147.

9. Lampe I: Radiation therapy of cancer of the buccal mucosa and lower gingiva. *AJR Am J Roentgenol* 1955;73:628–638.

10. Nair MK, Sankaranarayanan R, Padamnabhan K: Evaluation of the role of radiotherapy in the management of carcinoma of the buccal mucosa. *Cancer* 1988;61:1326–1331.

11. Urist MM, O'Brien CJ, Soong SJ, et al: Squamous carcinoma of the buccal mucosa; analysis of prognostic factors. *Am J Surg* 1987;154:411–414.

12. Fletcher GH: *Textbook of radiotherapy*, 2nd ed. Philadelphia: Lea & Febiger, 1973;240.

13. Ash CL: Oral cancer: a twenty-five year study. *AJR AM J Roentgenol* 1962;27:417–430.

14. Bakamjian VY: The surgical management of cancers of the cheek. *J Surg Oncol* 1974;6:255–267.

15. Paymaster JC: Cancer of the buccal mucosa. *Cancer* 1956;9:431.

F. CARCINOMA OF THE GINGIVA

Squamous cell carcinoma of the gingiva usually arises in the posterior portion of the lower dental arch and is commonly associated with leukoplakic changes. Most of these tumors are well differentiated squamous cell carcinomas. The mucous membrane is firmly attached to the underlying alveolar process of the maxilla and mandible. Although the periosteum tends to form a barrier for tumor spread, the presence of multiple tiny defects in the edentulous mandibular ridge facilitates tumor access for bone invasion. Therefore tumor arising from the gingiva is likely to invade the underlying occlusal surface of the jaw bone in its early stage of development.[1,2] Once the thin cortical bone is penetrated and the underlying cancellous bone or the neurovascular canal is involved, the cancer may extend approximately and distantly throughout the mandible beyond what can be demonstrated by radiographs.[3] Bone involvement occurs in approximately 50% of gingival carcinomas. The buccal plates and the inferior lingual plate and the cortical edge are relatively resistant and only involved in the late stage of the disease.

Approximately 80% of the gingival carcinomas arise from the lower gingiva, and of these 60% occur posterior to the bicuspid.[4] Carcinoma of the upper gingiva is an uncommon disease and should not be confused with tumors that originate from the maxillary sinus, secondarily extending to the gingiva. Radiographic examination of the paranasal sinuses and upper gingiva is helpful in differentiating between these two conditions and also allows a careful evaluation of the extent of bony involvement.

Lymphatic spread depends on whether the lesion arises from the buccal surface or lingual surface of the alveolar ridge. From the buccal side, metastases occur in the submandibular, submental, and subdigastric nodes. From the lingual side, metastases occur in the subdigastric, deep superior jugular, and retropharyngeal nodes. Both upper and lower gingival lesions follow similar patterns of spread, as shown in Figure 6F.1. Approximately one-third of patients present with nodal metastases at diagnosis, and less than 3% with contralateral metastases. This incidence is higher in lower gingival lesions than in the upper gingival lesions. Distant spread is most unusual.

Since bone involvement by carcinomas compromises radiotherapetuic results, careful radiographic examination of the mandible including Parorex, intraoral dental radiographs, and CT scans are essential as a pretreatment work-up. Special note should be made between a smooth, saucer-shaped pressure defect, as shown in Figure 6F.2, which results from a slowly pushing tumor, and the moth-eaten type of bone destruction, as shown in Figure 6F.2, which is caused by tumor infiltration with aggressive character. The former can be treated by radiation therapy with success, whereas the latter cannot.

SELECTION OF THERAPY

Treatment of carcinoma of the gingiva depends on the extent of the lesion, the status of the cervical lymph nodes, and, most importantly, the presence or absence of bone involvement. Small, T1, exophytic lesions without bone involvement can be

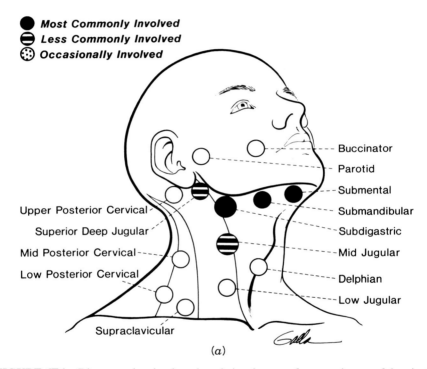

FIGURE 6F.1   Diagrams showing lymph node involvement from carcinoma of the gingiva: (a) tumor arising from the buccal aspect.

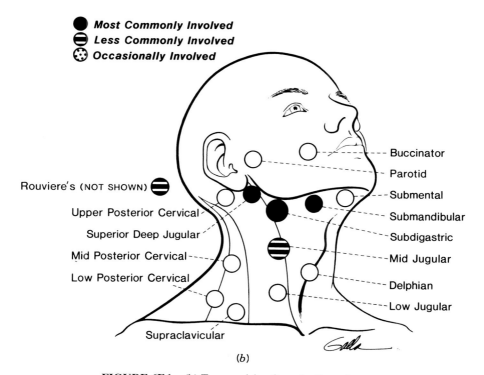

FIGURE 6F.1 (b) Tumor arising from the lingual aspect.

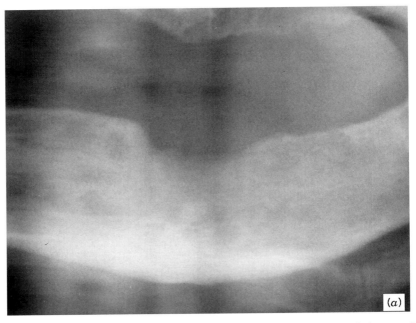

FIGURE 6F.2   (a) Radiograph showing saucer-shaped pressure defect of the mandible from slowly growing tumor.

managed by external beam therapy alone with success. Due to the mandible's low tolerance to high-dose radiation therapy, primary treatment by external beam is rarely successful for advanced T3–4 lesions, and therefore these tumors are treated by combined therapies. For advanced carcinoma of the lower gingiva, radical surgery is carried out. Lesions of the upper gingiva associated with bone destruction are treated by inferior maxillectomy and the surgical defect is managed by an obturator. All advanced lesions are further managed by postoperative RT.

For preservation of jaw continuity, marginal mandibulectomy or rim resection in properly selected patients has achieved satisfactory control and is believed as effective as segmental resection.[5–7] Contraindications for mandibular conservation procedure include extensive tumors enveloping the mandible, tumor invasion through the cortical plate, and recent tooth extraction proximal to the tumor. For close resection margins, a course of postoperative radiation therapy is often advised with a dose of 50–55 Gy.

RADIOTHERAPEUTIC MANAGEMENT

The small mucosal tumor can be treated satisfactorily by combined external beam radiation therapy and IOC boost if technically feasible. Radium mold was once

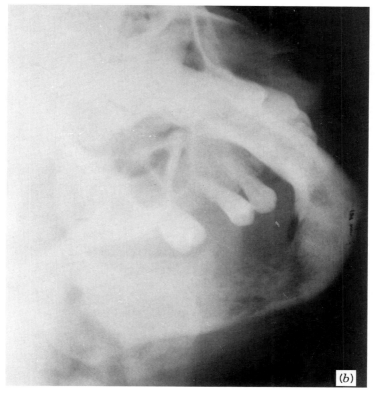

FIGURE 6F.2   (b) Radiograph showing moth-eaten bone destruction of the mandible from rapidly growing infiltrative carcinoma.

used but has entirely been replaced by modern megavoltage irradiation. Due to the proximity of bone to the tumors and resultant radionecrosis of the mandible, interstitial implant has no place in the management of this disease.

Because of the likelihood of local spread of the disease along the entire mandible, radiation therapy is delivered to the hemi-mandible from the mental symphysis to the temporomandibular joint, using ipsilateral and antertoposterior (AP) wedge pair technique, as shown in Figure 6F.3. Concurrently, the ipsilateral neck is irradiated if nodes are present or lesions are advanced. For primary radiation therapy, a basic tumor dose of 45 Gy in $4\frac{1}{2}$ weeks is planned, to be followed by localized boost either by IOC or appositional electron beam or ipsilateral oblique wedge pair portals for a total dose of 60 Gy in 6 weeks. For carcinoma of the upper gingiva treated by inferior maxillectomy and/or palatectomy, postoperative radiation therapy is carried out, and the first echelon lymphatic drainage nodes are treated by combined photons and electrons for approximately 55 Gy.

Because of the low tolerance of the mandible, most patients are referred to the radiation oncology department for postoperative radiation therapy. As an adjuvant

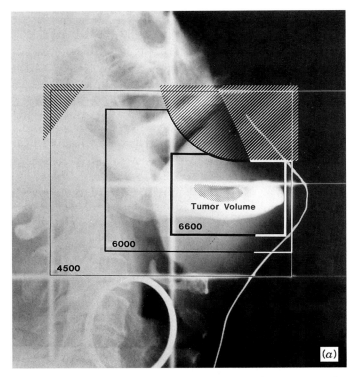

FIGURE 6F.3 Simulation film showing placement of portal for treatment of carcinoma of mandible: (a) lateral projection.

procedure, a dose of approximately 55 Gy is given, using the wedge pair technique, as shown in Figure 6F.4. The postoperative radiation therapy is begun approximately 3 weeks after surgery.

Technical Pointers

1. Patient is to lie supine and be immobilized with a face mask.
2. Use a bite block to depress the tongue and separate the upper lip and palate from the radiation beam; a dental roll is used to push the lower lip forward, away from the beam.
3. Radiation therapy portals cover the entire hemi-mandible, including the mental symphysis onto the temporomandibular joint (TMJ), using ipsilateral and AP wedge pair technique for 45 Gy.
4. Use a Cerrobend cutout to exclude the superior, anterior, and medial corners.
5. Use a shrinking field after 45 Gy to bring the dose to the tumor volume to 60 Gy.
6. Limit the dose to the entire mandible to 55–60 Gy.

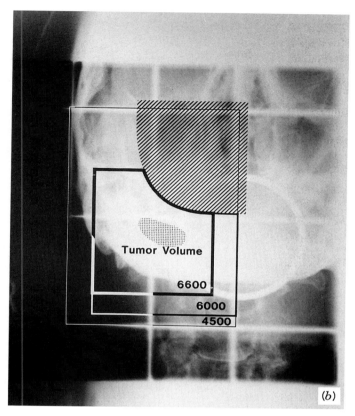

FIGURE 6F.3   Simulation film showing placement of portal for treatment of carcinoma of mandible: (b) anteroposterior view.

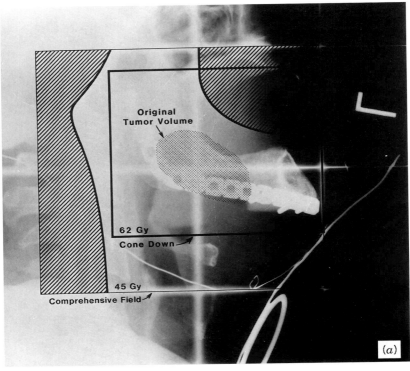

FIGURE 6F.4 Simulation film showing placement of postoperative portal: (a) lateral projection.

RESULTS OF TREATMENT

Combined mandibular resection and neck dissection can produce good local control and survival. Cady and Catlin[4] indicate that the most significant factors influencing survival rates are tumor size, evidence of mandibular invasion, and metastases in the neck. Of 557 patients treated for cure, the absolute survival rate was about 50%. Large tumors (i.e., >5 cm) with metastases below Level had a 0% survival rate, as compared 82% in patients with tumors <3 cm in size without node involvement. Adjuvant radiation therapy was recommended for large advanced lesions. Similarly, good results were reported by Byers et al.[8] with satisfactory local control and survival in patients with T1 and T2 lesions. In an attempt to preserve the integrity of the mandible, radiation therapy was tried but generally resulted in poor tumor control and morbidity. A few scattered reports in the literature indicate 5-year survival rates varying from 30% to 50%,[4,9,10] particularly for patients with small mucosal tumors without bone invasion.

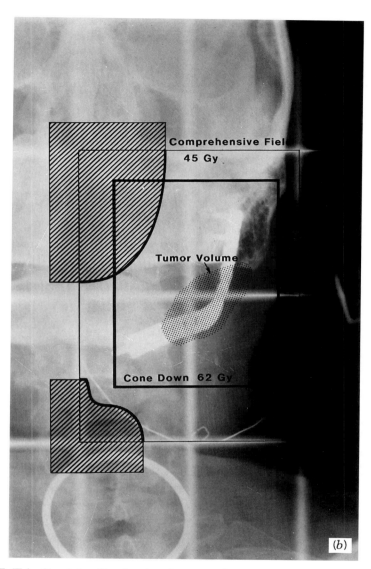

FIGURE 6F.4   Simulation film showing placement of postoperative portal: (b) anteroposterior view.

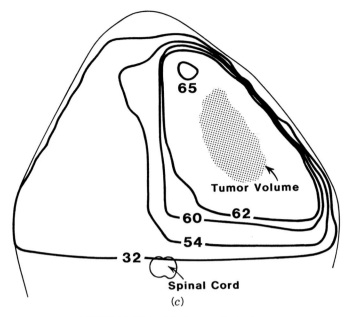

FIGURE 6F.4   (c) Composite isodoses.

MGH EXPERIENCE

From 1970 to 1994, a total of 50 patients were treated by radiation therapy and were available for evaluation. The 5-year actuarial local control and disease-specific survival rates for the entire group of patients were 63% and 61%, respectively, as shown in Table 6F.1. Of 30 patients with T1–2 lesions, the LC and DSS rates were 65% and 57%, respectively. For the T3–4 lesions, the rates were 64% and 70%, respectively.

Of 17 patients receiving a combination of surgery (mostly partial mandibulectomy) and radiation therapy, the local control and disease-specific survival rates for the T1–2 lesions were 83% and 83%, and for the T3–4 lesions the rates were 55% and 75%, respectively, as shown in Table 6F.2.

TABLE 6F.1   Five-Year Actuarial LC and DSS Rates After Radiation Therapy: 1970–1994

Lesions	n	LC (%)	DSS (%)
T1	15	65	72
T2	15	67	38
T1–2	30	65	57
T3–4	20	64	70
Total	50	64	62

**TABLE 6F.2   Five-Year Actuarial LC and DSS Rates
for T3–4 Carcinoma of the Gingival Ridge After
Combined Surgery and Postoperative Radiation
Therapy: 1970–1994**

Lesions	n	LC (%)	DSS (%)
T1–2	6	83	83
T3–4	11	55	75

RESULTS OF BID RADIATION THERAPY

From 1979 through 1994, a total of 30 patients received BID radiation therapy for squamous cell carcinoma of the gingival ridge. Of the entire group, the 5-year actuarial local control and disease-specific survival rates were 71% and 67%, as compared to 20 patients treated from 1970 to 1978, whose rates were 53% and 55%, respectively. For T1 and T2 lesions, the corresponding rates for BID and QD were 66% and 63%, respectively, $p = 0.68$. For T3 and T4 lesions, the rates were 78% and 33%, $p = 0.05$, as shown in Table 6F.3.

**TABLE 6F.3   Five-Year Actuarial LC and DSS Rates
After BID and QD Radiation Therapy: 1970–1994**

	n	LC (%)	DSS (%)
T1–2			
BID	16	66	60
QD	14	63	54
		$p = 0.68$	$p = 0.6$
T3–4			
BID	14	78	76
QD	6	33	53
		$p = 0.05$	$p = 0.45$
T1–4			
BID	30	71	67
QD	20	53	55
		$p = 0.15$	$p = 0.42$

SUMMARY

Squamous cell carcinoma of the gingiva is a relatively uncommon cancer. Surgical resection is generally considered to be the treatment of choice. However, in a small subset of patients in whom the lesions are small and exophytic without node involvement, T1N0 and T2N0, radiation therapy may play a curative role in the management of this disease with satisfactory cure rate. For extensive lesions, T3 and T4, with bone destruction and/or nodal metastases, the treatment of choice is a planned combination of surgery, reconstructive procedures, and postoperative radiation therapy.

Large, far advanced tumors, T4N1–3, with extensive bone destruction of the mandible and maxilla and with nodal metastases are rarely curable by either surgery or radiation therapy or combination of the two. High-dose radiation therapy or chemotherapy may offer some degree of palliation.

At the present time, accelerated hyperfractionation BID radiation therapy has not shown significant advantage over conventional QD radiation therapy for early lesions. In a small subset of patients with T3–4 lesions, a trend suggested some improvement in local control.

REFERENCES

1. McGregor AD, MacDonald DG: Routes of entry of squamous cell carcinoma to the mandible. *Head Neck Surg* 1988;10:294–301.
2. O'Brien CJ, Carter RL, Soo KC, et al: Invasion of the mandible by squamous carcinomas of the oral cavity and oropharynx. *Head Neck Surg* 1986;8:247–256.
3. Swearingen AG, McGraw JP, Palumbo VD: Roentgenographic pathologic correlation of carcinoma of the gingiva involving the mandible. *Radiology* 1966;96:15–18.
4. Cady B, Catlin D: Epidermoid carcinoma of the gum: a 20-year survey. *Cancer* 1969;23:551–569.
5. Porter EH: The local prognosis after radical radiotherapy for squamous carcinoma of the alveolus and of the floor of the mouth. *Clin Radiol* 1971;22:139–143.
6. Barttelbort S, Ariyan S: Mandible preservation with oral cavity carcinoma: rim mandibulectomy versus sagittal mandibulectomy. *Am J Surg* 1987;154:423–428.
7. Wald RM, Calcaterra TC: Lower alveolar carcinoma: segmental vs. marginal resection. *Arch Otolaryngol* 1983;109:578–582.
8. Byers RM, Newman R, Russell N, Yue A: Results of treatment for squamous carcinoma of the lower gum. *Cancer* 1981;47:2236–2238.
9. Lampe I: Radiation therapy of cancer of the buccal mucosa and lower gingiva. *AJR Am J Roentgenol* 1955;73:628–635.
10. Fayos JV, Lampe I: Treatment of squamous cell carcinoma of the oral cavity. *Am J Surg* 1972;124:493–500.

G. CARCINOMA OF THE SOFT PALATE

The palate forms the roof of the oral cavity and is divided into the hard and soft palates. Five pairs of muscles contribute to the structure of the soft palate. These are the (1) tensor veli palatini, (2) uvular, (3) palatoglossus, (4) palatopharyngeus, and (5) levator veli palatini muscles. The soft palate is attached anteriorly to the posterior border of the hard palate; posteriorly its border is free and is formed by the fusion of the anterior and posterior faucial pillars, both of which contribute to the formation of the central mass called the uvula. The soft palate therefore possesses dual biologic behavior, consisting of the clinicopathologic features of the oral cavity (the anterior pillar) and oropharynx (posterior pillar). The locations of tumors may affect different cell types, patterns of spread, management, and results of treatment. The structures of the soft palate are often collectively referred to as the *faucial arch*.[1]

Squamous cell carcinomas arising from the faucial arch are dissimilar and therefore it is not prudent to include all of these cancers in one category for general discussion. In this section an attempt is made to discuss only lesions of the soft palate and uvula as oral cancers. Lesions arising from the faucial tonsil and posterior pillars are included with the oropharyngeal cancers. The anterior pillar tumors are discussed under the heading of retromolar trigone lesions.

Sore throat and odynophagia are the common initial symptoms of this disease. Most tumors of the soft palate and uvula may be well differentiated to poorly differentiated squamous cell carcinomas, depending on the location of the lesions. Tumors arising from the anterior oral surface of the soft palate tend to be well differentiated while lesions originating from the free edge or involving the posterior pillar tend to be more undifferentiated, similar to the oral and oropharyngeal carcinomas, respectively. Soft palate carcinomas may be superficial and ulcerative with poorly defined borders and are often associated with widespread erythroplasia and in situ carcinoma and multiple primary lesions, either in the adjacent soft palate, pillars, hypopharynx, or floor of the mouth. Careful examination of the head and neck region to exclude multiple primary carcinomas should be carried out.

The incidence of nodal metastases for T1 and T2 lesions varies from 10% to 30%, and for advanced lesions from 60% to 70%. The principal group of nodes involved include the subdigastric, upper, and midjugular nodes, but the submandibular nodes may also be affected (Figure 6G.1). For midline lesions, metastases may be bilateral (20–50%).[2]

SELECTION OF THERAPY

Surgical resection of carcinoma of the soft palate is unsatisfactory, often resulting in recurrences at the margins. Strong[3] reported a 41% recurrence rate in 32 patients treated by surgery. For Stage I and II lesions, the recurrence rate was 46% (13/28).[3] Local control by surgery as reported by Ratzer et al.[4] was 38% for small lesions at 5 years. Even when surgery is successful, the impaired swallowing and speech functions are not acceptable.

T1 and T2 exophytic mucosal tumors generally respond to radiation therapy well and their treatment should be radiation therapy. For advanced T3 lesions, often associated with lymph node metastasis, radiation therapy may be given first with curative intent, and any residual disease at the primary site and in the neck may be dealt with by surgical resection. Massive squamous cell carcinoma of the soft palate, T4 with involvement of the entire oropharynx, base of the tongue, and tonsil,

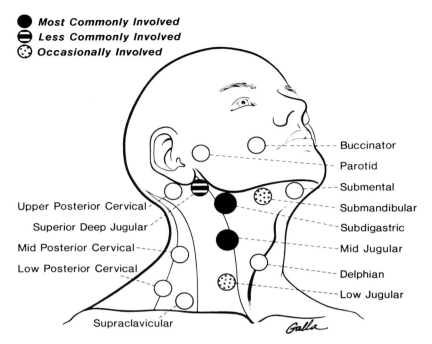

FIGURE 6G.1   Diagram showing lymph node involvement in carcinoma of the soft palate.

often associated with bilateral lymph node metastases, at present is incurable by any means. High-dose radiation therapy with or without chemotherapy may offer some palliation. Any attempt to eradicate such advanced tumors with primary surgery is rarely successful due to the uncontrolled primary lesion and metastatic disease in the neck.

RADIOTHERAPEUTIC MANAGEMENT

Squamous cell carcinomas of the soft palate tend to spread diffusely along the mucosal surface with poorly defined borders and escape detection by the naked eye. Toluidine blue staining and/or development of tumoritis after initial 20 Gy "mouth bath" may frequently delineate the tumor extent or in situ carcinoma or erythroplasia.

For small, well-defined, localized, superficial T1 lesions, a portion of the treatment may be given via the IOC electron beam technique followed by external beam radiation therapy. This may lessen significantly the radiation sequelae, such as dental caries and xerostomia. For large T2 and T3 lesions, external beam radiation therapy including the primary lesion and first echelon lymph nodes is used initially (Figure 6G.2). After the spinal cord tolerance is reached, "off-cord" radiation therapy via a boost technique to the primary site is given up to a total dose of 65–70

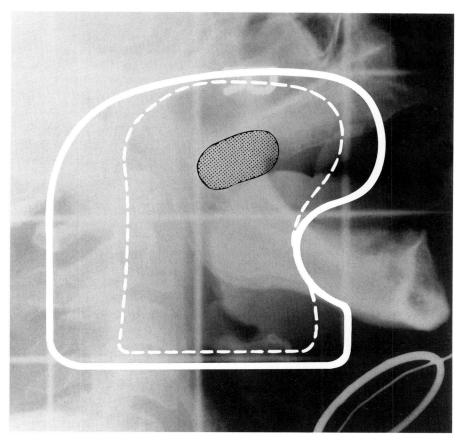

FIGURE 6G.2 Simulation film showing portal arrangement and shrinking field technique for RT of soft palate carcinoma. The final boost may be given by IOC if feasible after 65 Gy up to 72 Gy to the primary.

Gy over 6–7 weeks. Elective lower neck and supraclavicular irradiation is also given for 45 Gy over 5 weeks in those patients with an extensive primary lesion or lymph node disease.

Technical Pointers

1. Patient is to lie supine and be immobilized with a face mask. Cervical nodes are lead wired.
2. A bite block is used to depress the tongue and the FOM and a Cerrobend cutout is employed to shield the anterior tongue.
3. For poorly defined lesions, begin a "mouth bath" with the initial external beam radiation therapy through large opposing lateral portals with 1:1 loading for 20 Gy in 2 weeks for evaluation of tumoritis.

4. After the extent of the lesion is defined, its borders are tattooed for boosting purposes.
5. Radiation portals include the entire soft palate and posterior half of the hard palate and superiorly to the lower nasopharynx at the level of the tragus and inferiorly at the thyroid notch. The middle ear is shielded from the portal.
6. Nodal coverage includes the superior deep jugular lymph nodes (nodes between the angle of the jaw and the mastoid tip) and the subdigastric, submandibular, and midjugular nodes.
7. After 60 Gy, the gross residual lesion is boosted via IOC or three-field (right, left, and anteroposterior) technique or arc rotation to 70–72 Gy. If the lesion is obviously eccentric, us a lateral wedge pair boost after 50 Gy. The mandibular dose should be kept below 67 Gy.

RADIOTHERAPEUTIC RESULTS

For small T1 and T2 tumors, very good control rates (80–90%) have been achieved with radiation therapy, with excellent functional results.[5,6] Local control of advanced (T3) disease by radiation therapy is poor, approximately 10–20%. Far advanced (T4) lesions are inoperable and rarely curable and are treated with radiation therapy for palliation or with chemotherapy.

MGH EXPERIENCE

From 1970 through 1994 a total of 144 patients with squamous cell carcinoma of the soft palate and uvula were treated by radiation therapy. The 5-year actuarial lo-

TABLE 6G.1   Five-Year Actuarial LC and DSS Rates
After Radiation Therapy: 1970–1994

Lesions	n	LC (%)	DSS (%)
T1	39	96	86
T2	65	81	82
T3	27	55	40
T4	13	24	24
T3–4	40	45	34
Total	144	75	70
N0	107	85	81
N1	5	20	60
N2–3	32	55	40
		$p = 0.0001$	$p = 0.0001$

**TABLE 6G.2   Five-Year Acturial LC and DSS by
Stages After Radiation: 1970–1994**

Stages	n	LC (%)	DSS (%)
Stage 1	33	96	91
Stage 2	54	85	85
		$p = 0.13$	$p = 0.41$

cal control and disease-specific survival rates are shown in Table 6G.1. For T1 and T2 lesions, the LC rates were 96% and 81%, respectively, and the DSS rates were 86% and 82%. The rates for LC for the T3 and T4 lesions were 55% and 24%, respectively, and the DSS rates were 40% and 24%, respectively. The LC and DSS significantly improved in patients with no neck as compared with N1–3 disease.

The local control and disease-specific survival rates of patients with early lesions without node involvement are extremely satisfactory, as shown in Table 6G.2.

Salvage surgery was attempted in two patients but failed to control the disease. Most of the radiation therapy failures were due to uncontrolled disease at the primary site or lymph node disease in the neck. Distant metastasis rarely occurred except in far-advanced incurable lesions.

The value of routine elective neck radiation therapy or radical neck dissection was assessed. Of 47 patients without affected lymph nodes (T1N0 and T2N0) at the time of diagnosis and surviving 3 or more years after radiation therapy without disease at the primary site, only four (7%) underwent radical neck dissection for metastatic lymph nodes, and all four were salvaged by TND with no evidence of disease. Eight patients with T2N0 lesions died of the disease. Of these, four died of nodal disease within the irradiated portals; the others died of uncontrolled primary and nodal disease. Of this group of patients, only seven underwent elective neck irradiation. Therefore eight of 47 patients or 17% receiving partial or no neck radiation therapy failed in the neck only, and half were successfully salvaged by RND. It may be concluded that routine elective neck irradiation or elective neck dissection is not indicated for early well-differentiated lesions with N0 necks.

RESULTS OF BID RADIATION THERAPY

From 1979 through 1994, 99 patients received twice-daily (BID) radiation therapy. The 5-year actuarial local control and disease-specific survival rates for 14 patients were 91% and 81%, respectively. For T2 lesions, the rates were 79% and 82% and for T3 and T4 lesions the corresponding rates were 68% and 72%, respectively, as shown Table 6G.3.

Comparing these data with QD results, no significant difference was found with the exception that the QD local control was slightly higher, $p = 0.03$.

TABLE 6G.3 Five-Year Actuarial LC and DSS Rates
After BID Radiation Therapy: 1979–1994

Lesions	n	LC (%)	DSS (%)
T1	14	91	81
T2	51	79	82
T3–4	34	68	54

SUMMARY

Squamous cell carcinoma of the soft palate is a relatively less common cancer of the oral cavity. The early superficial mucosal lesions (T1N0 and T2N0) are highly amenable to treatment with radiation therapy, with extremely high cure rates and preservation of speech and swallowing mechanisms. For advanced disease, cure rates with radiation therapy are poor. The results after twice-daily radiation therapy are not significantly improved thus far. The presence of lymph node metastasis reduces survival to about half of that without node involvement. Elective lower neck irradiation does not seem to be indicated in patients with early superficial (T1N0) lesions; however, in patients with advanced disease and affected lymph nodes, aggressive radiation treatment to the primary site and neck may produce good local control and higher survival rates. Radical neck dissection for residual lymph nodes is efficacious for controlling neck disease. Primary surgery for carcinoma of the soft palate is not rewarding and often is unsuccessful because of the high incidence of tumor recurrence at the margins after surgery.

Squamous cell carcinoma of the soft palate tends to be associated with cancerous field diathesis and often with multiple primary lesions of the head and neck. Close follow-up of all treated patients is required. A few so-called local recurrences at the irradiated site or adjacent area may in fact be second or third primary carcinomas. Repeat irradiation of small recurrences or second primary lesions is feasible and occasionally successful with careful technique (i.e., IOC electron beam radiation therapy) because of the high tolerance of the mucomuscular structures of the soft palate, a fact rarely appreciated.

REFERENCES

1. Gelinas M, Fletcher GH: Incidence and causes of local failure of irradiation in squamous cell carcinoma of the faucial arch, tonsillar fossa and base of tongue. *Radiology* 1973; 108:383–387.

2. Lindberg R: Distribution of cervical lymph node metastases from squamous cell carcinoma of the upper respiratory ad digestive tracts. *Cancer* 1972;29:1446–1449.

3. Strong E: Sites of treatment failure in head and neck cancer. *Cancer Treat Symp* 1987;2:5–20.

4. Ratzer ER, Schweitzer RJ, Frazell EL: Epidermoid carcinoma of the palate. *Am J Surg* 1970;119:294–297.

5. Lindberg RD, Fletcher GH: The role of irradiation in the management of head and neck cancer. Analysis of results and causes of failure. *Tumori* 1978;64:313–325.

6. Chung CK, Constable WC: Treatment of squamous cell carcinoma of the soft palate and uvula. *Int J Radiat Oncol Biol Phys* 1979;5:845–850.

H. CARCINOMA OF THE HARD PALATE

The hard palate is developed by the horizontal plates of the palatine bones and forms the anterior rigid portion of the roof of the oral cavity and the base of the nasal cavity. The muscles of the soft palate attach to its posterior edge. The mucous membrane is firmly attached to the periosteum. Squamous cell carcinomas arising from this site, therefore, like cancer of the alveolar ridge, tend to invade the underlying bone in their early stage of development.[1]

The hard palate is the most common site for minor salivary gland tumors in the oral cavity. Squamous cell carcinomas arising from the hard palate are rare and are usually ulcerative and generally poorly defined. Most carcinomas are well differentiated with a low incidence (15–20%) of lymph node metastasis. The submandibular, upper jugular, and subdigastric lymph nodes are commonly involved.[1]

Painless irregularity or swelling with ill-fitting dentures is usually the only complaint of early carcinoma of the hard palate. As part of the physical examination, appropriate x-ray examination is mandatory, including CT and/or MR scans of the palatal bone and the maxillary antrum before a decision regarding management is made.

SELECTION OF THERAPY

Early squamous cell carcinoma, without radiographic bone involvement, can be treated satisfactorily with radiation therapy alone, and surgery is reserved for salvage after radiation failure. Advanced, deeply ulcerative, infiltrative lesions often associated with bone destruction are rarely curable with radiation therapy and should be treated with a planned combination of radiation therapy and surgery.[2] As long as a small band of free edge of the soft palate remains intact, subtotal palatectomy or inferior maxillectomy generally is not associated with great morbidity. The resulting bony defect can be corrected with an obturator. Malignant salivary gland tumors were traditionally treated with surgery alone but have been treated with increasing frequency with surgery followed by radiation therapy. Some inoperable malignancies of the minor salivary glands can be successfully treated and controlled with high-dose radiation therapy (see Chapter 12).

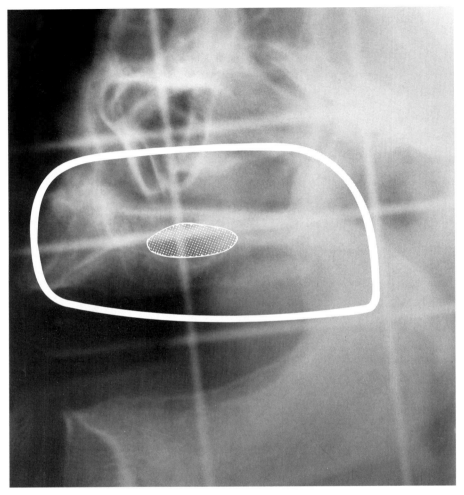

FIGURE 6H.1   Simulation film showing placement of treatment portal for T1N0 squamous cell carcinoma of the hard palate. No elective neck irradiation is required.

RADIOTHERAPEUTIC MANAGEMENT

Radiation therapy for early carcinoma of the hard palate is generally directed to treatment of the primary site if the neck is free from metastatic disease. A dose of 65–70 Gy over 7 weeks is required for good local control. For the well-defined primary lesion, IOC electron beam or wedge pair may be considered (Figure 6H.1). For advanced disease with bone destruction and affected lymph nodes, postoperative radiation therapy to approximately 60 Gy over 7 weeks is given following resection of the primary lesion and the involved palatal bone or radical neck dissection.

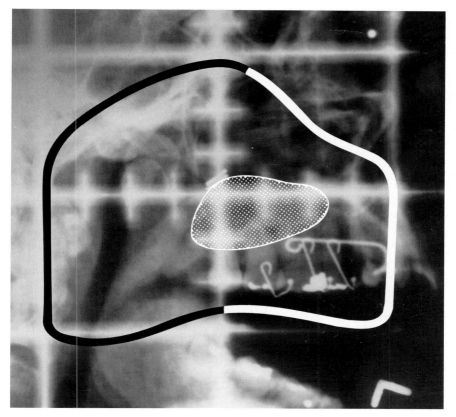

FIGURE 6H.2   Simulation film showing portal placement for treatment of adenocystic carcinoma with perineural spread; portal includes the primary site and its nerve onto the base of the skull.

Most malignant salivary gland carcinomas are treated by combined surgery and postoperative radiation therapy with a dose of approximately 60 Gy. For adenocystic carcinoma, the primary site and perineural spread are within the treatment field, as shown in Figure 6H.2.

Technical Pointers

1. Patient is to lie supine and be immobilized with a face mask.
2. A bite block is used to depress the tongue and a Cerrobend cutout shields the dorsum of the tongue and mandible.
3. Use opposing lateral portals to include the entire hard palate up to the premaxillary process and adjacent soft palate for the initial 50 Gy. Gross residual tumor is boosted with either IOC, wedge pair, or three-field technique to a total of 70 Gy.

4. Generally, a rectangular field is used to include tissue 3 cm above and below the hard palate bone and the alveolar ridge.
5. For N0 neck, no elective neck irradiation is given. Large nodes, however, are included in the large portals of 50 Gy and later treated with neck dissection.
6. For postoperative lesion, keep the obturator in situ to reduce dose inhomogeneity and to avoid the air-cavity effect.

RADIOTHERAPEUTIC RESULTS

Information regarding radiotherapeutic results for carcinoma of the hard palate is sparse because of the rarity of the disease. Scattered case reports suggest that local control rates can be achieved in approximately one-third to one-half of the lesions treated.[3] Those patients with bone destruction and affected lymph nodes are unlikely to be cured with radiation therapy, and a combination of radiation therapy and surgery has provided some improvement in local control and survival.

MGH EXPERIENCE

From 1970 to 1994, 23 patients with squamous cell carcinoma of the hard palate received radiation therapy. The 5-year actuarial local control and disease-specific survival rates were 49% and 79% after radiation therapy. For patients with T1–2 lesions, the rates were 60% and 84% and with T3–4 lesions, 100%, respectively, although the number of patients as small, as shown in Table 6H.1. Of five patients receiving a combination of surgery and radiation therapy, the LC and DSS rates were both 50%. Patients with cervical node metastases generally did very poorly with LC and DSS rates both about 50%.

TABLE 6H.1 Five-Year Actuarial LC and DSS Rates
for Patients Treated by Radiation Therapy: 1970–1994

Lesions	n	LC (%)	DSS (%)
T1–2	16	60	84
T3	3	33	100
T3–4	4	100	100
T1–4	23	49	79

SUMMARY

Squamous cell carcinoma of the hard palate is an uncommon cancer of the oral cavity. Traditional treatment is primarily with surgery. A small subgroup of patients with lesions limited to the mucosa without bone destruction and without affected lymph nodes may be treated successfully with irradiation, with good local control and long-term survival. Extensive lesions with bone involvement are best treated with a combination of radiation therapy and surgery, with improved results, and the resultant bone defect can satisfactorily be remedied with a prosthesis immediately after surgical resection.

REFERENCES

1. Ratzer ER, Schweitzer RJ, Frazell EL: Epidermoid carcinoma of the palate. *Am J Surg* 1970;119:294–297.
2. Konrad HR, Canalis RF, Calcaterra TC: Epidermoid carcinoma of the palate. *Arch Otolaryngol* 1978;104:208–212.
3. Schotlenfeld D: Cancer of the buccal cavity and pharynx: a review of end results of primary treatment of 2877 cases: 1947–1964. *Clin Bull* 1972;2:51–57.

CHAPTER 7

CARCINOMA OF THE OROPHARYNX

ANATOMICAL LANDMARKS

The oropharynx is continuous with the oral cavity anteriorly, with the nasopharynx superiorly, and with the hypopharynx inferiorly. It includes anteriorly the base of the tongue and circumvillate papillae, laterally the faucial tonsil, fossa, and glossopharyngeal sulcus, and inferiorly the glossoepiglottic fold and vallecula, lingual surface of the epiglottis, and epiglotticopharyngeal folds. The posterolateral wall is largely made up by the posterior tonsillar pillar and a short posterior wall and is related to the C2 and C3 vertebrae. Figure 7.1 shows the important anatomic structures of the oropharynx as seen from a lateral view. The anterior tonsillar pillar separates the oral cavity from the oropharynx, the circumvillate papillae divide the oral tongue and the base of the tongue, and the epiglotticopharyngeal fold is the border between the oropharynx and hypopharynx.

Embryologically, the tonsillar fossae, posterior faucial pillars, base of the tongue, and circumvillate papillae are derived from the oropharyngeal brachial arches, and these structures are innervated by the glossopharyngeal nerve. The retromolar trigone and anterior faucial pillars are embryologically connected to the oral cavity and innervated by the lingual nerve of the mandibular division of the trigeminal nerve.

The palatoglossus and palatopharyngeus are covered by mucosal folds, which form the anterior tonsillar and posterior pillars, respectively. The anterior pillars are inserted into the lateral tongue at the circumvillate papillae and the posterior pillars into the lateral pharynx.[1]

The faucial tonsil is a discrete mass of lymphoid tissue that fills the tonsillar fossae between the anterior and posterior pillars. It is covered by mucous membrane reflected off the pillars. The free surface consists of a large number of narrow ton-

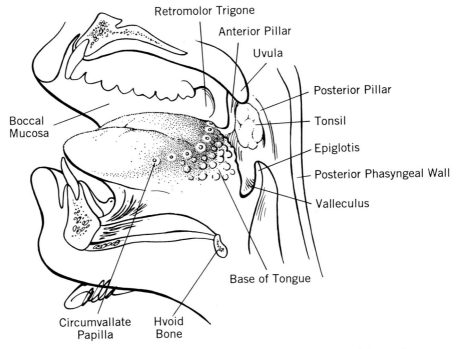

FIGURE 7.1 Diagram showing the important anatomic structures of the oropharynx.

sillar crypts. The deep surface is covered by a fibrous tissue capsule to which some fibers of the palatoglossus and palatopharvngeus are attached.

PARAPHARYNGEAL SPACE

The oropharynx is surrounded by the parapharyngeal space, which is bounded medially by the buccopharyngeal fascia overlying the superior constrictor muscle and laterally by the medial pterygoid muscle. Within this space lie the styloid process and its attached muscles, namely, the stylohyoid, stylopharyngeus, and styloglossus. The last four cranial nerves and the lingual nerve, external and internal carotid arteries, internal jugular vein, superior cervical sympathetic ganglion, and the retropharyngeal nodes including (Rouviere's node) are also found within this space. It is apparent from the anatomical aspect that some of these vital structures may be affected by an advanced tumor of the oropharynx, with manifestation of various signs and symptoms.

Squamous cell carcinomas arising from the tonsillar region tend to spread superiorly to the mucosal surface of the soft palate and infiltrate inferiorly the adjacent base of the tongue and glossopharyngeal sulcus. From the radiotherapeutic standpoint, the superficial components in the soft palate tend to be radioresponsive and curable, while the infiltrative elements in the base of the tongue are less curable

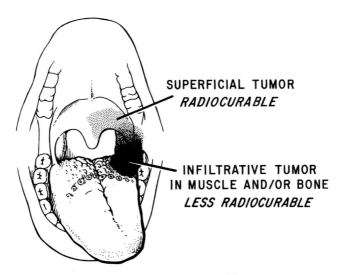

FIGURE 7.2 Diagram showing oropharyngeal tumor with various components of radioresponsiveness and radiocurability.

(Figure 7.2). Because of the various levels of radioresponsiveness, combined radiation and surgery may be beneficial to improve local control. (See Chapter 1 on combined therapies.)

COMMON FEATURES

The AJC staging of carcinoma of the oropharynx is the same as for oral cavity carcinomas, that is, according to tumor size[2]:

T1   Tumor 2 cm or less in greatest dimension
T2   Tumor more than 2 cm but not more than 4 cm in greatest dimension
T3   Tumor more than 4 cm in greatest dimension
T4   Tumor invades adjacent structures (e.g., through cortical bone, soft tissues of neck, deep (extrinsic) muscle of tongue)

SYMPTOMATOLOGY

Early lesions of the oropharynx are remarkably asymptomatic and are rarely recognized. As disease progresses, persistent unilateral sore throat, otalgia, dysphagia, odynophagia, dysarthria with difficulty in speech, and "hot potato" voice may indicate advanced stage and alert patients to seek medical attention. Not infrequently, the disease initially develops as a lump in the neck and is misdiagnosed as a case of "unknown primary."

CLINICAL EVALUATION

The oropharynx is a notoriously difficult area for examination. Many lesions have been overlooked on the part of clinicians who do not have the special skill or interest to exam this area for malignant disease. The faucial tonsil can be seen by direct inspection. The base of the tongue can only be examined by indirect and direct laryngoscopy. The mucosal surface of the tongue base is irregular and lumpy due to the lingual tonsils and it must be evaluated by digital palpation.

Radiographic imaging studies are useful in evaluating the extent of the disease. Lateral radiographs of the neck may show fissure-like defects in the base of the tongue and tumor extension to the nasopharynx, hypopharynx, and larynx. CT or MR scans are extremely informative to assess the primary tumors and the nodal status in the neck as well as for treatment planning purposes. Bone involvement of the base of the skull or the mandible by oropharyngeal carcinoma is unusual but should be looked for.

Pathologically, oropharyngeal carcinomas are generally nonkeratinizing or poorly differentiated squamous cell carcinomas, including a special variant of so-called lymphoepithelioma. Other tumors include adenocarcinoma, salivary gland tumors, and malignant lymphoma.

Oropharyngeal carcinomas are characterized by extensive primary disease and tend to spread extensively along the mucosal surface of the soft palate and lateral

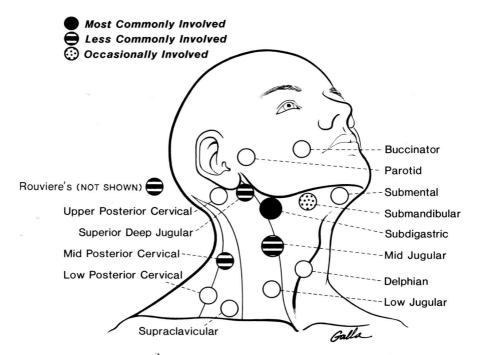

FIGURE 7.3 Diagram showing lymph node involvement in carcinoma of the faucial tonsil.

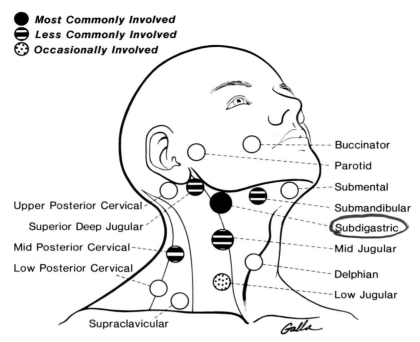

● **Most Commonly Involved**
⊜ **Less Commonly Involved**
⊙ **Occasionally Involved**

Buccinator
Parotid
Submental
Submandibular
Subdigastric
Mid Jugular
Delphian
Low Jugular

Upper Posterior Cervical
Superior Deep Jugular
Mid Posterior Cervical
Low Posterior Cervical

Supraclavicular

Galla

FIGURE 7.4   Diagram showing lymph node involvement in squamous cell carcinoma of the base of the tongue.

pharyngeal wall of the hypopharynx, as well as to the adjacent supraglottic larynx with a high incidence of cervical lymph node metastases[3] (60–75% at presentation). If the midline structures are involved, bilateral lymph node metastases occur, ranging from 20% to 30%. Approximately 50–60% of the clinically N0 necks are associated with occult metastases.

The principal lymph node commonly involved in oropharyngeal carcinoma is the subdigastric node, called the "tonsil" node. For carcinoma situated in the posterior oropharynx, the retropharyngeal nodes (Rouviere's node, the most superior lateral retropharyngeal node at the base of the skull), superior jugular nodes, and posterior cervical nodes are likely to be involved. For carcinoma situated anteriorly in the oropharynx at the base of the tongue, the subdigastric, midjugular, and low cervical nodes are frequently involved, as occasionally are the submandibular and posterior cervical nodes. Figures 7.3 and 7.4 show the principal groups of lymph nodes likely to be involved by carcinoma of the tonsil and base of the tongue, respectively.

TREATMENT OPTIONS

Early lesions may be treated by either surgery or radiation therapy with equally good local control. Primary surgery in the form of local excision, lumpectomy, or tonsillectomy is ineffective for early carcinoma. On the other hand, composite resection for the T1 and T2 lesions may be curative, but the procedure is attended by high functional and cosmetic morbidity and therefore is not a good choice. Since most of the oropharyngeal carcinomas are poorly differentiated and radiosensitive, and in the early stages highly radiocurable, radiation therapy is therefore the preferred treatment for T1 and T2 lesions. The advanced tumors, T3 and T4, are rarely curable by radiation therapy or surgery alone and therefore are better managed by combined therapies,[4,5] that is radical resection and postoperative radiation therapy. Undifferentiated or lymphoepitheliomatous tumors have high radiosensitivity and radiocurability, and surgery for the primary tumor or neck nodes is rarely justified. Massive tumors of the oropharynx, T4, with extensive nodal metastases currently are incurable by any means and are treated by palliative radiation therapy and/or chemotherapy.

RADIATION TECHNIQUES

Radiation therapy for oropharyngeal carcinoma is primarily by external beam radiation with large portals to include comprehensively the primary site and the adjacent structures as well as the regional lymph nodes. Figure 7.5 shows the arrangement of

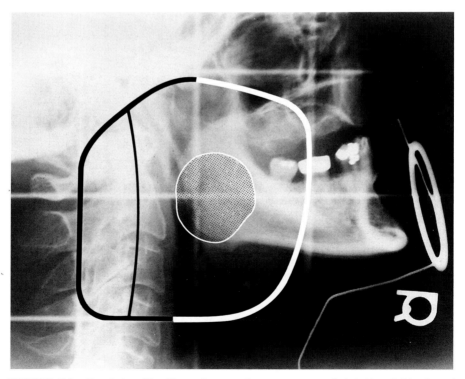

FIGURE 7.5 Simulation film illustrating portal arrangement and shrinking field off cord technique.

the portal for carcinoma of the tonsil. Technically, it is extremely difficult to obtain a satisfactory interstitial implant in lesions situated in the base of the tongue or tonsillar fossa. Likewise, it is difficult to deliver adequate homogeneous boost doses of radiation to these "hard to reach ares through the IOC technique.

A. CARCINOMA OF THE TONSIL

For early carcinoma of the tonsil, T1N0 and T2N0 without involvement of the base of the tongue, the initial dose of 20 Gy in 2 weeks is given as a "mouth bath" through opposing lateral portals to evaluate the extent of tumor in the adjacent soft palate or retromolar trigone by the development of tumoritis. If the lesion remains eccentric, further radiation therapy consisting of 45 Gy is given by ipsilateral–oblique wedge pair technique (Figure 7.6.) An additional boost dose of 6–7 Gy is

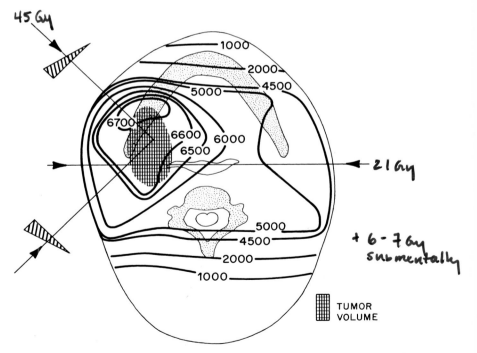

FIGURE 7.6   Composite isodoses for T1N0 carcinoma of the tonsil, using 21 Gy opposing lateral portals and ipsilateral oblique wedge pair technique, for 45 Gy, sparing the contralateral parotid from full dose.

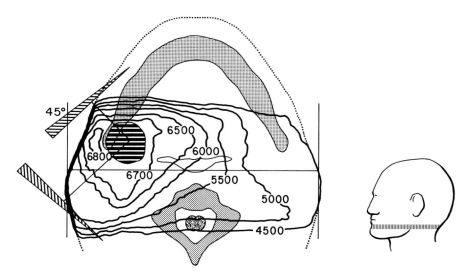

FIGURE 7.7 Composite isodoses for treatment of T3N0 carcinoma of the tonsil using opposing laterals for 45 Gy to be followed by ipsilateral oblique wedge pair technique. The contralateral parotid gland is spared from the full dose, thus xerostomia is lessened.

given through the submental route, bringing the dose to 72 Gy. This will spare the contralateral parotid glands form a full dose and avoid excessive xerostomia. For tumors involving the base of the tongue or soft palate, T3, most of the radiation therapy is given through opposed lateral portals, after the initial radiation therapy of 20 Gy, for approximately 65 Gy. A composite isodose plan is shown in Figure 7.7. An additional 5–10 Gy is given to the epicenter of the lesion through a submental approach. Care must be taken to keep the spinal cord dose within radiation tolerance. For patients with N2–3 disease, the posterior cervical nodes are "boosted" by separate "off cord" portals with low-energy electrons for 4 fractions of perfraction 2.5 Gy. Except for early and superficial T1N0 lesions, all patients with carcinoma of the oropharynx receive ipsilateral or bilateral elective low neck irradiation of 45–50 Gy.

Technical Pointers

1. Patient is to lie supine and be immobilized with a face mask. The anterior border of the lesion is marked by gold seeds. Lymph nodes are outlined by lead wire.
2. The anterior border is set at 2 cm from the seed; the posterior border includes the midspinal processes or vertebrae and the tip of the mastoid. The anterior oral tongue and mandible are shielded by a Cerrobend cutout.
3. The superior border lies 1–1.5 cm above the soft palate.
4. The inferior border lies at the thyroid notch, above the arytenoids, and always includes the entire vallecula as shown in Figure 7.5.

5. The middle ear is shielded but one must ascertain that coverage of the superior jugular nodes (nodes between angle of the jaw and mastoid tip) and posterior cervical nodes is adequate.

6. For boost to residual disease in the base of the tongue or tonsil, use submental photons, thus sparing the mandible, for additional 2.0 Gy × 4 after 64 Gy.

7. Use an accelerated hyperfractionated program to conclude RT with a minimum of 70 Gy in 6 weeks.

RADIOTHERAPEUTIC RESULTS

The results of treatment of carcinoma of the tonsil vary. In general, early carcinoma of the tonsil carries a highly favorable prognosis with local control rate better than 80%.[6-12] When the disease becomes massive, the results are poor, ranging from 15% to 20%. Interstitial brachytherapy boost after external beam radiation therapy did not improve the local control rates; particularly for T3 and T4 lesions.[13] N2a–3 disease may require neck dissection for residual nodes after a full course of radiation therapy. Since 80% of clinical N1 and N2b necks can be controlled by radiation therapy alone, routine elective neck dissection is not warranted.

MGH EXPERIENCE

From 1970 through 1994, a total of 288 patients with squamous cell carcinoma of the faucial tonsil received radiation therapy: 145 patients were treated with QD radiation therapy, 124 patients received BID radiation therapy, and 19 patients had a planned combination of radiation therapy and radical surgery.

Table 7.1 shows the results of radiation therapy for the entire group of 269 patients. For T1 and T2 lesions, the 5-year actuarial local control (LC) rates were 81% and 79%, respectively, and disease-specific survival (DSS) rates were 87% and 75%. For T3 and T4 lesions, the corresponding rates were 60% and 23% for LC and 48% and 22% for DSS.

Table 7.2 shows the LC and DSS rates at the primary sites related to the disease

TABLE 7.1   Five-Year Actuarial LC and DSS for Tonsillar Carcinoma Related to T Stage After Radiation Therapy: 1970–1994

T Stage	n	LC (%)	DSS (%)
T1	27	81	87
T2	111	79	75
T3	103	60	48
T4	28	23	22
		$p = 0.001$	$p = 0.0001$

TABLE 7.2   Five-Year Actuarial LC at the Primary Sites and DSS Rates for Tonsillar Carcinoma Related to N Stage After Radiation Therapy: 1970–1994

N Stage	n	LC (%)	DSS (%)
N0	114	79	76
N1	52	72	64
N2–3	103	49	41
		$p = 0.001$	$p = 0.001$

in the neck. There is no significant difference between the N0 and N1 necks, but the difference between N2–3 necks and N0–1 necks was significant: $p = 0.001$ (see Table 7.3).

Table 7.4 shows the results after QD radiation therapy. For T1–2 lesions, the 5-year actuarial LC and DSS were 75% and 69%, respectively. For T3 and T4 lesions, the corresponding rates were 45% and 17% for LC and 32% and 14% for DSS.

Table 7.5 shows the results after BID radiation therapy. For T1–2 lesions, the 5-year actuarial LC and DSS rates were 86% and 87%, respectively. For T3 and T4 lesions, the corresponding rates were 78% and 39% for LC and 41% and 47% for DSS.

Table 7.6 shows the comparison of BID and QD rates of LC and DSS. For the T2, T1–2, and T3 lesions, the difference is statistically significant. The difference for early T1 and T2 lesions and advanced lesions is not significant.

TABLE 7.3   Comparing LC and DSS Rates Related to Nodal Status

N Status	n	LC (%)	DSS (%)
N0	114	79	76
N1	52	72	64
		$p = 0.20$	$p = 0.14$
N0	114	79	76
N2–3	103	49	41
		$p = 0.002$	$p = 0.0001$
N1	52	72	64
N2–3	103	49	41
		$p = 0.006$	$p = 0006$

TABLE 7.4   Five-Year Actuarial LC and DSS Rates for Tonsillar Carcinoma Related to T Stage After QD Radiation Therapy: 1970–1994

T Stage	n	LC (%)	DSS (%)
T1	13	81	71
T2	66	73	68
T1-2	79	75	69
T3	51	45	32
T4	15	17	14

TABLE 7.5   Five-Year Actuarial LC and DSS Rates for Tonsillar Carcinoma Related to T Stage After BID Radiation Therapy: 1970–1994

T Stage	n	LC (%)	DSS (%)
T1	14	80	100
T2	45	88	83
T1-2	59	86	87
T3	52	78	41
T4	13	39	47

TABLE 7.6   Comparison of BID and QD Radiation Therapy Related to LC and DSS

T Stage	LC (%)	DSS (%)
T1	NS	$p = 0.06$
T2	$p = 0.02$	$p = 0.01$
T1–2	$p = 0.02$	$p = 0.002$
T3	$p = 0.01$	$p = 0.03$
T4	NS	$p = 0.07$

DISCUSSION AND SUMMARY

Squamous cell carcinoma of the tonsil is a fairly common malignant tumor of the head and neck. It should not be confused with squamous cell carcinoma of the retromolar trigone and anterior pillar. The latter would best be grouped with carcinoma of the oral cavity because of their similarity in terms of tumor growth and spread, prognosis, and therapeutic management.[7]

Early carcinoma of the tonsil is highly radiocurable. Of 27 patients with T1 lesion, 111 patients with T2, 103 patients with T3, and 28 patients with T4, the 5-year actuarial local control rates after radiation therapy alone were 81%, 79%, 60%, and 23%, respectively. The presence of early nodal disease (N1) did not affect survival—a typical feature of carcinoma of the oropharynx as compared to carcinomas of the oral cavity. The lymph node disease can be sterilized by radiation therapy with a high degree of success. Of 65 patients with T1–3N0, surviving after radiation therapy alone, only 3 or 5% required radical neck dissection. For patients dying of their disease, only 9% were due to failure in the neck alone. Most of the radiation failures were due to inability to control the primary sites with or without neck disease, particularly, the T3 and T4 lesions. Distant metastases alone occurred in 12 patients or 7% who died of the disease.

A planned combination of radiation therapy and surgery plays an important role in the treatment of advanced T3 and T4 lesions. Our past experience, however, was limited. With the advent of techniques of reconstructive surgery, more patients are subjected to radical resection first followed by high-dose postoperative radiation therapy (55–60 Gy) without significant complications. Massive disease, often associated with nodal metastases, is unlikely curable by either radiation therapy or surgery, and perhaps a combination of chemotherapy and radiation therapy may offer some palliation.

B. CARCINOMA OF THE BASE OF THE TONGUE

Squamous cell carcinoma arising from the base of the tongue is approximately one-fourth as common as in the oral tongue. The base of the tongue is supplied with rich lymphatics with multiple lymphatic crossings and three out of four patients when first seen have cervical lymph node metastases and of these one-third to one-half have bilateral cervical involvement. For a clinically negative neck (N0), 10–20% will have histologically occult metastasic disease.

RADIOTHERAPEUTIC MANAGEMENT

Radiation therapy for carcinoma of the tongue base must be comprehensive in nature. Generally, opposing lateral portals with equal loading are used for a tumor dose of 65 Gy with added submental boost dose of 7–8 Gy, as shown in Figure 7.8. The lower neck areas are irradiated electively for 50 Gy for microscopic disease. Gross disease is boosted for an additional 5–10 Gy. The spinal cord dose is limited to 45 Gy.

Technical Pointers

1. Patient is to lie supine, with chin hyperextended and immobilized with a face mask. Neck nodes are outlined by lead wire.
2. The anterior margin of the palpable lesion is outlined by gold seeds if possible. The base of the tongue lies vertically in the lateral projection.
3. The superior border of the portal is set below the auditory meatus and 1.5 cm above the dorsum of the tongue.
4. The anterior border is extended at least 2 cm anterior to the tumor or 2 cm anterior to the RMT.
5. The posterior border is at the spinous pedicles. The superior border includes the superior deep jugular nodes and nodes between the angle of the jaw and mastoid tip.
6. The inferior portal is at the thyroid notch, above the arytenoids, with full coverage of the vallecula, or 2–3 cm below the hyoid bone.
7. Boost radiation therapy to the primary site, sparing the mandible, is by submental photons after 64 Gy, to a total dose of 70–72 Gy in 6 weeks.
8. Use an accelerated hyperfractionated program.

RADIOTHERAPEUTIC RESULTS

The results of treatment of carcinoma of the base of the tongue by either radiation therapy or surgery generally were considered to be unsatisfactory. Most reported series often consisted of extensive T3 and T4 lesions with reputed poor local con-

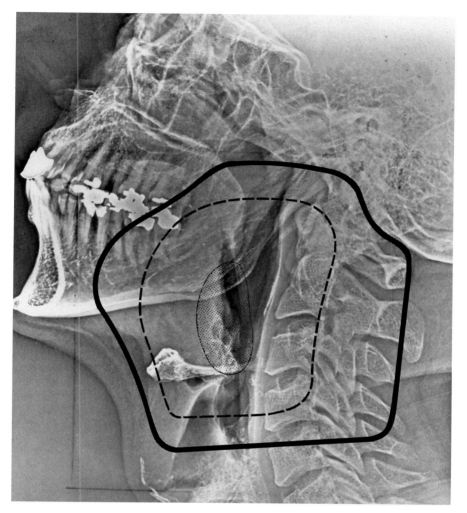

FIGURE 7.8   Radiograph showing radiation therapy portal arrangement for carcinoma of the base of the tongue.

trol and survival rates. Interstitial implant was used to boost the dose to the tumors but has not been found to be essential.[13] Whicker et al.[14] reported 57% NED (no evidence of disease) in 102 patients after surgery. Dalley[15] indicated that 12% of 102 patients were NED at 5 years, and 28% of 28 patients without node involvement were NED. The recent series of Spanos et al.[16] shows NED rate of 91% for T1, 71% for T2, and 78% for T3 after radiation therapy at 2 years. It is apparent that control of the small T1–2 lesions of the tongue can be achieved satisfactorily. Similarly, good local control resulted after hyperefractonated radiation therapy.[12]

MGH EXPERIENCE

From 1970 to 1994, a total of 224 patients with squamous cell carcinoma of the base of tongue received radiation therapy. Of these, 105 patients received once-daily radiation therapy and 119 received twice-daily RT. The 5-year actuarial local control (LC) and disease-specific survival rates (DSS) are shown in Tables 7.7 through 7.11.

Table 7.7 shows the LC and DSS rates for the entire group. For T1 and T2 lesions, the rates were 89% and 79% for LC and 78% and 76% for DSS, respectively. For T3 and T4 lesions, the corresponding rates were 48% and 21% for LC and 40% and 16% for DSS. The numbers were statistically significant with $p = 0.0001$.

Results after QD and BID radiation therapy are shown in Tables 7.8 and 7.9. The local control rates after QD and BID radiation therapy were high, with no significant difference in T1 and T2 lesions.

There is a statistical difference in the T3 and T4 lesions in favor of the BID group as shown in Table 7.10.

TABLE 7.7   Five-Year Actuarial LC and DSS Rates for Carcinoma of the Base of the Tongue Related to T Stage After Radiation Therapy: 1970–1994

Stage	n	LC (%)	DSS (%)
T1	40	89	78
T2	69	79	76
T3	78	48	40
T4	37	21	16
T3–4	115	39	32
		$p = 0.0001$	$p = 0.0001$
N0	75	71	67
N1	42	55	56
N2–3	107	55	42
		$p = 0.16$	$p = 0002$

TABLE 7.8   Five-Year Actuarial LC and DSS Rates for Carcinoma of the Base of the Tongue After QD Radiation Therapy: 1970–1994

T Stage	n	LC (%)	DSS (%)
T1	17	87	70
T2	33	74	70
T1–2	50	78	58
T3	32	28	19
T4	23	17	14

TABLE 7.9   Five-Year Actuarial LC and DSS Rates for Carcinoma of the Base of the Tongue After BID Radiation Therapy: 1970–1994

T Stage	n	LC (%)	DSS (%)
T1	23	90	87
T2	36	84	85
T1–2	59	87	85
T3	46	64	55
T4	14	28	16

TABLE 7.10   Comparison BID versus QD Related to LC and DSS Rates

T Stage	LC	DSS
T1	NS	NS
T2	NS	NS
T1–2	NS	NS
T3	$p = 0.0003$	$p = 0.004$
T4	$p = 0.0002$	$p = 0.005$

TABLE 7.11   Five-Year Actuarial LC and DSS Rates for Carcinoma of the Base of the Tongue related to N Stage After Radiation Therapy: 1970–1994

N Stage	n	LC (%)	DSS (%)
N0	75	71	67
N1	42	55	56
		$p = 0.24$	$p = 0.77$
N0	75	71	67
N2–3	107	55	42
		$p = 0.6$	$p = 0.0005$
N1	42	55	56
N2–3	107	55	42
		$p = 0.57$	$p = 0.007$

Lymph node metastases in the neck did not affect the local control of the primary lesions but influenced the disease-specific survival (DSS), as shown in Table 7.11. For patients with N0 and N1 necks, the DSS rates were 67% and 56%, $p = 0.77$. For patients with N2–3 disease, the rates of DSS were markedly decreased as compared to patients with N0–1 necks, $p = 0.0001$.

DISCUSSION AND SUMMARY

Squamous cell carcinoma of the base of the tongue is not accessible for casual clinical examination and tends to be advanced when the diagnosis is initially made. Traditionally, the prognosis of this disease is known to be notoriously poor after either radiation therapy or surgery. Primary surgery is rarely successful for this disease due to the extensive primary lesions and high incidence of marginal recurrence and nodal metastases, often bilateral. For early tumors, T1−2, the treatment of choice is radical comprehensive radiation therapy with surgery being reserved for salvage. For extensive disease, T3−4N2−3, multicycle chemotherapy may be used first, to be followed by radiation therapy and limited surgery.

Our experience, however, indicates that, stage for stage, the therapeutic results for carcinoma arising form the base of the tongue are favorably comparable to that of carcinoma of the oral tongue. Since a large group of patients can still be salvaged by carefully planned radiation therapy programs, a pessimistic approach to this disease is not justified.

REFERENCES

1. Paff GH: *Anatomy of the head and neck.* Philadelphia: Saunders 1973.
2. American Joint Committee on Cancer: *A manual for staging of cancer*, 4th ed. Philadelphia: Lippincott, 1992.
3. Perez CA, Mills WB, Ogura JH, et al: Carcinoma of the tonsil: sequential comparison of four treatment modalities. *Radiology* 1970;94:649−659.
4. Maltz R, Shumrick DA, Aron BS, et al: Carcinoma of the tonsil: results of combined therapy. *Laryngoscope* 1974;84:2172−2180.
5. Rolandier LL, Everts EC, Shumrick DA: Carcinoma of the tonsils: a planned combined therapy approach. *Laryngoscipe* 1971;81:1199.
6. Weller SA, Goffinet DR, Goode RL, et al: Carcinoma of the oropharynx: results of megavoltage radiation therapy in 305 patients. *Am J Roentgenol Radium Ther Nucl Med* 1976;126:236−247.
7. Wang CC: Management and prognosis of squamous cell carcinoma of the tonsillar region. *Radiology* 1972;104:667−671.
8. Shukovsky LJ, Fletcher GH: Time−dose and tumor volume relationships in the irradiation of squamous cell carcinoma of the tonsillar fossa. *Radiology* 1973;107:621−626.
9. Mendenhall WM, Parsons JT, Cassisi NJ, Million RR: Squamous cell carcinoma of the tonsillar area treated with radical irradiation. *Radiother Oncol* 1987;10:23−30.
10. Strong EW: Carcinoma of the tongue. *Otolaryngol Clin North AM* 1979;12:107−114.
11. Wong CS, Ang KK, Fletcher GH, Thames HD, Peters LJ, Byers RM, Oswald MJ: Definitive radiotherapy for squamous cell carcinoma of the tonsillar fossa. *Int I Radiat Oncol Biol Phys* 1989;16:657−662.
12. Wang CC, Montgomery W, Efird J: Local control of oropharyngeal carcinoma by irradiation alone. *Laryngoscope* 1995;105(5):529−533.
13. Foote RL, Parsons JT, Mendenhall WW, et al: Is interstitial implantation essential for

successful radiotherapeutic treatment of base of tongue carcinoma? *Int J Radiat Oncol Biol Phys* 1990;18:1293–1298.

14. Whicker JH, DeSanto IW, Devine KD: Surgical treatment of squamous cell carcinoma of the base of the tongue. *Laryngoscope* 1972;82:1853–1860.

15. Dalley VM. Cancer of the laryngopharynx. *J Laryngol Otol* 1968;82:407–419.

16. Spanos WT, Shukovsky LJ, Fletcher GH: Time, dose and tumor volume relationships in irradiation of squamous cell carcinomas of the base of the tongue. *Cancer* 1976;37:2591–2599.

CHAPTER 8

CARCINOMA OF THE HYPOPHARYNX

The hypopharynx is contiguous with the oropharynx superiorly and extends from the level of the hyoid bone and the epiglotticopharyngeal fold inferiorly to the cricoid cartilage and the esophageal introitus. It envelops the larynx and can be divided into three anatomic sites — the pyriform sinus, the posterior pharyngeal wall, and the postcricoid region. The pyriform sinus is bounded superiorly by the epiglotticopharyngeal fold and has three walls — anterior, lateral, and medial. The anterolateral wall is bounded by the thyroid cartilage and the thyrohyoid membrane; the posteromedial wall is bounded by the lateral surface of the arytenoid cartilage, quadrangular membrane, and aryepiglottic fold. The apex of the pyriform sinus extends slightly below the cricoid cartilage and usually extends below the level of the true vocal cords and corresponds approximately to the 6th cervical vertebra. The posterior pharyngeal wall extends from the level of the hyoid bone superiorly to the cricopharyngeal muscle inferiorly. It extends laterally to the posterior margins of the pyriform sinus. The postcricoid region is at the entrance to the cervical esophagus within the confines of the intraluminal projections of the cricopharyngeal muscle and the posterior lamina of the cricoid cartilage. Figure 8.1 shows the important anatomic structures of the hypopharynx. It is the junctional zone. There are no barriers to the spread of cancer from one anatomic site to another and the tumor often overlaps various sites. Squamous cell carcinomas arising from these sites are mostly moderately to poorly differentiated carcinomas. They tend to infiltrate the adjacent structures with involvement of the underlying cartilage and musculature with poorly defined borders. Owing to the extensive network of lymphatics in the area and the lack of severe symptoms, tumors arising from the hypopharynx tend to have extensive cervical lymph node metastases, often bilateral.[1] Occult metastases are present in approximately 50–80% of hypopharyngeal carcinoma.

The principal nodes of involvement are the subdigastric, superior deep jugular, and

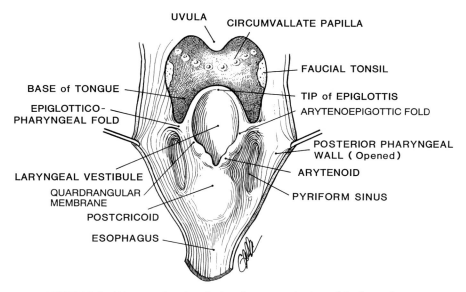

FIGURE 8.1 Diagram showing the interior anatomic sites of the hypopharynx.

midjugular nodes. Significant lymphatic drainage from the posterior pharyngeal wall communicates with the retropharyngeal nodes and Rouviere's node at the base of the skull.[2,3] Figures 8.2 and 8.3 show the principal group of lymph nodes likely to be involved by carcinoma of the pyriform sinus and posterior pharyngeal wall, respectively. The lymphatic vessels of the inferior portion of the pyriform sinus and the postcricoid drain to the inferior jugular and the paratracheal nodes. The upper portion of the pyriform sinus follows the pattern of spread as supraglottic carcinoma. Involvement of the nodes in the posterior cervical triangle is uncommon in hypopharyngeal carcinoma.[4]

The ominous premalignant "field change" seen elsewhere in the oral cavity is also significantly associated with carcinoma of the hypopharynx. Approximately 15–20% of patients have a second primary neoplasm, either concurrently or sequentially, the most frequent areas of involvement being in the upper aerodigestive tracts.

The symptoms of hypopharyngeal carcinoma consist of sore throat, dysphagia, odynophagia, and ipsilateral otalgia. Dysphagia is more common in patients with postcricoid and cervical esophageal carcinoma. When carcinoma of the pyriform sinus becomes extensive, symptoms are hoarseness, laryngeal stridor, and hemoptysis. Gross tumor in the upper pyriform sinus and posterior pharyngeal wall can easily be seen during indirect laryngoscopic examination. Indirect signs of tumor of the pyriform sinus are obliteration of the apex, arytenoidal edema, or pooling of secretions in the area of the pyriform sinus with or without fixation of the vocal cords. These may be the only clues to its presence. Postcricoid lesions may present edema and erythema of the arytenoid, loss of laryngeal crepitus, and, in the advanced stage, fixation of the hemilarynx.

The majority of hypopharyngeal tumors, 60–70%, arise from the pyriform si-

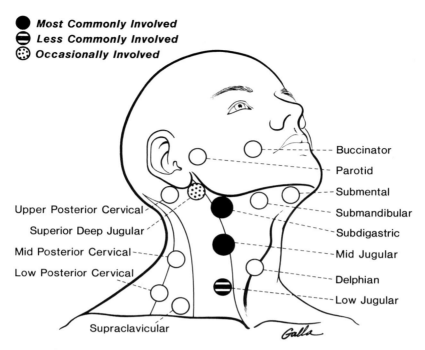

FIGURE 8.2 Diagram showing lymph node involvement in carcinoma of the pyriform sinus.

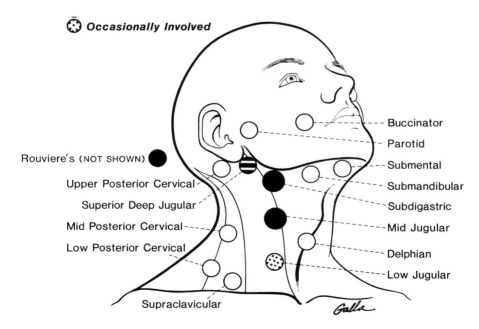

FIGURE 8.3 Diagram showing lymph node involvement in carcinoma of the posterior pharyngeal wall.

nus, and approximately 25–30% from the posterior pharyngeal wall. The post-cricoid tumors are the least common, approximately 5%, and in fact represent lesions of the upper cervical esophagus. Evaluation of the extent of the lesion calls for careful inspection of the hypopharynx by indirect and direct laryngoscopy and digital palpation of the lesion. Radiologic examinations, including plain film, contrast studies (Figure 8.4), polytomes (Figure 8.5), CT and/or MR scans, often yield

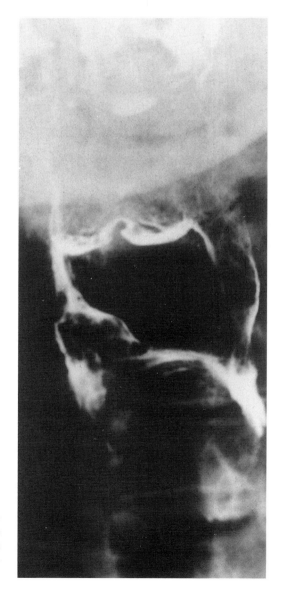

FIGURE 8.4   Radiograph with barium swallow shows a tumor in the right pyriform sinus, a filling defect indenting the adjacent contrast substance.

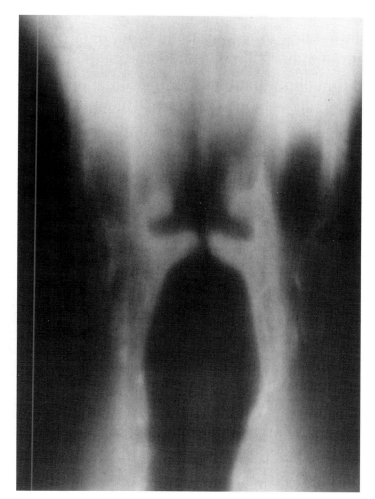

FIGURE 8.5   Anteroposterior tomogram showing obliteration of the air density in the right pyriform sinus, consistant with the barium image in Figure 8.4.

invaluable information as to the extent of the disease, particularly in lesions of the posterior pharyngeal wall and carcinomas of the pyriform sinus for parapharyngeal or subglottic extension. The mobility of the laryngeal structures and the pliability of the lateral pharyngeal walls likewise can be studied by appropriate radiological examinations.

The American Joint Committee system for hypopharyngeal carcinoma is defined by tumor extension to the adjacent sites and the status of mobility of the larynx, if involved, and is as follows[5]:

T1   Tumor limited to one subsite of hypopharynx

T2   Tumor invades more than one subsite of hypopharynx or an adjacent site, without fixation of hemilarynx

T3   Tumor invades more than one subsite of hypopharynx or an adjacent site, with fixation of hemilarynx

T4   Tumor invades adjacent structures (e.g., cartilage or soft tissues of neck)

Treatment of this group of tumors, either by surgery or radiation therapy, is unsatisfactory due to uncontrolled disease at the primary site and/or cervical lymph node metastases.[6-8] For advanced carcinoma, combined surgery and radiation therapy has been carried out with improved results.[9-11]

A. CARCINOMA OF THE PYRIFORM SINUS

These tumors are often extensive and frequently associated with cervical lymph node metastases. Approximately 70% of the patients have metastases to cervical nodes and two-thirds are palpable at presentation. The lymphatic drainage from the apex of the pyriform sinus enters the deep cervical lymphatics and the subdigastric and midjugular nodes. Of those with nodal disease, 10–20% show bilateral involvement. More than half of the patients, when first seen, present with T3 and T4 disease. Carcinomas arising from various portions of the pyriform sinus behave differently and therefore the management and therapeutic results may vary.[12]

Tumors originating from the apex of the pyriform sinus tend to be aggressive, infiltrative, and extensive, and the true tumor extent could be deceiving since iceberg presentation of the lesion often involves the adjacent cartilage, larynx, and upper trachea. To the contrary, lesions arising from the upper membranous lateral walls of the pyriform sinus tend to be less aggressive and exophytic with lesser incidence of node involvement.

SELECTION OF THERAPY

For T1–2N0 exophytic carcinomas arising from the membranous portion of the pyriform sinus, radiation therapy may be tried as a curative procedure and surgery is reserved for salvage. For extensive T3–4 lesions, particularly those arising from the apex of the pyriform sinus with node involvement, if operable, a combination of surgery and radiation therapy is preferred.

RADIOTHERAPEUTIC MANAGEMENT

Anatomically, the apex of the pyriform sinus lies below the level of the true vocal cords. Radiation therapy of carcinoma of the pyriform sinus therefore requires a large portal, including the primary site as well as the superior and midjugular and Rouviere's nodes, as shown in Figure 8.6. A total dose of 70–72 Gy in 7 weeks is given as a curative procedure. For postoperative radiation therapy, a dose of 50–55 Gy is planned to the neck and stoma following laryngopharyngectomy and recon-

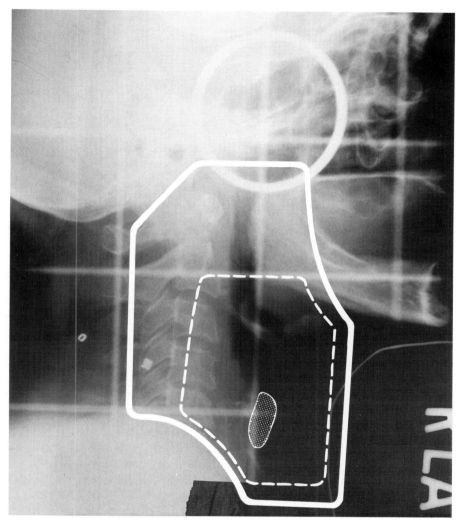

FIGURE 8.6   Simulation film showing radiation therapy portal arrangement for carcinoma of the pyriform sinus.

struction. Frequently, additional radiation therapy is given to the tracheal stoma using low-energy electrons as a boost, if the tumor is found to extend too close to the resection margins.

Technical Pointers

1. Patient is to lie supine and be immobilized with a face mask.
2. Use large portals with the superior border at the mastoid process, the inferior border including the subglottis and cricoid cartilage, and the posterior border including the spinous pedicles.

3. For N2–3 disease, the nodes outside the off-cord field are boosted with electrons to 60 Gy. For the N0 neck, electron boost to the posterior triangle is unnecessary.
4. Radical neck dissection is planned for any residual nodal disease.

RADIOTHERAPEUTIC RESULTS

Squamous cell carcinoma of the pyriform sinus is not reliably curable by radiation therapy alone except for exophytic T1–2 lesions arising from the membranous portion of the pyriform sinus. The 3-year local control rate after radiation therapy is approximately 20%.[7,9,13,14] Combined radiation therapy and surgery[11,15,16] has improved the rates to more than double in the T3 group and triple in lesions with metastatic nodes. The majority of therapeutic failures are due to uncontrolled nodal disease in the neck, recurrence in the base of the tongue or tracheal stoma, or tumor extension into the cervical esophagus or into the base of the skull. A small number of patients die with distant metastases.

MGH EXPERIENCE

From 1970 through 1994, a total of 186 patients with carcinoma of the pyriform sinus were treated by radiation therapy (RT) at the MGH. Of the entire group, T1–4, more than half of the patients presented with nodal metastases at diagnosis. The 5-year actuarial local control (LC) and disease-specific survival (DSS) rates are shown in Table 8.1.

For T1 and T2 lesions, the LC and DSS rates were 74% and 76%, respectively, and the DSS rates were 73% and 68%. For patients with T3–4 tumors, the corresponding rates were 32% and 28%.

From 1979 to 1994, 97 patients received BID radiation therapy; the LC and DSS rates were 74% and 71% for the T1–2 lesions. For 23 patients also with T1–2 lesions who received QD radiation therapy, the LC and DSS rates were 76% and 72%, respectively. When comparing LC rates for patients undergoing BID versus

TABLE 8.1   Five-Year Actuarial LC and DSS Rates After RT for Pyriform Sinus Carcinoma: 1970–1994

Stage	n	LC (%)	DSS (%)
T1	24	74	73
T2	51	76	68
T3–4	89	32	28
		$p = 0.0001$	$p = 0.0001$
N0	63	65	68
N1	32	46	41
N2–3	69	39	28
		$p = 0.04$	$p = 0.0001$

**TABLE 8.2   Five-Year Actuarial LC and DSS Rates
for Carcinoma of the Pyriform Sinus After BID and
QD RT: 1970–1994**

	n	LC (%)	DSS (%)
T1–2			
BID	52	74	71
QD	23	76	72
		$p = 0.85$	$p = 0.67$
T3–4			
BID	45	51	44
QD	44	17	15
		$p = 0.05$	$p = 0.09$

QD radiation therapy (RT). For advanced lesions, T3–4, the LC and DSS rates were significantly higher after BID programs ($p=0.05$), as shown in Table 8.2.

TREATMENT OF CARCINOMA OF THE PYRIFORM SINUS BY PLANNED COMBINED SURGERY AND RADIATION THERAPY

Seventy-five patients with carcinoma of the pyriform sinus were treated by planned combined therapies. For T1 and T2 lesions, the local control at the primary sites and DSS rates were 84% and 34%. For advanced tumors, T3–T4, the corresponding rates were 42% and 37% respectively. The difference is significant $p=0.005$.

For patients with N0 necks, the LC and DSS rates were 63% and 53% and for N1 and N2–3 disease the corresponding rates were 69% and 24% for local control, and 60% and 13% for DSS respectively, as shown in Table 8.3.

**TABLE 8.3   Five-Year Actuarial LC and DSS Rates
for Carcinoma of the Pyriform Sinus After Combined
Surgery and RT: 1970–1994**

Stage	n	LC (%)	DSS (%)
T1	3	100	67
T2	11	80	34
T1–2	14	84	34
T3–4	61	42	37
		$p = 0.005$	$p = 0.15$
N0	20	63	53
N1	18	69	60
N2–3	37	24	13
		$p = 0.04$	$p = 0.01$

B. CARCINOMA OF THE POSTERIOR PHARYNGEAL WALL

Carcinoma of the posterior pharyngeal wall is a less common tumor. The common symptoms are sore throat, dysphagia with foreign body sensation, and odynophagia. Occasionally, hemoptysis and ipsilateral otalgia are experienced by patients. Most of the lesions are quite large and exophytic and may extend laterally to involve the lateral pharyngeal wall, superiorly to the oropharynx, and inferiorly to the cervical esophagus. The prevertebral fascia hinders tumor extension posteriorly and therefore the vertebral bodies are involved only in the late stage of the disease. Approximately one or two patients, when first seen, present with cervical lymph node metastases and these are often bilateral. The involvement of the retropharyngeal nodes is rarely recognized clinically, except in the far advanced condition, but has been recognized more frequently by CT imaging studies.[17] Its incidence in patients is reported as high as 44%.[2,3] Therefore radiographs of the lateral pharynx, CT and MR scans of the neck and base of the skull, and a barium swallow are valuable investigative procedures to evaluate the extent of the primary lesions as well as the metastatic nodes.

SELECTION OF THERAPY

Because of the close proximity of the primary lesion to the adjacent fascia and muscles, surgical resection frequently is associated with local recurrence due to microscopic disease at resection margins. Therefore, like carcinoma of the nasopharynx, carcinoma of the posterior pharyngeal wall is rarely considered resectable and is best treated by radiation therapy.[16,18] Neck dissection is used for residual nodes postradiation. Extensive and massive T3–4 tumors currently are treated by combined therapies consisting of chemotherapy, surgery, and adjuvant postoperative radiation therapy. Surgery consists of laryngopharyngo-esophagectomy followed by reconstruction, and, in spite of such radical attempts, the rates for permanent cure are still poor, being in the neighborhood of one in four at 5 years.

RADIOTHERAPEUTIC MANAGEMENT

Because of the axial submucosal spread of the lesion along the prevertebral fascia, and the high likelihood of retropharyngeal lymph node metastases, radiation therapy calls for large portals, including the entire pharynx up to the base of the skull and upper cervical esophagus, to include the superior deep jugular nodes and Rouviere's node. The mid- and low jugular nodes are also irradiated. After 45 Gy, the portals are usually reduced to a long rectangular field, sparing the spinal cord, to boost the primary site for an additional 25 Gy, as shown in Figure 8.7. Because of the close proximity of the spinal cord to the tumor, care must be exercised not to exceed the tolerance of the spinal cord. In these circumstances, a "sharp edge" beam with small penumbra, that is, 4–6 MeV photons from an accelerator, is

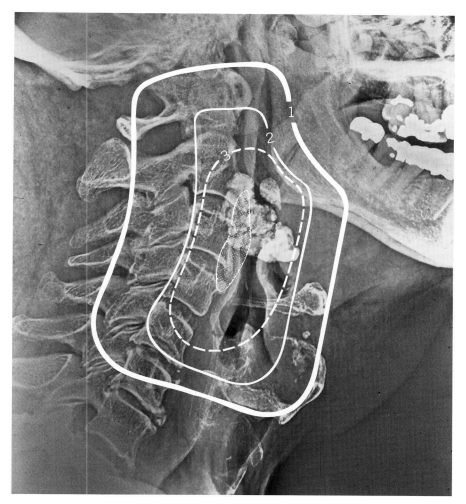

FIGURE 8.7   Radiograph showing placement of radiation therapy portal for carcinoma of the posterior pharyngeal wall with multiple shrinking fields: (1) comprehensive, (2) intermediate off-cord, and (3) final boost. (Position of calcified subdigastric node is seen.)

highly desirable. The posterior pharynx is a very radiosensitive structure and severe mucositis generally develops early with pain, dysphagia, and odynophagia interfering with the patient's nutrition. Close follow-up and monitoring of the patient's nutritional status are required during the entire course of radiation therapy.

Technical Pointers

1. Use a large rectangular portal to include the entire posterior pharynx.
2. The superior border is at the skull base or C1 vertebra.

3. The inferior border is 1 cm below the thyroid prominence.
4. The anterior border needs no fall-off approximately 1 cm posterior to the anterior skin.
5. The posterior border is at the spinous pedicles.
6. Use high-energy photons (i.e., 4×) to boost the primary site, including the entire width of the cervical vertebrae and the gross tumor.

RADIOTHERAPEUTIC RESULTS

The results following treatment of posterior pharyngeal carcinoma generally are poor. The reported 3-year determinate rates ranged from 15% to 30% by radiation therapy alone. For early T1 and T2 lesions, the radiotherapeutic results are approximately 50%.[18-20] Advanced tumors carry an approximately 10% cure rate after radiation therapy. Patients without node involvement generally do better than patients with nodal disease. Far advanced lesions and/or massive bilateral cervical metastases are rarely curable by radiation therapy or surgery and currently are treated for palliation.

MGH EXPERIENCE

From 1970 to 1994, 135 patients with carcinoma of the posterior pharyngeal wall were treated at the MGH. The local control (LC) and disease-specific survival (DSS) rates are shown in Table 8.4.

The local control rates of T1 and T2 lesions were 88% and 55% and the DSS rates were 83% and 57%. For advanced tumors, T3−4, the LC and DSS rates were 49% and 42%. The differences among various groups were significant, $p=0.03$. For patients without node involvement, the local control at the primary sites was 67% as compared to patients with node involvement, which was about 30−50%. The DSS rates likewise were inferior in patients with cervical metastases.

TABLE 8.4   Five-Year Actuarial LC and DSS Rates for Carcinoma of the Posterior Pharyngeal Wall After RT: 1970–1994

Stage	n	LC (%)	DSS (%)
T1	18	88	83
T2	46	55	57
T3−4	41	49	42
		$p=0.03$	$p=0.03$
N0	69	67%	66%
N1	17	31%	39%
N2−3	19	52%	46%
		$p=0.019$	$p=0.03$

TABLE 8.5 Five-Year Actuarial LC and DSS Rates for Carcinoma of the Posterior Pharyngeal Wall After BID and QD RT: 1970–1994

	n	LC (%)	DSS (%)
T1–2			
BID	37	74%	71%
QD	27	55%	60%
		$p = 0.08$	$p = 0.53$
T3–4			
BID	19	70%	53%
QD	22	33%	35%
		$p = 0.01$	$p = 0.16$
Total			
BID	56	72%	64%
QD	49	45%	49%
		$p = 0.0\,1$	$p = 0.13$

From 1979 to 1994, 56 patients received BID radiation therapy and the local control rates were 74% for T1–2 lesions and 70% for T3–4 lesions. For patients treated by QD programs, the rates were 55% for T1–2 and 33% for T3–4 lesions. The BID rates were significantly higher than the QD rates with $p=0.01$ for advanced tumors and $p=0.08$ for early lesions, as shown in Table 8.5.

Carcinoma of the posterior wall is rarely considered operable at the MGH and MEEI. Therefore the number of patients treated by combined surgery and radiation therapy is infinitely small. No meaningful data are available.

C. POSTCRICOID CARCINOMA

Squamous cell carcinomas of the postcricoid area are usually well differentiated and are considered to represent iceberg presentation of carcinoma of the upper cervical esophagus.[13,21,22] They are uncommon in the United States. These lesions infiltrate insidiously through the anterior wall of the esophagus and in late stages may become annular and descend into the esophagus proper. The larynx and trachea are displaced forward. Lateral radiographs of the neck and a barium swallow demonstrate a soft tissue mass of the cervical esophagus arising from the anterior wall, confirming the diagnosis (Figure 8.8).

Although surgical resection consisting of laryngopharyngo-esophagectomy and plastic closure is often considered the preferred procedure, the overall control rates of the disease remain dismal, with 5-year survival rates of approximately 10–20%.[21,22] Many of the failures are due to spread of disease beyond the scope of surgical resection.

The experience for treatment of these lesions with primary radiation therapy is

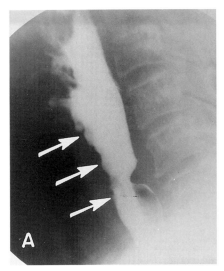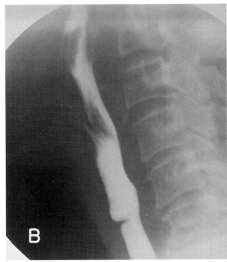

FIGURE 8.8 Radiograph with barium swallow showing typical appearance of post cricoid carcinoma. (a) Pretreatment appearance showing an irregular tumor involving the anterior wall of the cervical esophagus. (b) Post-treatment appearance—5 years after BID radiation therapy; patient is NED.

limited. The experience at Edinburgh[23] showed improved local control and survival after radical radiation therapy with a 5-year NED rate of 35%. These results, however, have not been duplicated elsewhere.

Our experience with squamous cell carcinomas of the postcricoid area was scarce. Only 17 patients received radiation therapy, and of these three (18%) were NED at 24 months. Seven patients had combined preoperative radiation therapy and resection and none survived at 24 months.

SUMMARY

Carcinoma of the hypopharynx is a silent disease, and the tumors frequently are advanced and bulky, with extensive lymph node metastases. Carcinoma of the pyriform sinus has various biologic behavior in regard to the location of the tumor. For early T1–2 lesions arising from the membranous portion of the pyriform sinus, a trial course of high-dose radiation therapy is worthwhile, with surgery being reserved for salvage. For lesions arising from the apex of the pyriform sinus or large, bulky tumors, the local control rates after QD radiation therapy are low and a planned combination as radiation therapy and surgery therefore had been used conventionally.

For early (T1–2) posterior pharyngeal wall lesions, radiation therapy is the reasonable treatment modality with one-third being salvaged. For those without node involvement, approximately two-thirds are expected to do well. Far-advanced lesions with extensive nodal disease currently are rarely curable by radiation therapy, and perhaps combined therapies including chemotherapy, radical surgery, and postoperative radiation therapy, at the expense of functional and anatomic mutilation, may offer a glimpse of hope of improved results.

Postcricoid carcinoma is a rare disease. No meaningful data are available. Treatment by a combination of radiation therapy and surgery is advocated although the therapeutic results have been dismal.

The results of treatment of carcinoma of the hypopharynx remain a challenge to radiation oncologists and head and neck surgeons. Our data thus far indicate that local control rates of this disease after BID radiation therapy are somewhat higher as compared to previous QD radiation therapy experience, but the p values have not reached statistical significance though the trend suggests some improvement. Because of these findings, all patients with this disease are currently managed by accelerated hyperfractionation radiation therapy in our institution with some improvement.

REFERENCES

1. Lindberg R: Distribution of cervical lymph node metastases from squamous cell carcinoma of the upper respiratory and digestive tracts. *Cancer* 1972;29:1446–1449.

2. Ballantyne AJ: Significance of retropharyngeal nodes in cancer of the head and neck. *Am J Surg* 1964;108:500.

3. Guillamondegui OM, Meoz R, Jesse RH: Surgical treatment of squamous cell carcinoma of the pharyngeal walls. *Am J Surg* 1978;136:474–476.

4. Byers RM, Wolf PF, Ballantyne AJ: Rationale for elective modified neck dissection. *Head Neck Surg* 1988;10:160–167.

5. American Joint Committee on Cancer: *A manual for staging of cancer*, 4th ed. Philadelphia: Lippincott, 1992.

6. Carpenter RJ III, DeSanto LW: Cancer of the hypopharynx. *Surg Clin North Am* 1977; 57:723–735.

7. McGavran MH, Bauer WC, Spjut HJ, et al: Carcinoma of the pyriform sinus: the results of radical surgery. *Arch Otolaryngol* 1963;78:826.

8. Shah JP, Shaha AR, Spiro RH, et al: Carcinoma of the hypopharynx. *Am J Surg* 1976; 132:439–443.

9. Byers RM, Krueger WW, Saxton J: Use of surgery and postoperative radiation in the treatment of advanced squamous cell carcinoma of the pyriform sinus. *Am J Surg* 1979;138:597–599.

10. Vandenbrouck C, Sancho H, LeFur R, et al: Results of a randomized clinical trial of preoperative irradiation versus postoperative in treatment of tumors of the hypopharynx. *Cancer* 1977;39:1445–1449.

11. Wang CC, Schulz MD, Miller D: Combined radiation therapy and surgery for carcinoma of the supraglottis and pyriform sinus. *Laryngoscope* 1970;82:1883–1890.

12. Inoue T, Shigematsu Y: Hypopharyngeal carcinoma. Long-term survivors following radical radiation therapy. *Acta Radiol Ther* (*Stockh*) 1976;15:201–208.

13. Dalley VM: Cancer of the laryngopharynx. *J Laryngol Otol* 1968;82:407–419.

14. Kirchner JA: Pyriform sinus cancer: a clinical and laboratory study. *Ann Otol Rhinol Laryngol* 1975;84:793–803.

15. Ballantyne AJ: Principles of surgical management of cancer of the pharyngeal walls. *Cancer* 1967;20:663–667.

16. Briant TD, Bryce DP, Smith TJ: Carcinoma of the hypopharynx—a five year follow-up. *J Otolaryngol* 1977;6:353–362.

17. Mancuso AA, Harnsberger HR, Muraki AS, Stevens MH: Computed tomography of cervical and retropharyngeal lymph nodes: normal anatomy variants of normal, and applications in staging head & neck cancer. Part II: Pathology. *Radiology* 1983;148:715–723.

18. Wang CC: Radiotherapeutic management of carcinoma of the posterior pharyngeal wall. *Cancer* 1971;27:894–896.

19. Meoz-Mendez RT, Fletcher GH, Guillamondegui OM, Peters LJ: Analysis of the results of irradiation in the treatment of squamous cell carcinomas of the pharyngeal walls. *Int J Radiat Oncol Biol Phys* 1978;4:579–585.

20. Marks JE, Freeman RB, Lee F, et al: Pharyngeal wall cancer: an analysis of treatment results, complications and patterns of failure. *Int J Radiat Oncol Biol Phys* 1978;4:587–593.

21. Burdette WJ, Jesse R: Carcinoma of the cervical esophagus. *J Thorac Cardiovasc Surg* 1972;63:41–53.

22. Harrison DFN: Role of surgery in the management of postcricoid and cervical esophagus neoplasms. *Ann Otol Rhinol Laryngol* 1972;81:465–468.

23. Pearson JG: The present status and future potential of radiotherapy in the management of esophageal cancer. *Cancer* 1977;39:882–890.

CHAPTER 9

CARCINOMA OF THE LARYNX

New laryngeal cancers in the United States for the year 1995 number 11,600—approximately 4.6 per 100,000 population—with a mortality rate of 1.9 per 100,000.[1] Males more commonly present than females with a ratio of 4:1 for all laryngeal cancers. Most patients are in the fifth to seventh decade of life. Patients in their twenties and thirties are seen with increasing frequency due to the change in American life-style.

The risk of laryngeal cancer related to cigarette smoking is well established. Alcohol alone does not appear to enhance cancer development but its excessive use has been found synergistically to increase the risk factors to a significant degree.[2]

Anatomically, the larynx is a cartilaginous framework held in position by intrinsic and extrinsic musculature and ligaments.[3] The thyroid cartilage encloses the larynx anteriorly and laterally. The cricoid cartilage lies directly below the thyroid cartilage, forming a complete ring around the larynx below the true vocal cord. It is wider and thicker posteriorly, giving the appearance of a signet ring. The thyroid and cricoid cartilages are connected anteriorly by the cricothyroid ligament. The arytenoid cartilages, roughly pyramidal in shape, are superimposed on the cricoid cartilage, lying side by side posteriorly. Two cuneiform cartilages lie within the arytenoepiglottic folds and two corniculate cartilages lie on top of each arytenoid cartilage. The remaining cartilage of the larynx is the unpaired, slightly curled, spoon-shaped epiglottis, which arches diagonally upward and backward from the posterior surface of the thyroid cartilage to which it is attached by the thyroepiglottic ligament. The superior limit of the larynx is generally accepted to be the hyoepiglottic ligament, while the anterior border is the thyrohyoid membrane and thyroid cartilage; the inferior limit is the bottom of the cricoid cartilage and the posterior limit is the arytenoid cartilages. The hyoid bone and the mucosal surface of the vallecula are considered extralaryngeal.

The quadrangular membrane (QM)[4,5] has four borders and consists of a sheet of elastic tissue, connecting the lateral border of the epiglottic cartilage anteriorly, the arytenoid cartilage posteriorly, and the ventricular ligament inferiorly. The superior border is free, and, with the overlying mucosa, this border forms the arytenoepiglottic (AE) fold. This membranous structure separates the laryngeal vestibule and the hypopharynx, as shown in Figure 9.1. The conus elasticus is a bilateral membrane consisting of fibers attaching inferiorly to the arch and lamina of the cricoid and superiorly to the vocal ligament and the vocal process of the arytenoid cartilage. It is an important barrier to tumor spread, as most of the glottic tumors with a mobile cord remain superficial to it. There are no intrinsic muscles of the larynx inferior to the conus. Below the conus is the elastic lamina of the trachea.

The epiglottic cartilage has numerous dehiscences that facilitate tumor spread into the pre-epiglottic space, which is a fat-filled funnel-shaped space, bounded anteriorly by the upper thyroid cartilage and thyrohyoid membrane, superiorly

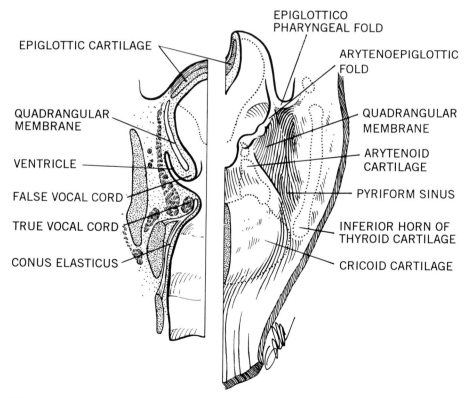

FIGURE 9.1 Diagram shows the various anatomic structures of the larynx: left half with mucosa removed, revealing the QM, ventricle, false and true vocal cords, and conus elasticus; right half with mucosa intact showing various anatomic parts.

by the hyoepiglottic ligament, and posteriorly by the epiglottic cartilage. It extends in a horseshoe fashion posterolaterally and merges with the paraglottic space.

The paraglottic space is the portion of the larynx bounded by the thyroid ala anterolaterally, conus elasticus inferiorly, quadrangular membrane medially, and pyriform sinus mucosa laterally. This space may be involved by extensive tumor from the supraglottic larynx or the pyriform sinus and can be evaluated by CT or MR scan.

Both the true and false vocal cords are mucosal folds overlying the vocal ligament and ventricular ligament, respectively; they attach to the inside of the thyroid cartilage anteriorly and the vocal process of each arytenoid cartilage posteriorly. Lying between the true and false vocal cords is the laryngeal ventricle or recess (sinus of Morgagni). Since the laryngeal ventricle is not protected by the quadrangular membrane laterally, this area is vulnerable for easy spread of tumors into the space and invasion of the thyroid cartilage.

The larynx is innervated by the 10th cranial nerve, consisting of the superior laryngeal and its internal branch entering the larynx through the thyrohyoid membrane, and the recurrent laryngeal nerves to the intrinsic muscles and the vocal cords.

The larynx can be divided into three separate regions, supraglottic, glottic, and subglottic,[6] as shown in Figure 9.2. Embryologically, the supraglottis is derived from the buccogingival anlagen (arches III and IV) and the glottic and subglottic portions are derived from the tracheobronchial anlagen (arches V and VI). These embryologic derivations serve as compartmental barriers to the vertical spread of

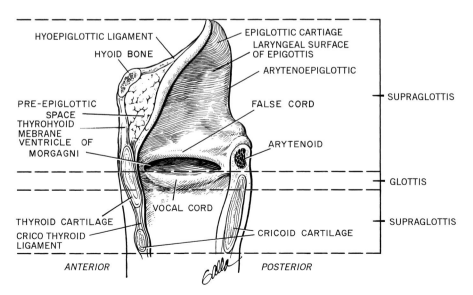

FIGURE 9.2   Anatomic subdivisions of the larynx: supraglottis, glottis, and subglottis.

tumors, account for the differences in the growth behavior and incidence, and determine the pattern of lymphatic spread at each anatomic region.[7,8] Therefore, infrahyoid epiglottic carcinomas very rarely spread below the true vocal cord into the subglottis until late in the disease. This phenomenon is the basis of surgical treatment of a selected group of patients with supraglottic laryngectomy. The supraglottic tumors include the lesions arising from the laryngeal surface or the rim of the epiglottis, arytenoepiglottic fold, arytenoid, false cord, and laryngeal ventricle. The glottic tumors originate from the vocal cord and commissures. The subglottic lesions arise from the area approximately 5 mm below the true cord, and caudally to the inferior border of the cricoid cartilage. In this region, the larynx is considerably smaller than in the supraglottic region and is relatively rigid because of the heavy cricoid cartilage that surrounds it. The supraglottic larynx is lined with a very low stratified squamous epithelium, and the free round border of the true cord has no submucosa and is covered with very thick stratified squamous epithelium, which is firmly attached to the underlying vocal ligament. The subglottis is lined with ciliated columnar epithelium. The most common cancer of the larynx is squamous cell carcinoma of varying degrees of malignant potential, ranging from in situ carcinoma to poorly differentiated carcinoma. Other cell types include verrucous carcinoma, adenocystic carcinoma, neuroendocrine carcinoma, oat cell carcinoma, and lymphoma.[9]

STAGING SYSTEM

The tumor staging system for laryngeal carcinoma as recommended by the American Joint Committee in 1992 is as follows:[10]

Glottis

Tis   Carcinoma in situ
T1   Tumor limited to vocal cord(s) (may involve anterior or posterior commissures) with normal mobility
    T1a   Tumor limited to one vocal cord
    T1b   Tumor involves both vocal cords
T2   Tumor extends to supraglottis and/or subglottis, and/or with impaired vocal cord mobility
T3   Tumor limited to the larynx with vocal cord fixation
T4   Tumor invades through thyroid cartilage and/or extends to other tissues beyond the larynx (e.g., oropharynx, soft tissues of neck)

Supraglottis

Tis   Carcinoma in situ
T1   Tumor limited to one subset of supraglottis with normal vocal cord mobility

T2   Tumor invades more than one subsite of supraglottis or glottis with normal vocal cord mobility

T3   Tumor limited to larynx with vocal cord fixation and/or invades postcricoid area, medial wall of the pyriform sinus, or pre-epiglottic tissues

T4   Tumor invades through thyroid cartilage and/or extends to other tissues beyond the larynx (e.g., oropharynx, soft tissues of neck)

Subglottis

Tis   Carcinoma in situ

T1   Tumor limited to subglottis

T2   Tumor extends to the vocal cord(s) with normal or impaired mobility

T3   Tumor limited to larynx with vocal cord fixation

T4   Tumor invades through cricoid or thyroid cartilage and/or extends to other tissues beyond the larynx (e.g., oropharynx, soft tissues of neck)

As is common in any staging system, there are weaknesses of the AJC's tumor–node–metastasis (TNM) system. The T2 glottic lesions include tumors with both mobile cord and impaired cord mobility. As seen from the available data, it would be desirable to subdivide T2 lesions into T2a (mobile cord) and T2b (impaired cord mobility). Transglottic lesion[11] denotes tumor arising above and below the laryngeal ventricle with involvement of the true and false vocal cords and is not recognized in the AJC staging system. Likewise, for supraglottic carcinoma, the AJC system includes multiple subsites, which are not readily identifiable clinically. The tumors arising from the tip of the epiglottis (AE fold) are unlikely to involve the vocal cord, causing fixation, in spite of extensive primary disease.

Clinical Examination

Thorough understanding of the anatomic structures of the larynx and careful evaluation of the extent, growth pattern, and spread of a laryngeal tumor is *sine qua non* for successful therapies. Examination of the larynx by indirect laryngoscopy is the most informative, inexpensive, and readily available clinical procedure. More than 90% of the patients can easily be examined by laryngeal mirrors. In occasional instances, when the epiglottis is slit-like (i.e., fish mouth deformity) or when gagging reflexes are unusually active, examination of the larynx can be carried out with ease by fiberoptiscope, and very few patients require direct laryngoscopy under general anesthesia just for the purpose of routine observation.

During laryngoscopic examination, the extent of the tumor, ulceration, swelling, and mobility of the involved part and its adjacent structures must be carefully diagrammed and recorded. The anterior commissure must be clearly seen; otherwise, the examination is incomplete.

Careful palpation of the neck should be carried out to assess the presence or absence of cervical adenopathy, which has a great bearing on the treatment outcome. The absence of "laryngeal click" or thyrovertebral crackle indicates either extralaryngeal tumor invasion posteriorly and/or associated edema or infection.

Radiologic examination of laryngeal cancer[12] includes (1) soft tissue films of the neck in anteroposterior (AP) and lateral projections, which can detect tumor involvement of the base of the tongue, epiglottis, AE fold, arytenoid, posterior pharyngeal wall, and thyroid cartilage destruction; (2) AP tomograms of the larynx (Figure 9.3), which can show the normal anatomic structures and any tumor of the larynx (Figure 9.4); (3) conventional barium swallow, which can allow evaluation of any pyriform sinus involvement, permit Valsava maneuver dynamic study of the larynx, and study of the pharyngo-esophageal junction by fluoroscopy, spot films, and a complete esophagogram; (4) chest radiographs; and (5) CT and MR scans. CT scans in axial projection are valuable in evaluating the lateral paraglottic extent, as well as vertical extension of tumor spread, and pre-epiglottic space invasion. MR scans are not very useful in

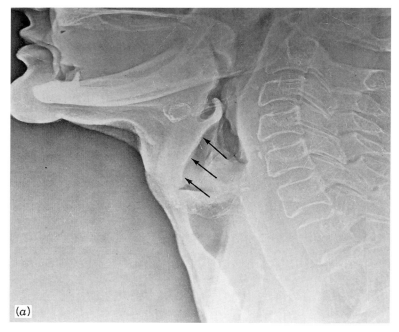

(a)

FIGURE 9.3   (a) Xerogram shows normal pre-epiglottic space with intact epiglottic white line (*black arrows*). (A posterior pharyngeal wall tumor is also apparent.) (b) Pre-epiglottic space involvement with destruction of epiglottis. Note irregular epiglottis with absence of epiglottic white line (*black arrows*) and tumor in the pre-epiglottic space bulging into the anterior neck.

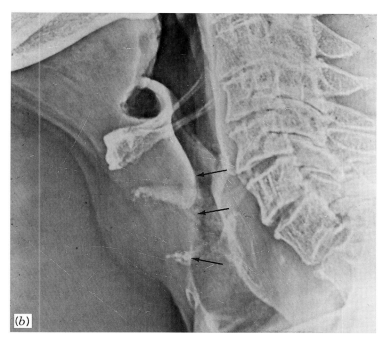

FIGURE 9.3   *Continued*

the early stage of the disease, that is, T1 and T2 tumors, but they are helpful for T3 and T4 tumors. With the availability of CT imaging and the fiberoptis-cope, the laryngogram is no longer routinely performed. For T1 glottic lesions, additional in-formation from these radiological studies is unlikely to be sig-nificant. From the cost and effect standpoint, therefore, routine radiographic imaging studies for T1 glottic lesions are not advised. For more advanced tumors, these up-to-date investigations may yield invaluable information as to the extent of the lesion, mobility of the involved part, presence or absence of cartilaginous destruction, and subglottic extension of glottic tumor and may pro-foundly influence the decision-making in the management of carcinoma of the larynx.

Tissue Confirmation of Malignancy

Before definitive treatment is planned, biopsy and mapping of the lesion by direct laryngoscopy are indicated for confirmation of and extent of malignant disease. If the patient presents with a large, bulky tumor and marginal glottic rima, one must be prepared to perform a tracheostomy due to the risk of additional edema causing laryngeal obstruction after biopsy and instrumentation.

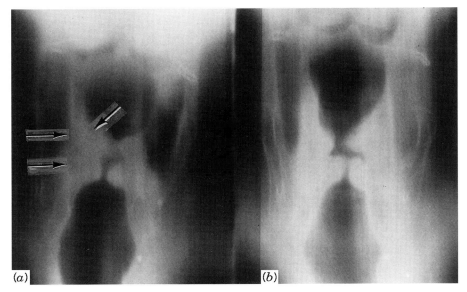

FIGURE 9.4 Anteroposterior tomograph showing normal left hemilarynx and tumor in the right supraglottic extension, (a) before and (b) after RT.

A. CARCINOMA OF THE GLOTTIS

Cancer of the vocal cord is the most common form of laryngeal cancer and the majority of cases are well differentiated squamous cell carcinoma. Owing to its manifestation of disease by hoarseness of voice, glottic carcinoma is often discovered early and is therefore a highly curable malignant tumor. The majority of tumors arise from the anterior half of the membranous portion of the vocal cord. As the disease progresses, the lesion extends anteriorly toward and/or around the anterior commissure to the opposite cord. This forms a "horseshoe" lesion but rarely invades the thyroid cartilage to such an extent as to be of therapeutic importance. The tumor may also extend posteriorly toward the vocal process and arytenoid, supraglottically into the laryngeal ventricle and false cord, and inferiorly into the infraglottic space. Tumors arising primarily de novo in the anterior and posterior commissures are uncommon.

Distinction must be made among the various tumor sites, growth characteristics, stage of the primary, nodal status, mobility of the involved cord, and sex of the patient,[13] as these may affect significantly the treatment outcome. Generally, exophytic and superficial lesions are more readily controlled by radiation therapy with lesser incidence of nodal metastases. Deeply ulcerative and endophytic lesions tend to represent advanced disease. Superficial tumors extensively involving the cord or pericordal structures, with the mobility of the involved cord remaining intact, are highly curable by radiation therapy. Small infiltrating tumors of limited extent, but with impairment of mobility of the involved cord or cord fixation, represent advanced disease with poor local control by radiation therapy.

Owing to the lack of extensive lymphatics, the incidence of lymph node metastases for glottic carcinoma generally is low.[14-16] With tumor confined to the cord with normal mobility, T1, the incidence ranges from 0% to 2%.[17,18] For advanced disease, T2-3, the rate was 11%.[15] Daly and Strong[19] reported the rate of metastases for T1 as 5%, for T2 as 8%, and for T3 as 15%. For far-advanced lesions, T4, the rate was 20-30%. The pattern of nodal metastases follows the secondarily involved site; that is, with supraglottic extension, the upper and midneck nodes, and for infraglottic extension, the inferior jugular, Delphian, and paratracheal nodes may be involved.

SELECTION OF THERAPY

T1 Lesions

Treatment of early glottic carcinomas, T1, can be by either radiation therapy or surgery with comparably good results. In our experience, radiation therapy is considered to be the treatment of choice. It not only provides excellent control of disease but also preserves a good, useful voice in approximately 90-95% of patients. If radiation therapy fails to control the disease, the patients still have a second chance of lasting cure by surgery, either hemi- or total laryngectomy, since the success of salvage surgery is extremely high—approximately 80%.[7,20] Conservation surgery[7,21,22] such as laryngofissure and cordectomy, laser excision,[23] or hemilaryngectomy in experienced hands can control early glottic lesions in highly selected patients but the functional results and voice quality are inferior to those achieved by radiation therapy. Hemilaryngectomy is not suitable for tumors with diffuse in situ carcinoma, for lesions that cross the anterior commissure to the opposite cord, or in patients of advanced age (i.e., 60 years or older) or with chronic obstructive pulmonary disease (COPD).

T2a Lesions with Normal Mobility

T2 lesions represent mucosal spread of glottic carcinoma without significant muscle invasion with tumor extension above and/or below the vocal cord superficially. Such lesions are generally amenable to treatment by radiation therapy with good local control—approximately 70-80%. Failures after radiation therapy can often be salvaged by surgery with a success rate of 70%. In our experience, treatment of these lesions is by radiation therapy with surgery as salvage.

T2b Lesions with Impaired Cord Mobility

Impairment of cord mobility generally indicates considerable depth of invasion of the intrinsic muscle by the carcinoma. Occasionally, the impairment may be due to the bulk of the growth or trauma after instrumentation for biopsy. For this stage of the disease, total laryngectomy would certainly rid the patient of the disease with lasting cure but at the expense of the larynx and is ill-advised. Another treatment option is "conservation" surgery as the definitive treatment.[7,22] However, if the extent of the lesion precludes hemilaryngectomy, it is justified to proceed with curative radiation therapy first, with surgery in the form of total laryngectomy reserved for salvage. The local control rate for such lesions is 60–70% after conventional radiation therapy and the rate of salvage surgery is approximately 60–70%. Another option is to irradiate the tumor first; if the lesion shows good regression and/or return of normal cord mobility after a dose of 45 Gy, treatment may then be continued to a curative dose level of about 65 Gy. On the other hand, if the mobility of the involved cord remains impaired or fixed, conservation surgery may still be considered.

T3 Fixed Cord Lesions

Fixation of the vocal cord is a grave prognostic sign indicating extensive disease with deep infiltration of the thyroarytenoid muscle. Management of such advanced lesions should be individualized. If the lesion is limited to the cord or its adjacent supraglottic structures, vertical hemilaryngectomy may be considered with local control rates ranging from 60% to 70% and voice preservation in two out of three patients.[14] If the extent of the lesion calls for initial total laryngectomy, one may try radiation therapy first, with laryngectomy being reserved for salvage for failure. The success rate after conventional radiation therapy ranges from 35% to 50%[24,25] and 60–70% after accelerated hyperfractionated radiation therapy; the surgical salvage rate is approximately 40–50%.

T4 Extensive Lesions

Far-advanced carcinoma of the vocal cord (T4) is most uncommon. The lesions of such extent most likely represent extensive supraglottic or pyriform sinus carcinomas with secondary involvement of the glottis. Treatment of this condition is a combination of laryngectomy with or without neck dissection to be followed by postoperative radiation therapy.

MANAGEMENT OF PREMALIGNANT LESIONS

Leukoplakia and in situ carcinoma of the glottis are premalignant lesions and are not clinically distinguishable from invasive cancers except by histopathologic examination. Carcinoma in situ may occur de novo on the cord or may represent an intramucosal peripheral spread at the border of an invasive carcinoma present in an adjacent area. These tumors may recur either as in situ carcinoma or as invasive carcinoma.

Therapeutic options include the following:

1. Careful observation after stripping. Since cord stripping alone can control 75–80% of cases, this procedure may be used in patients who present with a completely normal-appearing larynx after the procedure with reliable follow-ups. If the lesion recurs, radiation therapy can be considered as for invasive carcinoma because of the malignant potential.

2. Definitive radiation therapy. In situ carcinoma of the vocal cord has been managed and treated as invasive carcinoma, although the results of radiation therapy generally are not as good as invasive T1 lesions. The "failure" may be due to inherent radioinsensitivity of intramucosal lesions or, not infrequently, may be due to a second carcinoma developing from a mucosa with "field malignant diathesis."

3. Other options include cordectomy[26] and laser excision therapy,[27,28] with local control rates of 80–90%. These procedures often remove some normal tissue of the cord and result in permanent residual hoarseness and therefore are often reserved for radiation failures.

RADIOTHERAPEUTIC MANAGEMENT

Because of the low incidence of lymph node metastases, the treatment of early T1–2a lesions does not include treatment of cervical disease and calls for careful simulation and localization of normal laryngeal structures and tattooing for accurate daily radiation therapy. The sagittal position of the level of the vocal cords is approximately 1.0–1.2 cm below the thyroid notch, as shown by Figure 9.5. Our policy for irradiation of T1 lesions is to deliver a uniform dose throughout the entire glottis with inclusion of the anterior half of the arytenoids; this is particularly necessary for lesions arising from the posterior cord or involving the entire cord. This can be accomplished by employing two opposing open lateral portals and two anterior oblique wedge pairs with equal weighting, the so-called four-field technique, with the 95–97% isodose line bisecting the arytenoids. The dose variation is not greater than 3–5%, as shown in Figure 9.6a. An alternative approach is to employ two opposing lateral portals with wedges, as seen in Figure 9.6b. A tumor dose of 65–66 Gy is delivered by QD program in 6-½ weeks.

The cobolt-60 unit is most suited for vocal cord irradiation. Unfortunately, it is out of vogue. The alternative photon machines are 4–6 MV linear accelerators. Due to the excessive D_{max} of 4–6 MV x-rays, care must be taken to avoid underdosing of the anterior commissure, and some bolus must be added during treatment to avoid any "cold spot" in this area. Although a recent report indicates no significant decrease of local control in patients treated with 6 MV radiations,[29] the use of 6 MV photons for treatment of T1 glottic carcinoma must be considered with caution.

For T2a lesions, RT is given by opposing lateral portals, by a QD program, for 66–70 Gy in 7 weeks. For thicker lesions, use BID programs.

For T2b and T3 lesions, the treatment portals include the entire larynx and the subdigastric and midjugular nodes with the accelerated RT programs (BID) through

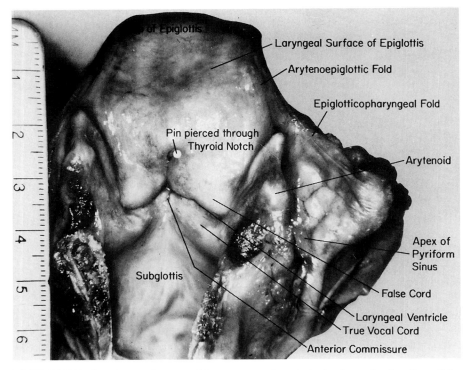

FIGURE 9.5 Specimen of a normal larynx opened posteriorly shows the location of the false and true vocal cords in relation to the pin pierced through the thyroid notch. The thyroid notch is useful for placement of radiation portal for T1–2 glottic carcinoma.

opposing lateral portals, with shrinking field, for a total dose to the primary site of up to 70 Gy in 6 weeks. If the lesions show significant subglottic extension, the inferior and supraclavicular nodes are also irradiated.

Technical Pointers

1. Patient is to lie supine, with the chin extended and the head immobilized and supported by straps or a face mask, depending on circumstances. A cross-tabletop beam is employed (Figure 9.7).

2. Palpate the thyroid notch, and place the field center at 1.2–1.5 cm inferior to the notch. *Note:* The position of the female larynx may be high up in the neck, and the prominence of the cricoid can be confused with the thyroid prominence.

3. For T1–2 lesions, the posterior border is at the prevertebral fascia, the su-

POS: .00 cm T=1

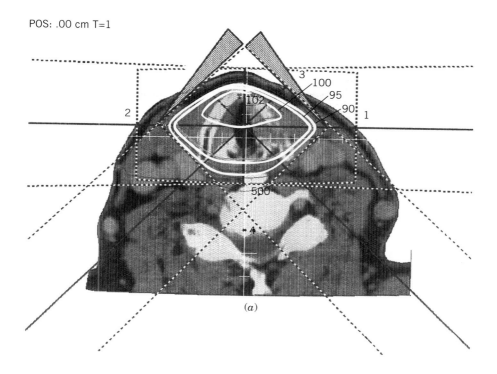

(a)

POS: .00 cm 4 T=1

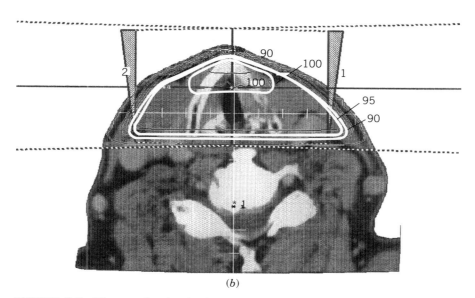

(b)

FIGURE 9.6 Diagram showing isodose distribution in various radiation therapy techniques for T1 glottic carcinoma: (a) four-field technique, that is, opposing open lateral and anterior oblique wedge pair (45°) and (b) opposing laterals with 30° wedges.

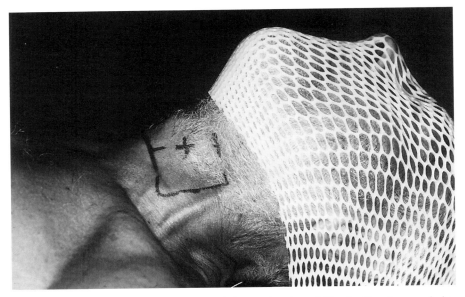

FIGURE 9.7 Photograph showing patient lying supine, immobilized with a face mask, being treated with cross-tabletop photon for glottic carcinoma.

perior border is below the hyoid bone, the inferior border is below the cricoid, and the anterior border falls off the anterior neck for 1.5–2 cm. The field size is 5.0 cm×5.0 cm or 4.5 cm×4.5 cm as shown in Figure 9.8.

4. The recommended total dose is 10 Gy per week with 2 Gy per fraction, as smaller fraction size may inversely affect local control.[30,31]

5. For T2a lesions with supraglottic extension, the treatment portals include the entire larynx, from the tip of the epiglottis to the subglottis or the superior border is lengthened for 2 cm. *Note:* The vocal cords radiate from the bottom of "figure 8" calcification toward the arytenoids. A portal size of 7 cm × 5 cm should suffice.

6. During radiation therapy, symptoms of severe sore throat or dysphagia with bullous edema of the arytenoids call for some adjustment of the "iso" anteriorly or slight field reduction posteriorly, that is, 5 mm, respectively.

7. For T2b and T3 lesions, use accelerated hyperfractionated programs (BID). The superior border is at the angle of the jaw, the posterior border is at the vertebral pedicles, the inferior border is below the cricoid, and the anterior border falls off the skin (Figure 9.9). Use wedges, to create uniform doses, and a shrinking field technique. The posterior triangle and submandibular nodes need not be included.

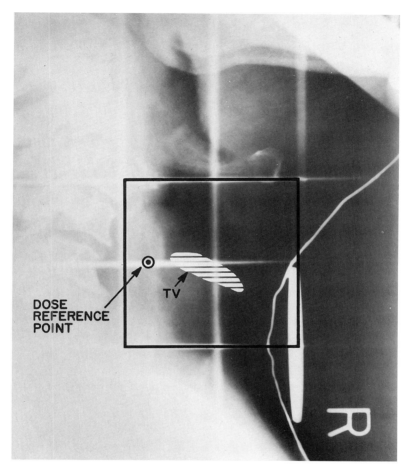

FIGURE 9.8 Simulation radiograph showing portal arrangement for radiation therapy of T1 glottic carcinoma in lateral projection.

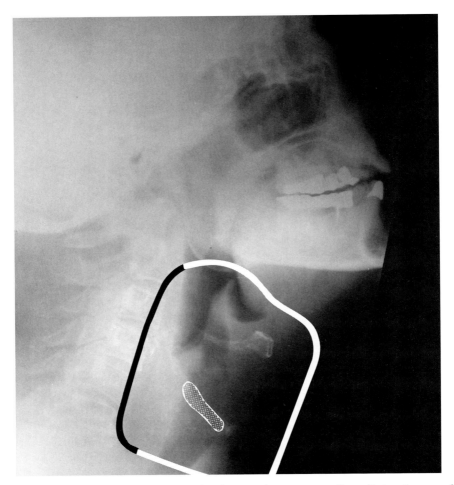

FIGURE 9.9 Simulation radiograph showing portal arrangement for radiation therapy of T2 glottic carcinoma in lateral projection.

RADIOTHERAPEUTIC RESULTS

The results of treatment of early T1 glottic carcinoma by irradiation as reported in the literature show excellent local control, ranging from 80% to 90%,[24,32–35] and, including surgical salvage from 95% to 98%. This is comparable to that achievable by hemilaryngectomy, laser excision,[23,28] or laryngofissure and cordectomy.[14]

For T2 lesions, the results are still quite high, approximately 70–80%[24,33–35] for RT alone and approximately 90% when surgical salvage follows. For the T3 fixed cord lesion, the results of local control following radiation therapy are not entirely satisfactory, being approximately 30–65%;[24,33,34] when surgical salvage follows RT, the LC rates ranged from 40% to 70%.

MGH EXPERIENCE

From 1970 through 1994, a total of 970 patients with glottic carcinoma were treated by radiation therapy at the MGH. There were 665 patients with T1, 145 patients with T2a, 92 patients with T2b, 65 patients with T3, and 3 patients with T4. The incidence of nodal metastases at diagnosis was less than 1% for T1, 4% for T2a and T2b, and 5% for T3.

Owing to the low incidence of lymph node metastases, the treatment results were analyzed according to the lesions at the primary site (T stage), the degree of mobility of the involved cord, and the treatment programs employed (i.e., BID versus QD). The results of radiation therapy for in situ carcinoma and of combination surgery and radiation therapy for a few patients are also presented in Table 9.1.

TABLE 9.1   Five-Year Actuarial Local Control (LC) and Disease-Specific Survival (DSS) Rates Related to T Stage of Cancer of Glottis After BID and QD Radiation Therapy: MGH 1970–1994

Stage[a]	n	LC (%)	DSS (%)
T1	665	93	98
T2a	145	77	92
T2b	92	71	84
T3	65	57	75
T4	3	67	33
	$p = 0.0001$	$p = 0.001$	

[a]Comparing T Stages: T1 versus T2a, $p = 0.0001$; T2a versus T2b, $p = 0.59$; T2a versus T3, $p = 0.004$.

Since 1979, BID radiation therapy was offered to patients with T2–3 disease. Most patients with T1 lesions were managed by QD programs. The results of the BID program are shown in Table 9.2.

TABLE 9.2   Five-Year Actuarial LC and DSS Rates After BID Radiation Therapy for Glottic Carcinoma: MGH 1979–1994

Stage	n	LC (%)	DSS (%)
T2a	76	83	93
T2b	61	72	87
T3	41	67	85

TABLE 9.3 Five-Year Actuarial LC and DSS Rates After QD Radiation Therapy for Glottic Carcinoma

Stage	n	LC (%)	DSS (%)
T2a	69	70	91
T2b	31	67	76
T3	24	42	60

The results of the QD programs are shown in Table 9.3.

The results after BID therapy as compared to the QD programs are shown in Table 9.4.

TABLE 9.4 Five-Year Actuarial LC and DSS Rates After Radiation Therapy: Comparing QD and BID Programs

T2a	$p = 0.07$
T2b	$p = 0.66$
T3	$p = 0.03$

Salvage surgery was carried out for radiation failures at primary sites. The rate of success was 82% for T1 lesions, 63% for T2a lesions, and 50% for T2b and T3 lesions.

In Situ Carcinoma

Our experience in the management of in situ carcinoma of the vocal cord was previously reported. Unfortunately, some in situ carcinomas may in fact be sampling errors of the peripheral population of invasive squamous cell carcinoma. Radiotherapeutically, therefore, the treatment of in situ carcinoma of the glottis should be radical and is identical to that of invasive carcinoma in terms of radiation therapy dosages and portal techniques.

Recent review of the experience of radiation therapy for in situ carcinoma of the glottis at the MGH is indicated in Table 9.5.

These data indicate similar local control of in situ carcinoma as compared to invasive lesions.

TABLE 9.5 Five-Year Actuarial LC and DSS Rates for Tis of the Glottis After Radiation Therapy: MGH 1970–1995

n	LC (%)	DSS (%)
60	92	98

COMBINED THERAPIES FOR GLOTTIC CARCINOMA

A small number of patients were treated by a combination of surgery and radiation therapy related to various stages of glottic carcinoma, and the local control (LC) and disease-specific survival (DSS) rates are shown in Table 9.6.

These results of combined therapies did not show any significant improvement when compared to those after primary radiation therapy with surgical salvage.

TABLE 9.6   Five-Year Actuarial LC and DSS Rates After Combined Surgery and Radiation Therapy for Glottis Carcinoma

Stage	n	LC (%)	DSS (%)
T2N0	9	78	89
T3N0	25	73	72
T4N2	1	100	100

Complications of Radiation Therapy for Glottic Carcinoma

Radiation complications vary from edema of the arytenoids to laryngeal chondritis and necrosis, but fortunately they are extremely rare, less than 1%. These complications are primarily due to excessively high total dose and increased daily fraction size, faulty treatment technique (i.e., single portal for entire course), and/or large radiation portals to the larynx and neck. With careful radiation therapy planning and technique, the "usual" postradiation edema of the arytenoids[36] following treatment of T1 glottic carcinoma is mostly eliminated. In our experience, edema of the laryngeal structures after radiation therapy should arouse the suspicion of tumor recurrence.[36] On the other hand, a minimal degree of swelling of the arytenoids and arytenoepiglottic folds after radiation therapy for advanced glottic lesions occurs quite frequently. If the mobility of the laryngeal structures remains normal and without mucosal ulceration, the probability of recurrence is low and the patients should be kept under observation only. Frequent laryngoscopies and biopsies may induce the risk of infection and/or necrosis in the heavily irradiated larynx.

Late radiation sequelae consist of telangiectasis, subcutaneous fibrosis, and, in extreme cases after high-dose radiation therapy, an immobile, functionless larynx requiring permanent tracheostomy. With modern radiation therapy principles and techniques and the aid of dedicated computers, these complications are reduced to a minimum.

Necrosis of the larynx, persistent edema of the arytenoids, and functionless larynx were uncommon. Our series consisted of eight patients with necrosis of the larynx, four in T1, two in T2, and two in T3, and all were due to faulty radiation therapy technique with excessive total dosages, high daily radiation therapy fractions, and single lateral and/or overly large irradiated portals, and all occurred prior to 1970.

B. CARCINOMA OF THE SUPRAGLOTTIS

Carcinoma of the supraglottis ranks second to glottic carcinoma in incidence and generally is associated with a poorer prognosis. Most of these tumors are relatively poorly differentiated squamous cell carcinomas and biologically aggressive. Patients may initially experience foreign body sensation and sore throat, hemoptysis, and, later on, odynophagia and pain referred to the ear. Hoarseness of the voice is not an initial manifestation of this disease but denotes advanced condition when the lesion has extended to the vocal cord. Owing to the abundant supply of submucosal lymphatics and poorly differentiated cellular nature, supraglottic carcinoma is characterized by a high incidence of cervical lymph node metastases. As a rule, as the lesions arise further from the glottis toward the base of the tongue, or further posteriorly toward the esophagus, there is a higher incidence of lymph node metastases. The difference in the incidence may vary from 25% to 50%, depending on the stage and location of the primary lesions.[37,38] For T1–2 lesions, the incidence of metastases ranged from 27% to 40%[39,40]; for T3–4 lesions, the rates ranged from 55% to 65%. Suprahyoid, arytenoid, and AE fold lesions presented with higher rates of metastases than the infrahyoid lesions, that is, 36% versus 15%.[41] Bilateral cervical lymph node metastases are not uncommon, either overt or occult, and occur in 13% for T1, 23% for T2, 33% for T3, and 50% for T4 lesions.[7] The rates ranged from one-quarter to one-third of the patients in whom ipsilateral metastases are present.[42]

The lymphatics from the supraglottis drain through the thyrohyoid space to the upper cervical lymph nodes. The principal nodes involved by supraglottic carcinoma, as shown in Figure 9.10, include the subdigastric, superior deep, and midjugular nodes. Rouviere's node is occasionally involved. Metastases to the posterior cervical triangle are most unusual in spite of the presence of metastases in the anterior cervical triangle.[42,43] Likewise, metastatic involvement of the submandibular group of lymph nodes rarely occurs.

The hyoid bone is connected to the thyroid cartilage by the thyrohyoid membrane and divides the epiglottis into suprahyoid and infrahyoid portions. Carcinomas arising from the suprahyoid epiglottis tend to be bulky and exophytic and may involve the base of the tongue and vallecula and resemble oropharyngeal carcinoma, with increased incidence of lymph node metastases, often bilateral. Early lesions often regress after radiation therapy and the normal epiglottis is reinstituted. Occasionally, the residual epiglottis is markedly deformed or autoamputated. Large tumors may destroy the epiglottic cartilage, resulting in autoamputation after healing takes place. Lesions originating from the infrahyoid epiglottis are prone to invade the pre-epiglottic space[13] but rarely extend inferiorly into the subglottis and have fewer lymph node metastases as compared to suprahyoid epiglottic lesions.

False vocal cord carcinomas may be exophytic or ulcerative. The deeply invasive lesions may involve the adjacent thyroid cartilage.

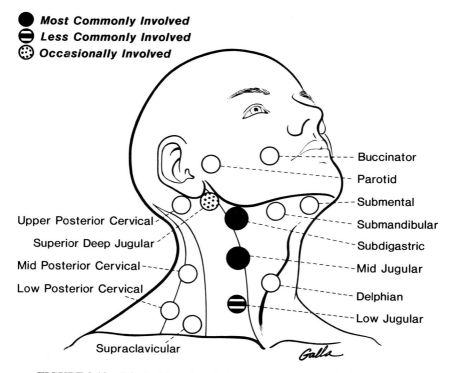

FIGURE 9.10   Principal lymph node involvement in supraglottic carcinoma.

Carcinomas arising from the laryngeal ventricle cannot be seen by indirect laryngoscopy. Clinically, this lesion presents as a smooth, nonulcerated tumefaction of the adjacent false vocal cord. It tends to invade the adjacent thyroid cartilage early.

Among the various anatomic sites of the supraglottis, the epiglottis is most commonly involved, reportedly as high as 50%; the false cord is involved 25% of the time, to be followed by the AE fold at 20%. The laryngeal ventricle and arytenoids are the least frequent sites of origin. Approximately one-quarter of the supraglottic carcinomas were midline situated.[37]

SELECTION OF THERAPY

Management of supraglottic carcinoma is extremely controversial. Some advocate total laryngectomy,[37,44] others select radiation therapy alone,[45,46] and still others recommend partial supraglottic laryngectomy.[47,48] The selection of method of treatment depends on the extent, anatomic location, and growth pattern of the primary lesion; nodal status; availability and skill of the surgeon and radiation oncologist; and last, but not least, the risk, physical condition, and wishes of the patient.

In general, for a superficial, exophytic, early lesion, T1 or T2, without node involvement, radiation therapy is as effective as surgery and should be considered as the initial method of treatment of choice.[35,39] This is particularly true for tumors arising from the tip of the epiglottis and the arytenoepiglottic fold. For more advanced, deeply ulcerative lesions and/or extensive cervical lymph node metastases (i.e., T3 or T4, N2 or N3), the treatment is combined laryngectomy with neck dissection,[21,27] to be followed by postoperative radiation therapy.[39,44,49] Other options are conservative supraglottic laryngectomy. For a small subset of female patients with T3N0 exophytic growths, radiation therapy may be tried with total laryngectomy being reserved for salvage.

RADIOTHERAPEUTIC MANAGEMENT

Radiation therapy for supraglottic carcinomas must include treatment of the primary lesions and regional nodes in the neck even in T1N0 lesions, because of the propensity for nodal metastases. Generally, large opposing lateral portals are employed to include the whole larynx and the regional lymphatics through a shrinking field technique for a total dose of approximately 70–72 Gy in 6 weeks, following a BID program.

For extensive disease, T3–4 with nodal metastases, postoperative radiation therapy is given through opposing large lateral portals for 55–60 Gy, with cord dose limited to 45 Gy. The tracheal stoma can be irradiated through an open, low anterior neck portal without cord block for 45 Gy. Another option is to employ a "mini-mantle" technique, delivering 45–50 Gy to the prevertebral fascia. Both techniques include electron beam boost to the tracheal stoma and the high risk areas in the neck with additional 10 Gy using 9 MeV electrons.

Technical Pointers

A. Primary Radiation Therapy

1. Lead wire the cervical node(s). Patient is to lie supine, with the chin extended and the head and neck immobilized by clamps, tapes, or a face mask.

2. The comprehensive portals include superiorly the superior jugular and subdigastric nodes 2–3 cm above the angle of the mandible, posteriorly the spinous pedicles, inferiorly the true vocal cord, and anteriorly the skin of the anterior neck. For N0 neck, the posterior cervical and submandibular nodes need not be included.

3. The anterior commissure, the pre-epiglottic space, the lymphatics in the thyrohyoid membrane, and the Delphian node are close to the skin of the anterior neck. "Fall off" of the anterior neck for 1–2 cm is required (Figure 9.11).

4. Use the accelerated hyperfractionated radiation therapy program, with opposing lateral portals and shrinking field to the primary only up to 70–72 Gy in 6 weeks. The angle of the mandible is to be excluded after 60 Gy. The isodose distribution is shown in Figure 9.12.

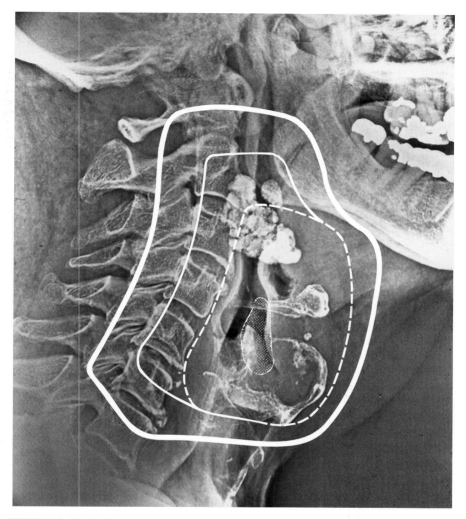

FIGURE 9.11   Radiograph showing portal arrangement with shrinking field technique for radiation therapy of supraglottic carcinoma. (Calcified subdigastric node is shown.)

5. Use wedges to avoid excessive "hot spots" in the anterior neck.
6. For patients with N2–3 nodal disease, the residual neck nodes posterior to the spinal cord are boosted with low-energy electrons up to 60 Gy. Consider neck dissection if the primary tumor is under control.

B. Postoperative Radiation Therapy

1. Patient is to lie supine, with the chin extended and immobilized. The incision scars and tracheostomy are outlined with lead wire.

POS: .00 cm T=1

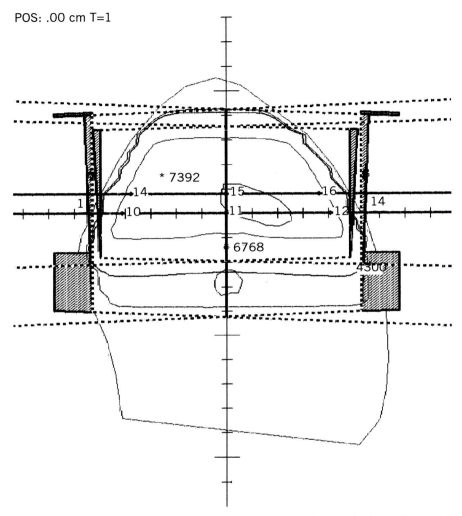

FIGURE 9.12 Isodose distribution for radiation therapy of supraglottic carcinoma with wedges to create uniform dose distribution through opposing lateral portals. Dose is cGy.

2. Use large lateral portals to include the base of tongue and the superior jugular, subdigastric, and midjugular nodes. The superior border is at the mastoid tip, the posterior border at the spinous pedicles, the inferior border includes the stoma, and the anterior border falls off the anterior neck. The angle of the mandible can be partially shielded from the lateral portals.

3. Use a QD or BID program for 40–45 Gy, then off-cord to 60 Gy in 5–6 weeks.

4. For N2–3 neck, the lower inferior and supraclavicular nodes and tracheal

stoma (if not included by the lateral portals) are treated by open anterior portal without midline cord block for 45 Gy. Under such circumstances, the posteroinferior corner of the lateral portals must be "cut off" in order to avoid a hot spot over the spinal cord and adjacent esophagus from the three convergent beams (i.e., two laterals and one anterior).

5. After the basic dose of 45 Gy is delivered, the high-risk areas in the neck and the tracheal stoma are boosted with electrons for an additional 10–15 Gy.

6. An alternative approach is to employ a "mini-mantle" technique as discussed in Chapter 2.

RADIOTHERAPEUTIC RESULTS

The NED (no evidence of disease) rates following radiation therapy vary depending on the extent of the primary tumor and the status of the cervical nodes. For T1N0 and T2N0 lesions, the local control (LC) rates are approximately 80% and 60%, respectively, following radiation therapy alone.[33,35,50–53] For T3 and T4 lesions with or without node involvement, the rates were 37% and 23%, respectively, following radiation therapy. The rates after a combination of surgery and radiation therapy[35,49,53,54] are considerably higher, approaching 50–60%.[44,46,48,50]

The results of once-daily radiation therapy for advanced supraglottic carcinoma have not been highly satisfactory. At the present time, hyperfractionated radiation therapy programs are extensively used with considerable promise, especially for T3–4 tumors.[55,56]

MGH EXPERIENCE

From 1970 through 1994, a total of 566 patients with supraglottic carcinoma were treated at the MGH. Of these, 244 patients received once-daily (QD) radiation therapy and 322 patients received twice-daily (BID) RT. There were 114 T1 (20%), 211 T2 (37%), 183 T3 (32%), and 58 T4 (10%). The incidence of nodal status was as follows: N0, 72%; N1, 10%; and N2–3, 19%.

The results of treatment of this group are shown in Table 9.7.

TABLE 9.7   Five-Year Actuarial LC and DSS Rates of Supraglottic Carcinoma Related to T Stage After QD Radiation Therapy: 1970–1994

Stage	n	LC (%)	DSS (%)
T1	72	74	76
T2	85	61	70
T3	47	56	56
T4	40	29	21
T1–4	244	58	60

The presence of cervical metastases indicates advanced disease and adversely affects local control and disease-specific survival, as shown in Table 9.8.

TABLE 9.8 **Five-Year Actuarial LC and DSS Rates of Supraglottic Carcinoma Related to N Stage After QD Radiation Therapy: 1970–1994**

Stage	n	LC (%)	DSS (%)
N0	169	69	76
N1	24	43	40
N2–3	51	27	20

RESULTS OF BID RADIATION THERAPY

From 1979 through 1994, a total of 322 patients with supraglottic carcinoma received BID radiation therapy. The results related to T and N stages are shown in Tables 9.9 and 9.10.

TABLE 9.9 **Five-Year Actuarial LC and DSS Rates of Supraglottic Carcinoma Related to T Stage After BID Radiation Therapy: 1979–1994**

Stage	n	LC (%)	DSS (%)
T1	42	84	90
T2	126	83	88
T3	136	71	70
T4	18	84	74
T1–4	322	78	80

TABLE 9.10 **Five-Year Actuarial LC at Primary Sites and DSS Rates of Supraglottic Carcinoma Related to N Stage After BID Radiation Therapy: 1979–1994**

Stage	n	LC (%)	DSS (%)
N0	232	82	87
N1	32	73	63
N2–3	58	63	56

The comparison of QD versus BID results indicates significant improvement related to T and N stages with T2–3–4 ($p=0.005$), N0 ($p=0.008$), and N2–3 ($p=0.0001$).

The results of treatment related to AJC stages are shown in Table 9.11.

TABLE 9.11 Five-Year Actuarial LC and DSS Rates of Supraglottic Carcinoma Related to AJC Stages: 1970–1994

Stage	n	LC (%)	DSS (%)
I	96	85	91
II	167	77	86
III	162	69	71
IV	141	47	38

The patients who failed radiation therapy underwent salvage surgery. The success was not as high as for glottic carcinomas; the rates are shown in Table 9.12.

TABLE 9.12 Incidence of Surgical Salvage at the Primary Site Related to T Stage of Supraglottic Carcinoma

Stage	n	Local Failure	Salvage NED (%)
T1	114	21/114 (18%)	56%
T2	211	49/211 (23%)	46%
T3	183	49/183 (27%)	50%
T4	58	30/58 (52%)	25%

Supraglottic carcinomas are known to spread to the cervical nodes. In spite of routine coverage of nodal areas during radiation therapy, nodal failure is still quite high, as shown in Table 9.13, related to the T stages. Over one third and one half of the patients with T3 and T4 lesions failed in the neck after radiation therapy respectively.

TABLE 9.13 Incidence of Nodal Metastases in Supraglottic Carcinoma Related to T Stage

Stage	n	RND Cases	Neck Metastases
T1	114	5	19/114 (17%)
T2	211	9	52/211 (25%)
T3	183	7	71/183 (39%)
T4	58	4	38/58 (66%)

PLANNED COMBINED RADIATION THERAPY AND SURGERY FOR SUPRAGLOTTIC CANCER

A combination of radiation therapy and surgery was carried out for advanced supraglottic carcinoma. From 1950 through 1994, a total of 187 patients were available for analysis. The 5-year actuarial local control (LC) and disease-specific survival

(DSS) rates are compared with QD radiation therapy alone and are shown in Table 9.14:

Failures after combined therapies were mostly due to regional recurrent disease at the resection margins and stomal site and nodal disease in the neck. Distant metastases only occurred in one in five failures. These data indicate higher local control of the T3 lesions by combined surgery and radiation therapy, but the DSS rates showed no significant difference. More than half of the patients treated only by radiation therapy retained their voice.

TABLE 9.14 Five-Year Actuarial LC and DSS Rates of Supraglottic Carcinoma After RT and Combined RT and Surgery: 1950–1994

	n	LC (%)	DSS (%)
T2 lesions			
RT	252	72	76
SR or RS	47	79	77
		$p = 0.13$	$p = 0.76$
T3 lesions			
RT	230	60	60
SR or RS	140	95	66
		$p = 0.0001$	$p = 0.24$

Tracheal Stoma Recurrence

Tracheal stoma recurrence following laryngectomy is an ominous complication of treatment of laryngeal carcinoma. The incidence averages approximately 5%. The occurrence is often due to extensiveness of the lesion with submucosal extension or lymphatic spread, paratracheal nodal metastases, most commonly found with advanced glottic tumor extending to the subglottic area, subglottic carcinoma, or extensive carcinoma of the supraglottis and pyriform sinus.

It has been postulated that the incidence of tracheal stoma recurrence following preliminary emergency tracheostomy was increased in patients with laryngeal stridor. The increase is probably due to the extensiveness of the lesion with paratracheal nodal metastases rather than prelaryngectomy tracheostomy per se. Likewise, the development is unlikely to be due to tumor implant at the time of surgery. It is remarkable to note that tracheal stoma recurrence rarely occurs following elective tracheostomy for composite resection for cancer of the oral cavity or oropharynx; whereas constant contamination of the tracheostomy site by tumor cells during intubation occurs, in spite of the propensity for tumor seeding in some other sites.

Distinction must be made between recurrence at the tracheal stoma ring or adjacent to but not involving the ring. The latter may be localized and radiocurable; the former is not.

In general, treatment of stomal ring recurrence is unsatisfactory with extremely poor local control either by surgery or radiation therapy. Most failures are due to inability to achieve local control and/or due to distant metastases in the mediastinum and lungs. Only a few patients were salvaged by combined surgery and radiation therapy.

The most important concept for treatment of stomal recurrence is its prevention. Patients with extensive laryngeal or pyriform sinus carcinoma with subglottic extension treated by laryngectomy would benefit from a course of postoperative radiation therapy to the neck and stoma with a dose of 55 Gy. For the past 20 years very few patients have developed this complication after laryngeal surgery.

C. CARCINOMA OF THE SUBGLOTTIS

Malignant tumors arising de novo from the subglottic region are rare—averaging 1–2% of all laryngeal cancers. Most so-called subglottic lesions are extensions of lesions from the glottis. Subglottic lesions are relatively asymptomatic in their early stage and are commonly situated in the anterior half of the subglottis as a submucosal tumefaction without obvious ulceration. Because of the narrow and relatively rigid subglottic space, tumor arising in the subglottis is often heralded by airway obstruction and laryngeal stridor. Over one-third of the patients required emergency tracheotomy. Extensive tumor may secondarily involve the true vocal cord, resulting in hoarseness of voice and vocal cord fixation. Most lesions, when diagnosed, are often extensive and far advanced and may invade the adjacent thyroid cartilage. The arytenoid cartilage is rarely involved. The lymphatics of the subglottic area originate in the undersurface of the true vocal cords. The lymphatic trunk pierces the cricothyroid membrane and terminates in the lower deep jugular chain and/or Delphian (prelaryngeal) nodes, as shown in Figure 9.13. Drainage proceeds to the pretracheal, supraclavicular, and paratracheal nodes. Other lymphatic drainage proceeds posterolaterally through the cricotracheal membrane to paratracheal and superior mediastinum.

The incidence of lymph node metastases varies from 5% to 20%.[16,57,58] When the subglottis is involved by glottic carcinoma, the incidence of metastases ranged from 5% to 19%.[58]

SELECTION OF THERAPY

Since most lesions are diagnosed initially with laryngeal stridor and dyspnea requiring emergency tracheostomy,[58] the patients are best dealt with by laryngectomy first followed by postoperative radiation therapy. The early lesions, T1 and T2, though rare in occurrence, can be treated successfully by radiation therapy alone,[6,15] with preservation of normal voice; surgery is reserved for failure.

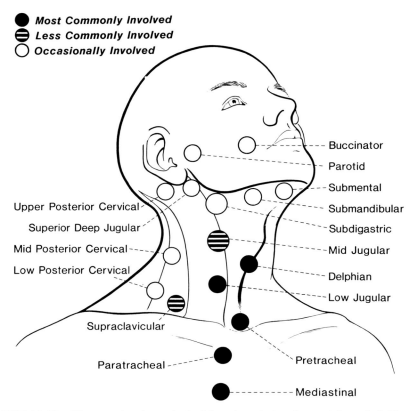

● *Most Commonly Involved*
⊜ *Less Commonly Involved*
○ *Occasionally Involved*

Upper Posterior Cervical
Superior Deep Jugular
Mid Posterior Cervical
Low Posterior Cervical

Supraclavicular

Paratracheal

Buccinator
Parotid
Submental
Submandibular
Subdigastric
Mid Jugular
Delphian
Low Jugular

Pretracheal

Mediastinal

FIGURE 9.13 Diagram showing principal lymph node involvement for subglottic carcinoma.

RADIOTHERAPEUTIC MANAGEMENT

Radiation therapy for subglottic carcinoma should include the primary site, the inferior jugular and supraclavicular nodes, the upper trachea, and the upper mediastinum. This can best be achieved by the so-called mini-mantle technique using high-energy radiation therapy, for example, 10 MV x-rays. After 45 Gy, the portals are reduced to spare the spinal cord and the larynx and upper trachea are irradiated through lateral boost portals for an additional dose up to a total of 65 Gy. An evaluation of the primary lesion after radiation therapy must be made by careful radiographic examination as well as by direct laryngoscopy. Any residual nodes are treated by neck dissection after the primary lesion is controlled.

RADIOTHERAPEUTIC RESULTS

Information related to radiation therapy results for subglottic cancer is sparse due to the rarity of the disease. Generally, the local control is not as good as glottic carcinoma, with local control rates ranging from 40% to 60%.[58-60] Most failures are due to local recurrence with high incidence of distant metastases, mostly to the bone, lung, and mediastinum.

MGH EXPERIENCE

Subglottic carcinoma is an extremely rare disease. Only four patients with this diagnosis were treated by radiation therapy in the past 25 years. Two patients were treated definitively by radiation therapy and two received preoperative radiation therapy followed by laryngectomy. All four were NED and three of the four were females. Of this group, one had T1N0, two had T2N0, and one had T3N1 lesions. No meaningful local control and survival data are available.

SUMMARY

Radiation therapy, surgery, and a combination of the two procedures remain the principal treatment of laryngeal carcinoma. The current concept maintains that radiation therapy failures, often due to uncontrolled primary disease, can be successfully salvaged in a high percentage of incidence. On the other hand, surgical failures are primarily the result of peripheral recurrence, that is, in the base of the tongue or tracheal stoma, and/or in the neck and are rarely amenable to treatment by further surgery and are not salvageable by radiation therapy. The choice between radiation therapy and surgery is determined largely by mobility of the involved structures, degree of invasion of underlying muscle or cartilage, as well as to a lesser extent, by the vertical mucosal extension of the tumor.

For glottic lesions with normal cord mobility, T1 and T2a, radiation therapy is preferred and achieves high local control. On the other hand, if mobility of the involved cord becomes impaired (T2b) or completely fixed (T3), the prognosis for such lesions is guarded following conventional radiation therapy. At the present time, such lesions are treated by BID radiation therapy with improved local control. If the patient opts for radiation therapy first, total laryngectomy may be reserved for radiation failure.

For the small, exophytic supraglottic carcinoma without node involvement,T1N0 and T2N0 lesions, radiation therapy is curative. For early T3 tumors, a trial course of radiation therapy may be attempted and surgery is then reserved for radiation failure. For the large, extensive, or deeply infiltrative T3 and T4 lesions with extensive nodal disease, a planned program of combined therapies including multidrug, multicycle chemotherapy, radical surgery, and postoperative radiation therapy is advised.

Tracheal stoma irradiation should be part of the integrated postoperative radiation therapy procedure for the management of advanced laryngeal carcinoma. Its routine use has practically eliminated stomal recurrence.

Subglottic carcinoma is a most unusual form of laryngeal cancer. The early lesions can be and have been controlled by radiation therapy alone, however.[61] If the lesions are extensive with laryngeal stridor, requiring emergency laryngectomy, postoperative radiation therapy to the low neck, tracheal stoma, upper trachea, and mediastinum is indicated as an adjuvant procedure to prevent stomal recurrence.

The management of laryngeal carcinoma is complex and calls for intimate cooperation among the surgeon, radiation oncologist, and medical oncologist. The primary aim is to eradicate the cancer with maximal preservation of the larynx with useful voice. For the past 16 years, a hyperfractionated accelerated radiation therapy program has been used at the MGH, showing improved local control of advanced laryngeal cancers with preservation of patients' larynges and voices without sacrificing survival. The results thus far are gratifying.

REFERENCES

1. *CA Cancer Clin* Jan/Feb, 1995;45:12–13.
2. Rothman KJ: Epidemiology of head and neck cancer. *Laryngoscope* 1978;88:435–438.
3. Saunders WH: The larynx. *Clin Symp* 1964;16(3):67–99.
4. Last RJ: *Anatomy—regional and applied.* Boston: Little, Brown, 1954.
5. Paff GH: *Anatomy of the head and neck.* Philadelphia: Saunders, 1973.
6. Lederman M: Cancer of the larynx. I: Natural history in relation to treatment. *Br J Radiol* 1971;44:569–578.
7. Biller HF, Ogura JJ, Pratt L: Hemilaryngectomy for T2 glottic cancers. *Arch Otolaryngol* 1971;93:238–243.
8. Goepfert H, Jesse RH, Fletcher GH, et al: Optimal treatment for technically resectable squamous cell carcinoma of the supraglottic larynx. *Laryngoscope* 1975;85:14–32.
9. Batsakis JG: *Tumors of the head and neck,* 2nd ed. Baltimore: Williams & Wilkins, 1979.
10. American Joint Committee on Cancer Staging. *Manual for staging of cancer,* 4th ed. Philadelphia: Lippincott, 1992.
11. Kirchner JA, Cornog JL, Holmes RE: Transglottic cancer: its growth and spread within the larynx. *Arch Otolaryngol* 1974;99:247–251.
12. Jing BS: Roentgen examination of laryngeal cancer: a critical evaluation. In: Alberti PW, Bryce DP, eds. *Workshops from the Centennial Conference on Laryngeal Cancer.* New York: Appleton-Century-Crofts, 1976;232–241.
13. Wang CC: Factors influencing the success of radiation therapy for T2 and T3 glottic carcinoma. Importance of cord mobility and sex. *Am J Clin Oncol* 1986;9:517–520.
14. Kirchner JA: Staging as seen in serial sections. *Laryngoscope* 1975;85:1816–1821.
15. Kirchner JA, Owen JR: Five hundred cancers of the larynx and pyriform sinus. Results of treatment of radiation and surgery. *Laryngoscope* 1977;87:1288–1303.
16. Lederman M: Radiotherapy of cancer of the larynx. *J Laryngol Otol* 1970;84:867–896.
17. Jakobsson PA: Histologic grading of malignancy and prognosis in glottic carcinoma of the larynx. In: Alberti PW, Bryce DP, eds. *Workshops from the Centennial Conference on Laryngeal Cancer.* New York: Appleton-Century-Crofts, 1976;847–854.
18. Leroux-Robert J IV: A statistical study of 620 laryngeal carcinomas of the glottic region personally operated upon more than five years ago. *Laryngoscope* 1975;85:1440–1452.

19. Daly CJ, Strong EW: Carcinoma of the glottic larynx. *Am J Surg* 1975;130:489–492.

20. Bataini JP, Ennuyer A, Poncet P, et al: Treatment of supraglottic cancer by radical high dose radiotherapy. *Cancer* 1974;33:1253–1262.

21. Ogura JH, Marks JE, Freeman RB: Results of conservation surgery for cancers of the supraglottis and pyriform sinus. *Laryngoscope* 1980;90:591–600.

22. Ogura JH, Sessions DG, Spector GJ: Conservation surgery for epidermoid carcinoma of the supraglottic larynx. *Laryngoscope* 1975;85:1808–1815.

23. Strong MS: Laser excision of carcinoma of the larynx. *Laryngoscope* 1975;85: 1286–1289.

24. Harwood AR, Beale FA, Cumming BJ, et al: T3 glottic cancer: an analysis of dose–time–volume factors. *Int J Radiat Oncol Biol Phys* 1980;6:675–680.

25. Hawkins NV: The treatment of glottic carcinoma: an analysis of 800 cases. *Laryngoscope* 1975;85:1485–1493.

26. Lillie J, DeSanto L: Transoral surgery of early cordal carcinoma. *Trans Am Acad Ophthal Otolaryngol* 1973;77:92–96.

27. Bryce D: The management of carcinoma-in-situ and microinvasive carcinoma of the larynx. In: Bailey B, Biuer HF, eds. *Surgery of the larynx*. Philadelphia: Saunders, 1985; 229–242.

28. Wetmore S, Key M, Suen J: Laser therapy for T1 glottic carcinoma of the larynx. *Arch Otolaryngol Head Neck Surg* 1986;112:853–855.

29. Foote RL, Grado GL, Buskirk SJ, et al: Radiation therapy for glottic cancer using 6-MV photon. *Cancer* 1996;77(2):381–386.

30. Schwaibold F, Scariato A, Nunno M, et al: The effect of fraction size on control of early glottic cancer. *Int J Radiat Oncol Biol Phys* 1988;14:451–454.

31. Kim RY, Marks ME, Salter MM: Early stage glottic cancer: importance of dose fractionation in radiation therapy. *Radiology* 1990;182:273–275.

32. Wang CC: Treatment of glottic carcinoma by megavoltage radiation: therapy and results. *Am J Roentgenol Radium Ther Nucl Med* 1974;120:157–163.

33. Mendenhall WM, Parsons JT, Million RR, et al: T1–2 squamous cell carcinoma of the glottic larynx treated with radiation therapy: relationship of dose-fractionation factors to local control and complications. *Int J Radiat Oncol Biol Phys* 1988;15:1267–1273.

34. Woodhouse RJ, Quivey JM, Fu KK, et al: Treatment of carcinoma of the vocal cord: a review of 20 years experience. *Laryngoscope* 1981;91:1155–1162.

35. Fletcher GH, Jesse RH, Lindberg RD, et al: The place of radiotherapy in the management of the squamous cell carcinoma of the supraglottic larynx. *Am J Roentgenol* 1970; 108:19–26.

36. Kagan AR, Calcaterra T, Ward P, et al: Significance of edema of the endolarynx following curative irradiation for carcinoma. *Am J Roentgenol* 1974;120:169–172.

37. Coates HL, DeSanto LW, Devine KD, et al: Carcinoma of the supraglottic larynx: a review of 221 cases. *Arch Otolaryngol* 1976;102:686–689.

38. Hansen HS: Supraglottic carcinoma of the aryepiglottic fold. *Laryngoscope* 1975;85:1667–1681.

39. Cachin Y: Supraglottic carcinomas: the early cases. *Laryngoscope* 1975;85:1617–1623.

40. Shah JP, Tollefsen HR: Epidermoid carcinoma of the supraglottic larynx. Role of neck dissetion in initial surgical treatment. *Am J Surg* 1974;128:494–499.

41. Jankovic I, Merkas Z: Radiotherapy as the primary approach in the treatment of laryngeal cancer. In: Alberti PW, Bryce DP, eds. *Workshops from the Centennial Conference on Laryngeal Cancer.* New York: Appleton-Century-Crofts, 1976; 881–888.

42. McGavran MH, Bauer WC, Ogura JH: The incidence of cervical lymph node metastases from epidermoid carcinoma of the larynx and their relationship to certain characteristics of the primary tumor. A study based on the clinical and pathological findings for 96 patients treated by primary en bloc laryngectomy and radical neck dissection. *Cancer* 1961;14:55.

43. Skolnik EM, Yee KF, Friedman M, Golden TA: The posterior triangle in radical neck surgery. *Arch Otolaryngol* 1976;102:1–4.

44. Flynn MB, Jesse RH, Lindberg RD: Surgery and irradiation in the treatment of squamous cell cancer of the supraglottic larynx. *Am J Surg* 1972;124:477–481.

45. Fletcher GH, Lindberg RD, Hamberger A, et al: Reasons for irradiation failure in squamous cell carcinoma of the larynx. *Laryngoscope* 1975;85:987–1003.

46. Wang CC: Megavoltage radiation therapy for supraglottic carcinoma: result of treatment. *Radiology* 1973;109:183–186.

47. Taskinen PJ: The early case of supraglottic carcinoma. *Laryngoscope* 1975;85: 1643–1649.

48. Reddi RP, Mercado R Jr: Low-dose preoperative radiation therapy in carcinoma of the supraglottic larynx. *Radiology* 1979;130:469–471.

49. Wang CC, Schulz MD, Miller D: Combined radiation therapy and surgery for carcinoma of the supraglottis and pyriform sinus. *Am J Surg* 1972;124:551–554.

50. Weems DH, Mendenhall WM, Parsons JT, Cassisi NJ, Million RR: Squamous cell carcinoma of the supraglottic larynx treated with surgery and/or radiation therapy. *Int J Radiat Oncol Biol Phys* 1987;13:1483–1487.

51. Goldman JL, Zak FG, Roffman JD, et al: High dosage preoperative radiation and surgery for carcinoma of the larynx and laryngopharynx. *Ann Otol Rhinol Laryngol* 1972;81:488–495.

52. Fu KK, Eisenberg L, Dedo HH, et al: Results of integrated managements of supraglottic carcinoma. *Cancer* 1977;40:2874–2881.

53. Ghossein A, Bataini JP, Ennuyer A, et al: Local control and site of failure in radically irradiated supraglottic cancer. *Radiology* 1974;112:187–192.

54. Kumar PP, Good RR, Epstein BE, Yonkers AJ, Ogreen FP, Moore GF: Outcome of locally advanced stage III and IV head and neck cancer treated by surgery and postoperative external beam radiotherapy. *Laryngoscope* 1987;97:615–620.

55. Wang, CC, Suit HD, Blitzer PH: Twice-a-day radiation therapy for supraglottic carcinoma. *Int J Radiat Oncol Biol Phys* 1986;12:3–7.

56. Wendt CD, Peters LJ, Ang KK, et al: Hyperfractionated radiotherapy in the treatment of squamous cell carcinomas of the supraglottic larynx. *Int J Radiat Oncol Biol Phys* 1989;17:1057–1062.

57. Pietrantoni L, Agazzi C, Fior R: Indications for surgical treatment of cervical lymph nodes in cancer of the larynx and hypopharynx. *Laryngoscope* 1962;72:1511.

58. Stell PM, Tobin KE: The behavior of cancer affecting the subglottic space. In: Alberti PW, Bryce DP, eds. *Workshops from the Centennial Conference on Laryngeal Cancer.* New York: Appleton-Century-Crofts, 1976;620–625.

59. Vermund H: Role of radiotherapy in cancer of the larynx as related to the TNM system of staging. A review. *Cancer* 1970;25:485–504.

60. Harrison DFN: The pathology and management of subglottic cancer. *Ann Otol Rhinol Laryngol* 1971;80:6–12.

61. Goellner JR, Devine KD, Weiland LH: Pseudosarcoma of the larynx. *Am J Clin Pathol* 1973;59:312–326.

CHAPTER 10

CARCINOMA OF THE NASOPHARYNX

Anatomically, the nasopharynx is a cubical chamber that has four walls. The superior and posterior walls are bordered by the base of the skull and floor of the sphenoid sinus, sloping downward and backward continuously to the second cervical vertebra at the level of the uvula. The anterior wall communicates with the choanae divided by the nasal septum. The lateral walls are perforated by the cartilaginous portion of the eustachian tube, which enters the nasopharynx through the sinus of Morgagni. The latter is a gap between the uppermost fibers of the superior pharyngeal constrictor muscle and the base of the skull. The gap is closed by a fascia known as the pharyngobasilar fascia, which is attached to the base of the skull superiorly and passes inferiorly deep to the constrictor muscles. The raised anterior portion of the cartilaginous portion of the eustachian tube is termed the torus tubarius, lying posteriorly to the eustachian tube orifice. The lateral nasopharyngeal recess or the fossa of Rosenmüller lies posterosuperiorly to the torus. The inferior wall of the nasopharynx is the dorsal surface of the soft palate and its posterior portion opens into the oropharynx at the isthmus.

Figure 10.1 shows the relative positions of various structures of the nasopharynx as seen in the lateral view. Figures 10.2a and 10.2b demonstrate the important parts as seen by CT scans in axial and coronal projections, respectively.

The nasopharyngeal structures are supported by the pharyngobasilar fascia, which is continuous with the foramen lacerum and in close proximity with the eustachian tube and foramina in the base of the skull, including the ovale, spinosum, carotid, jugular, and hypoglossal,[1] which provide routes of direct tumor intracranial extension and access to the carotid canal, middle ear, and petro-occipital suture. Other routes of tumor spread may occur into the nasal cavity anteriorly and the oropharynx posteriorly.

The superior and lateral walls of the nasopharynx are lined by respiratory cili-

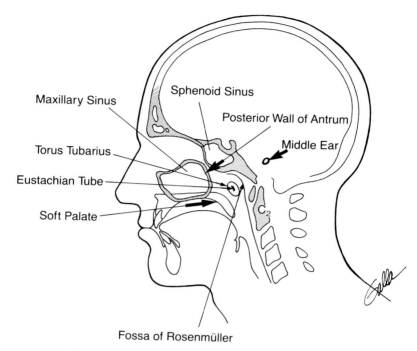

Fossa of Rosenmüller

FIGURE 10.1 Diagram showing various anatomic structures adjacent to the nasopharynx. Note position of fossa of Rosenmüller, torus tubarius, and eustachian tube.

ated pseudostratified epithelium, and the posterior wall is lined by stratified squamous epithelium.

Owing to the rich lymphatic supply, carcinoma of the nasopharynx is notoriously known to have a high incidence of regional cervical lymph node metastases: 70–90% of patients will have developed metastatic nodes during the course of the disease and of these 30–50% are bilateral.[2,3] The first echelon of nodes to be involved are the deep upper jugular, subdigastric, posterior cervical, and retropharyngeal nodes, as shown in Figure 10.3. The uppermost node in the lateral group situated at the skull base is known as Rouviere's node.[2,3] The submandibular and submental nodes are rarely involved and therefore these nodes need not be included during elective irradiation.

In order to assess and evaluate the extent and location of the tumor spread, a basic review of various clinical nerves is highly desirable. Table 10.1 shows various anatomic cavities or foramina of the base of the skull through which the cranial nerves traverse.

Squamous cell carcinoma is the most common malignant tumor and includes a large variety of histologic cell types ranging from undifferentiated carcinomas, to well differentiated keratinizing and nonkeratinizing squamous cell carcinomas, including transitional cell carcinoma to undifferentiated carcinoma. The latter includes lymphoepithelioma, so-called Schmincke's or Regaud's tumor, which is

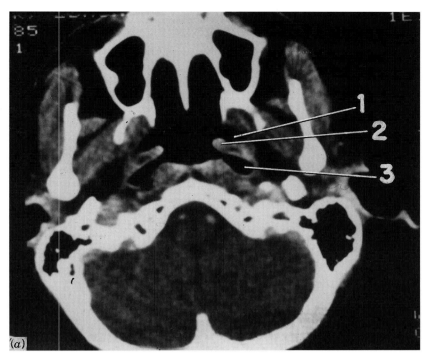

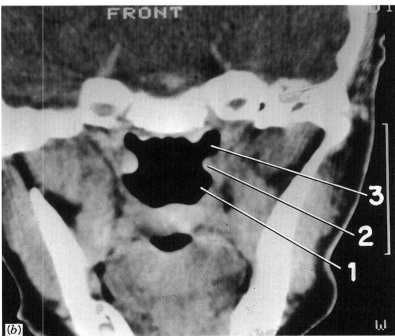

FIGURE 10.2 Computed tomography scan of the nasopharynx in (a) axial view and (b) coronal view, showing (1) eustachian tube opening, (2) torus tubearius, and (3) fossa of Rosenmüller.

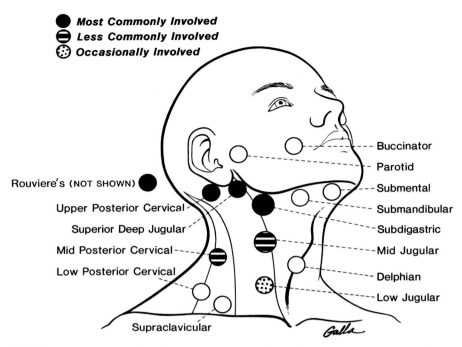

FIGURE 10.3 Diagram showing important group of lymph nodes involved by nasopharyngeal carcinoma.

TABLE 10.1 Exit Sites of Cranial Nerves from Skull[a]

	Cranial Nerve	Exit Site
I	Offactory	Cribriform plate of ethmoid bone
II	Optic	Optic canal
III	Oculomotor	Superior orbital fissure
IV	Trochlear	Superior orbital fissure
V	Opthalmic division	Superior orbital fissure
	Maxillary division	Foramen rotundum
	Mandibular division	Foramen ovale
VI	Abducens	Superior orbital fissure
VII	Facial	Stylomastoid foramen
VIII	Auditory	Confined to petrous portion of temporal bone
IX	Glossopharyngeal	Jugular foramen
X	Vagus	Jugular foramen
XI	Accessory	Jugular foramen
XII	Hypoglossal	Hypoglossal canal

[a]The middle meningeal artery passes through the foramen spinosum. No major nerves or blood vessels pass through the foramen lacerum. Since the roof of the fossa of Rosenmüller is closely related to the foramen lacerum, tumor arising from this site has ready entry into the cranial cavity.

composed of squamous cell carcinoma accompanied by lymphoid infiltration. The lymphoid component of this tumor is benign, but the epithelial element is malignant, and such lesion can also be diagnosed even in metastatic nodes. The pattern of spread may be different. In general, lymphoepitheliomas are likely to metastasize to the bones, lungs, and liver, whereas keratinizing squamous cell carcinomas tend to be localized, with invasion of the surrounding structures.

The World Health Organization (WHO) classification of nasopharyngeal carcinoma (NPC) is as follows[4]:

Type 1   Well to moderately differentiated carcinoma with obvious keratin production
Type 2   Nonkeratinizing carcinoma, including transitional carcinoma
Type 3   Undifferentiated carcinoma, including lymphoepithelioma, with anaplastic, clear cell, and spindle cell variants

Carcinoma of the nasopharynx is a common malignant tumor among the Chinese in southern China.[5] It has been shown to be associated with high titers of antibody to Epstein–Barr virus, particularly for the lymphoepitheliomatous cell type.[6-8]

Carcinoma of the nasopharynx frequently presents as a painless swelling in the neck. It is not surprising that this lesion, in addition to those of the tonsil, base of tongue, supraglottis, and pyriform sinus, is responsible for a large number of so-called unknown primaries with metastatic nodes in the neck.

Various patterns of spread may develop various symptoms and signs in patients with NPC[2,9-12] and these are presented in Table 10.2.

The nerves most commonly involved by nasopharyngeal carcinoma are the fifth and the sixth (16% and 14%, respectively), followed by the third, fourth, tenth, and eleventh cranial nerves. Various neurologic syndromes have been recognized and may provide valuable clues as to the location of the lesion and these are listed in Table 10.3.

Other symptoms may be periorbital pain or pain distributed over the cutaneous territory of the fifth cranial nerve; unilateral anesthesia of the tongue, floor of the

TABLE 10.2   Symptoms and Signs of NPC

Cervical	Mass in the neck, 30–50%
Otic	Unilateral hypoacusis or otitis media, 40%
Nasal	Nasal obstruction, epistaxis, difficult breathing, or nasal twang in speech, 30%
Ophthalmic	Loss of sight, corneal reflex, palpebral ptosis, fixation of the eyeball, or isolated paralysis of ocular muscles
Neurologic	Various cranial nerves affected either by direct tumor extension into the base of the skull or into the intracranial cavity or by compression of cranial nerves from retropharyngeal lymph node metastases, 15–30%

TABLE 10.3 Syndromes Resulting from Cranial Nerve Involvement of Nasopharyngeal Carcinoma

Syndrome	Mode of Tumor Spread	Cranial Nerve												Cervical Sympathetic Nerve
		I	II	III	IV	V	VI	VII	VIII	IX	X	XI	XII	
Jacod's syndrome (petrosphenoid)	Compression from direct tumor spread		X	X	X	X	X							
St. Villaret's syndrome (retroparotid space)	Compression from metastasis to retropharyngeal lymph nodes (Rouviere's node)									X	X	X	X	X
Jackson's syndrome	Metastasis to lymph nodes in base of skull											X	X	
Vernet's syndrome (jugular foramen)	Metastasis to lymph nodes in base of skull									X	X	X		
Collet–Sicard syndrome	Metastasis to lymph nodes in base of skull									X	X	X	X	
Horner's syndrome	Metastasis to lymph nodes in base of skull													X

Source: Modified from Ackerman LV, del Regato JA: *Cancer,* 3rd ed. St Louis: CV Mosby, 1962.

mouth, soft palate, or buccal mucosa; and muscular atrophy and paralysis of the pterygoid, masseter, trapezius, and sternomastoid muscles.

Careful diagnostic work-up prior to definitive radiation therapy is essential and should include inspection by indirect and direct nasopharyngoscopy, including fiberoptiscopy, and palpation of the primary site and the neck. Radiographic studies are most important to determine the extent of the lesion. CT and MR scans[13] in coronal and sagittal projections are most useful in definition of skull base erosion and destruction; cervical node status is best determined by CT, white parapharyngeal tumor extension and CSF space and cavernous sinus involvement can be determined by MRI. The incidence of skull base involvement at diagnosis is approximately 25–30%.

Tumor staging of carcinoma of the nasopharynx, as recommended by the American Committee on Cancer Staging in 1992, is as follows[14]:

T1	Tumor limited to one subsite of nasopharynx
T2	Tumor invades more than one subsite of nasopharynx
T3	Tumor invades nasal cavity or oropharynx
T4	Tumor invades skull or cranial nerve(s)

SELECTION OF THERAPY

Because of the inaccessible location of the nasopharnx and lack of clean resection margins and mode of spread of the disease, surgical resection of a primary lesion is rarely successful. Routine radical neck dissection is likewise seldom effective, because (1) metastasis to lymph nodes frequently is extensive and bilateral and, with few exceptions, most of these nodes are radiosensitive and often radiocurable; (2) the commonly involved Rouviere's node cannot be surgically removed and accounts for most recurrences in the base of the skull; and (3) the patients with extensive metastatic lymph nodes in the neck are highly prone to develop distant metastases. Radiation therapy is therefore considered the most viable treatment for regional and local control of this disease.

However, in highly selected patients, limited neck dissection may be carried out for residual lymph node disease after a course of radical radiation therapy and after the primary lesion is controlled.

RADIOTHERAPEUTIC MANAGEMENT

Because of the many vital structures surrounding the nasopharynx, treatment with radiation therapy calls for careful, well-planned techniques. Recent approaches with particle radiation and three-dimensional (3-D) treatment planning are emerging rapidly in hope of improved local control.[15,16] Because of the high incidence of overt and occult cervical lymph node metastasis, irrespective of T stage, the treatment of carcinomas of the nasopharynx must be directed to both the primary lesion and the neck, even in patients without palpable nodal disease. Radiation therapy with large opposing lateral portals to include the nasopharynx and whole neck en bloc from the base of the brain to the supraclavicular fossae for the entire course of treatment to 70–75 Gy is dangerous and should be discouraged because of the possibility of major, irreversible radiation therapy complications involving the soft tissues, jaw, temporal lobes of the brain, and spinal cord.[17–19,21,22]

The primary lesion and the base of the skull, sphenoid sinuses, cavernous sinuses, eustachian tubes, middle ears, posterior nasal cavity, and upper neck, as shown in Figure 10.4, are treated in continuity, first through opposed lateral portals. A special cutout made with Cerrobend material is used to shape the irradiated portal for maximum shielding of normal structures such as the pituitary gland, eyes,

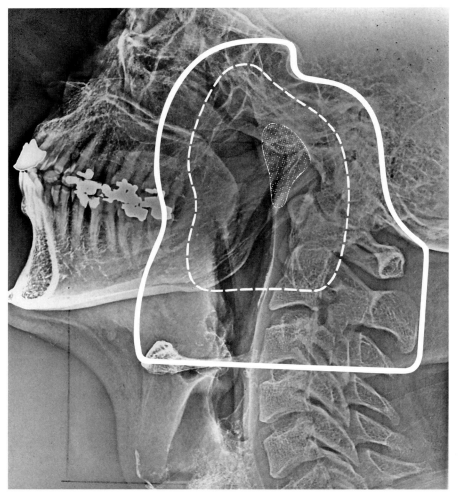

FIGURE 10.4 Radiograph showing placement of comprehensive portal for the primary site and bilateral neck for treatment of carcinoma of the nasopharynx. Dashed-line circle identifies "off cord" portal for boosting dose to the primary site.

oral tongue, anterior mandible, and submental and submandibular glands. With conventional fractionation, when a dose of 45 Gy is reached, the primary lesion is boosted separately by a 270° arc or two anterior infraorbital oblique portals to an additional 25 Gy over 2.5 weeks, making a total dose to the primary up to 70 Gy; the neck lymph nodes, including the subdigastric and submastoid nodes, are treated through anterior and posterior portals with midline spinal cord block to a combined dose of approximately 60–65 Gy to the upper neck and 50 Gy to the lower neck and supraclavicular areas (Figure 10.5). The spinal cord and base of the brain, middle ears, temporal lobes, and temporomandibular joints are excluded from further

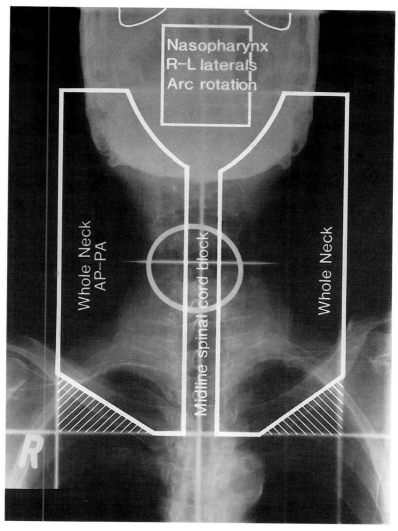

FIGURE 10.5 Simulation film showing placement of nasopharyngeal portal for "cone down" arc rotation. The bilateral neck is treated by split fields.

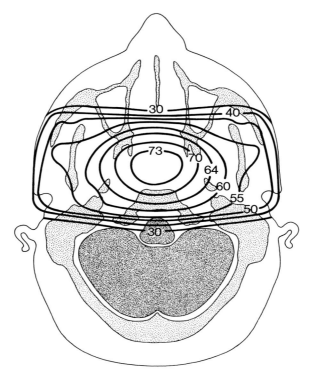

FIGURE 10.6 Composite isodoses at the level of the nasopharynx after 45 Gy delivered by opposed lateral portals, arc rotation of 20 Gy, and 7 Gy intracavitary implant.

radiation therapy, and the dose to these structures is limited to approximately 50–55 Gy. After this procedure is completed, the primary lesion in the nasopharynx is boosted by an intracavitary isotope implant for an additional 6–7 Gy. Figures 10.6, 10.7, and 10.8 show the composite isodoses of radiation therapy at the primary site and midneck and supraclavicular level. For lesions invading the base of the skull or extending into the cranial cavity (T4) an intracavitary implant is not advisable, and the dose to the nasopharynx is carried to 72–75 Gy through an external beam technique. Table 10.4 summarizes the doses currently used at the MGH to various sites in the treatment of carcinoma of the nasopharynx.

Since lymphoepithelioma represents a variant of undifferentiated squamous cell carcinoma, there is no allowance for adjustment of radiation dose, although the radiation response may be quite prompt.

Technical Pointers

External Beam Therapy
1. Lead wire the nodes in the neck.
2. Immobilize the head with a face mask and depress the tongue and jaw with a bite block. A lead marker is placed at the outer canthi of the eyes.

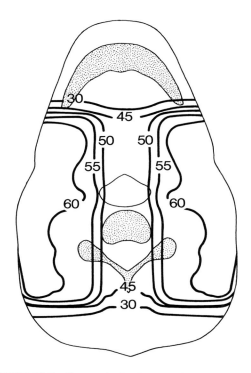

FIGURE 10.7   Composite isodoses at the level of midneck.

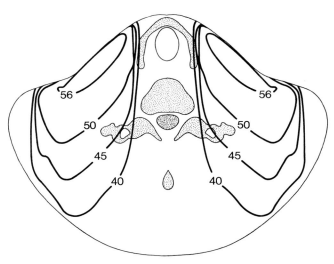

FIGURE 10.8   Composite isodoses at the level of lower neck.

TABLE 10.4 **Doses for Various Sites in Treatment of Carcinoma of the Nasopharynx at MGH**

Site	Opposed Laterals	AP	AP–PA	Arc Rotation	Implant	Total Dose (Gy)
Nasopharynx	38.4			31.6	7	76
Upper neck	38.4[a]		25.6[b]			60 (N0)
Lower neck		43.2[c]		6.8		70 (N1–3)

[a] 1.6 Gy/fraction twice a day.
[b] Additional 5 Gy to bulky nodes.
[c] 1.8 Gy/fraction twice a day.

3. The lateral portals include the external auditory meatus, the base of the skull, and the sphenoid sinus over the floor of the pituitary fossa superiorly; 2 cm from the posterior wall of the maxillary antrum anteriorly; midway between the hyoid and the thyroid notch inferiorly; and the mastoid tip and spinous processes posteriorly.

4. A Cerrobend cutout shields the pituitary gland, optic chiasm, mid- and anterior oral tongue, hard palate, mandible, and submandibular and submental glands.

5. After 45 Gy conventional RT and 38.4 Gy BID RT, off-cord, the pituitary gland, middle ears, and spinal cord are excluded during the boost RT.

6. Use arc rotation to boost the primary tumor through the infraorbital route, sparing both eyes. The head is hyperextended or infraorbital oblique portals are used.

7. Neck disease is treated by anteroposterior–posteroanterior (AP–PA) photons or by appositional electrons to the desired doses.

Intracavitary Nasopharyngeal Brachytherapy

Afterloading intracavitary brachytherapy with cesium-137 or high-dose rate (HDR) [192]Ir sources can be achieved with relative ease. The procedure uses two pediatric endotracheal tubes with inner and outer diameters of 5 mm and 6.8 mm, respectively, each afterloaded with two 20-mg radium-equivalent ^{137}Cs slugs. Figure 10.9 shows the accessories for intracavitary brachytherapy for NPC. After topical anesthesia of the nasal and nasopharyngeal mucosa using cocaine and mild analgesics, endotracheal tubes are introduced into the nasopharynx via the nares. With fluoroscopic control using a simulator, the distal tip of the dummy slugs are placed at the free edge of the soft palate posteriorly and at the posterior wall of the maxillary sinus anteriorly. The inflated balloon, which is attached to the distal end of the endotracheal tube, is used for anchoring purposes and to create a distance between the radiation sources and the nasopharyngeal vault to gain better depth dose. The dose reference point is 0.5 cm below the vault mucosa at the midline. The isodose distribution to the nasopharynx is shown in Figure 10.10. The entire implant treatment can be performed as an outpatient procedure.

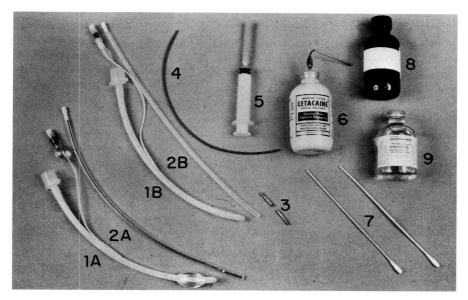

FIGURE 10.9   Diagram shows various items for nasopharyngeal implant: (1A) pediatric endotracheal tube with inflated balloon; (1B) pediatric endotracheal tube with deflated balloon (available commercially); (2A) source carrier with cesium-137 slugs in place; (2B) unloaded source carrier; (3) cesium-137 slugs, 20 mg radium equivalent each, two slugs to be loaded into each pediatric tube; (4) pediatric rubber catheter occasionally used to guide insertion of pediatric tube; (5) 5-cm syringe; (6) Cetacaine spray to anesthetize the oropharyngeal mucosa; (7) cotton swabs; (8) cocaine solution to anesthetize and shrink nasal mucosa prior to insertion of pediatric tubes; and (9) Renografin to fill balloon.

Technical Pointers

A. Intracavitary Implant

1. Use 5% cocaine to shrink the mucous membranes of the nasal cavity.
2. Use meperidine (Demerol) 75 mg and hydroxyzine (Vistaril) 25 mg IM for medication.
3. Hyperextend the chin and head for endotracheal insertion.
4. If the angiocath can not "bend" at the basi-spinal juncture, use the following maneuver, as shown in Figure 10.11.

B. Procedure to Facilitate Insertion of Endotracheal Tube[19]

1. Insert rubber catheter through the nostril into the oral cavity as a guide.
2. Slide pediatric endotracheal tube into the catheter.
3. With the catheter under tension, move the endotracheal tube into the oropharynx.
4. After the endotracheal tube is correctly positioned, retrieve the rubber catheter guide.

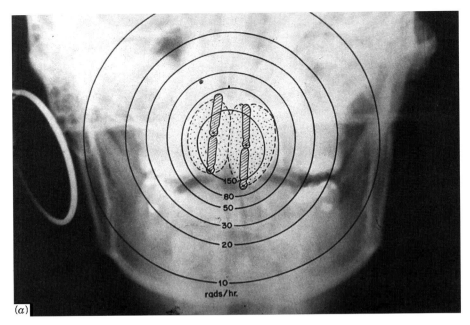

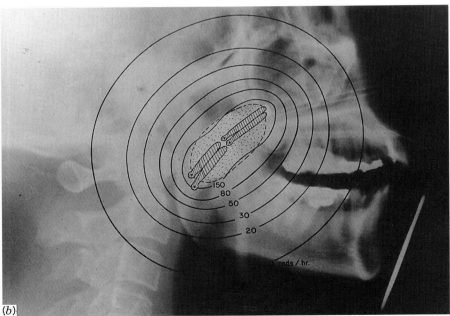

FIGURE 10.10 Simulation film with intracavitary implant in place showing isodose distribution in (a) anteroposterior (AP) projection and (b)lateral projection.

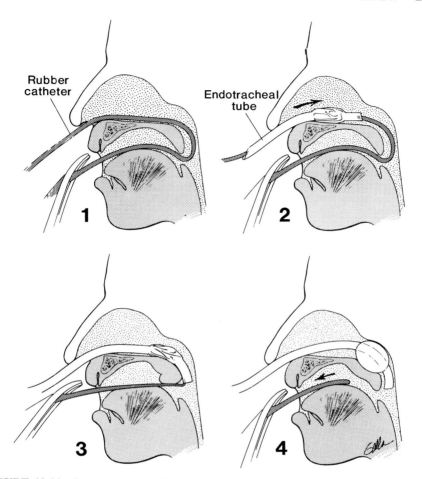

FIGURE 10.11   Procedure to facilitate correct placement of endotracheal tube: (1) insert the rubber catheter through the nostril into the oral cavity as a guide; (2) slide the pediatric tube into the catheter; (3) with the catheter under tension, move the endotracheal tube into the oropharynx; (4) after the endotracheal tube is correctly positioned, inflate the balloon and retrieve the rubber catheter, as shown.

5. Insert dummy sources for simulation and adjustment of position of sources.
6. Inflate each balloon with 4 mL Renografin.

Reirradiation of Recurrent Carcinoma of the Nasopharynx

Retreatment for locally recurrent carcinoma of the nasopharynx at the primary site by a second course of radiation therapy is possible with meticulous technique and can produce good results.[20–25] Although the risk of necrosis is high, it should be accepted for salvage of a seemingly lethal condition. Radiation therapy for most recurrent lesions, if small (T1 or early T2), relies greatly on the use of intracavitary implant in combination with external beam therapy. Therefore it is most important that the patient have nonobstructed nasal passages bilaterally. If the nostril is markedly narrowed by a deviated nasal septum, submucosal resection of the deviated septum should be carried out prior to a definitive course of repeat irradiation. In general, approximately 40 Gy in 4–5 weeks is given through a small 6×5 cm^2 portal by rotational technique, followed by 2–3 fractionated intracavitary implants to deliver an additional 20 Gy. Recurrent cervical metastatic lymph nodes are managed by neck dissection. For extensive recurrences (T4), reirradiation is not curative and the condition is best managed by palliative radiation therapy for symptoms and/or by chemotherapy.

RADIOTHERAPEUTIC RESULTS

The radiotherapeutic results for carcinoma of the nasopharynx are influenced by the extent of the primary tumor and lymph node status, the treatment programs, brachytherapy boost techniques, and others.

For T1–2 lesions, local control rates range from 70% to 90%; for T3 and T4 tumors, the rates are 50–65% and 30–40%, respectively.[26-28]

Survival rates range from 40% to 60%, and the disease-free rate is approximately 55%.[26,28,30-32] Local control rates of metastatic nodes in the neck by radiation therapy are remarkably satisfactory. For N0–1 nodes, local control rates are over 90%. For the N2 neck, the rates range from 80% to 90%, and for N3 disease, the rate is about 50%.[26-29]

Although local control rates in the neck are high, the presence of extensive disease in the neck influences patients' survival. For N0–1 disease, the 5-year survival rates range from 60% to 75%, and for patients with N2–3 nodes, the survival rates drop to 40–50%.[26,33-35]

Carcinoma of the nasopharynx has a propensity for local recurrence,[21,22,36] sometimes 5 or more years after the initial radiation therapy.[20] This has been shown to be related to the radiation dose and occurs in approximately one-third of patients after radiation therapy. Routine supplemental therapy with intracavitary cesium implant as part of the overall treatment program for T1–3 lesions has been found to reduce the incidence of local recurrence.[20]

The results of reirradiation for recurrent NPC vary and generally are not entirely satisfactory. For T1 and T2 locally recurrent carcinoma, the 5-year local control and survival rates are 30–50%;[20,32,34] for extensive recurrence with invasion of the base of the skull and cranial nerve deficits, the rates are approximately 20–25%. Far advanced recurrences after high-dose radiation therapy rarely salvageable by reirradiation.

MGH EXPERIENCE

From 1970 through 1994, 259 patients with squamous cell carcinoma of the nasopharynx received radical radiation therapy. Of this group, 125 received QD and

TABLE 10.5   Five-Year Actuarial LC and DSS Rates After Radiation Therapy: 1970–1994

Stage	n	LC (%)	DSS (%)
T1–2	148	72	65
T3	46	66	58
T4	65	49	42
T3–4	111	56	50
		$p = 0.006$	$p = 0.02$
T1–4	259	65	59
N0	92	62	63
N1	23	63	63
N2–3	144	67	56
		$p = 0.58$	$p = 0.20$

134 BID radiation therapy. Of the 259 patients, 171 were male and 88 were female, with a M:F ratio of 2:1.

Table 10.5 shows the 5-year actuarial rates related to stage of disease. Of the entire group, the local control (LC) and disease-specific survival (DSS) rates were 65% and 59%, respectively. The LC rates for T1, T2, T3, and T4 lesions were 67%, 73%, 66%, and 49%, respectively. The corresponding DSS rates were 63%, 66%, 58%, and 42%. The patients without affected lymph nodes had a 5-year actuarial LC of 62% and DSS of 63% as compared to about 50% for those with N1–3 disease.

The results after once-daily (QD) and twice-daily (BID) radiation therapy are shown in Tables 10.6 and 10.7.

TABLE 10.6   Five-Year Actuarial Rates After QD Radiation Therapy for NPC: MGH Experience, 1970–1994

Stage	n	LC (%)	DSS (%)
T1–2	71	71	60
T3–4	54	47	35
T1–4	125	60	49
N0–1	58	57	52
N2–3	67	64	47

TABLE 10.7   Five-Year Actuarial Rates After BID Radiation Therapy for NPC: MGH Experience, 1979–1994

Stage	n	LC (%)	DSS (%)
T1–2	77	72	70
T3–4	57	65	70
T1–4	134	69	69
N0–1	57	68	76
N2–3	77	68	63

These data indicate some improvement of local control and disease-specific survival after BID RT in the advanced T stages (i.e., T3–4) and nodal disease (i.e., N2–3), as shown in Table 10.8.

TABLE 10.8 Comparing QD and BID Radiation Therapy Results Related to Stages of the Primary and Nodal Status

Stage	LC (%)	DSS (%)
T1–2	p = NS	p = 0.09
T3–4	p = 0.0009	p = 0.0002
T1–4	p = 0.008	p = 0.0001
N0–1	p = NS	p = 0.01
N2–3	p = 0.04	p = 0.003

Squamous cell carcinomas of the nasopharynx are mostly poorly differentiated, and the metastatic lymph nodes in the neck generally are radiosensitive and locally radiocurable. Following a therapeutic dose of radiation therapy, the neck failure rates for N0–1 and N2 necks are 0% and 4%, respectively, and for N2–3 necks, the rate is 19%, as shown in Table 10.9.

Neck Failures and Effects of RND on Patients' Survival: 1970–1994

Metastatic cervical nodes of the squamous cell carcinomas of the nasophargnx are quite radio responsive and often controllable by radiation therapy alone. As shown in Table 10.9, for the N and N2-3 neck, the rates of neck failure after irradiation were 4% and 19% respectively.

TABLE 10.9 Neck Failures After Radiation Therapy Related to Neck Status (Control of Neck Disease), T1–3: 1970–1994

Status	n	Patients with RND	# Patients Died of Neck Disease Only	Total[a]
N0	63	0	0	0%
N1	17	1	0	4%
N2–3	114	14	8	19%

[a]Of 15 Patients with RND, 8 or 53% died with the disease locally and/or distantly.

Although radical neck dissection (RND) is often used for head and neck squamous cell carcinomas, for nasopharyngeal carcinoma it is only indicated for any residual lymph nodes after radical radiation therapy. The efficacy of radical neck dissection is only marginal. Of 114 patients with T1, T2, and T3 with N2–3 lesions, 14 underwent radical neck dissection for positive lymph nodes; only 6 (43%) had no evidence of disease after the surgical procedure. Most patients requiring radical neck dissection had extensive disease and often died of local failure or distant failures. This may indicate that failures to control neck disease carry a rather poor prognosis.

Carcinoma of the nasopharynx tends to develop distant metastases.[37,38] Their incidence is related to the extent of the primary and the status of the neck nodes, increasing with increasing T and N status. Of the entire group of patients, the incidence of distant metastases (DM) was 19.3%, as shown in the Table 10.10. The use of chemotherapy for extensive NPC should be considered.[38]

TABLE 10.10 Incidence of Distant Metastases Related to the Primary Lessions and Nodal Status: 1970–1994

Stage	n	Number with DM	DM (%)
T1	46	6	13
T2	102	20	19.6
T3	46	9	19.5
T4	65	15	23
T1–4	259	50	19.3
N0	92	16	17.3
N1	23	0	0
N2	128	29	22.6
N3	16	5	31
N0–3	259	50	19.3

Another factor affecting local control and survival of patients with nasopharyngeal carcinoma is the historical cell types, shown in Table 10.11. Of 76 patients with a diagnosis of lymphoepithelioma, the 5-year actuarial LC and DSS rates were 79% and 69%, compared with 98 patients with keratinizing squamous cell carcinoma, who had LC and DSS rates of 68% and 68%, respectively. Those with undifferentiated carcinoma had LC and DSS rates of 54% and 41%, respectively, with $p=0.0004$.

TABLE 10.11 Five-Year Actuarial Rates After Radiation Therapy for NPC Related to Cell Types: 1970–1994

Cell Types	n	LC (%)	DSS (%)
Lymphoepithelioma	76	79	69
Squamous cell carcinoma	98	68	68
Undifferentiated carcinoma	51	54	41
		$p=0.0004$	$p=0.0001$

Reirradiation of Recurrent Carcinoma of the Nasopharynx

From 1950 through 1994, 38 patients received reirradiation. The 5-year actuarial rates after high-dose radiation therapy were approximately 40% LC and 59% DSS. Seven patients lived more than 10 years, and of these, three lived more than 20 years, one of whom had no evidence of disease but had radiation complications of central nervous system injuries. For patients with T3 or T4 lesions, the corresponding rates were poor. Those patients in whom tumor recurred 24 months or longer after initial radiation therapy had a better survival rate than those in whom disease recurred in less than 24 months.[20]

Low-dose radiation therapy is rarely effective, and the benefits of palliation are often short-lived (Table 10.12).

TABLE 10.12 Five-Year Actuarial Rates After Reirradiation for Recurrance of NPC and Versus Dose

	n	LC (%)	DSS (%)
1950–1994	38	40	59
Dose			
≥ 60 Gy	30	52	55
< 60 Gy	8	21	71
		$p = 0.31$	$p = 0.33$

Brachytherapy Boost to Nasopharyngeal Carcinoma

Since 1974, afterloading intracavitary implant as a routine procedure to deliver a dose of 7–12 Gy 0.5 cm below the mucosa as a boost to the nasopharynx has been carried out for most T1 and T2 and occasionally T3 lesions.[20] Table 10.13 shows the 5-year actuarial local control (LC) and disease-specific survival (DSS) rates after the boost technique (i.e., brachytherapy versus external beam radiation therapy). For T1 and T2 lesions ($n=146$) the LC and DSS rates after brachytherapy boost were 82% and 78%, compared with 55% and 43%, respectively, for lesions treated with external beam (no brachytherapy) boost. The difference was statistically significant ($p=0.0001$). Twenty patients with T3 lesions who had brachytherapy boost had LC and DSS rates of 74% and 74%, compared with 60% and 46%, respectively, in 26 patients with external beam boost ($p=0.25$). For the entire group T1–3, the LC and DSS rates after brachytherapy boost for 112 patients were 81% and 78%; for 82 patients without brachytherapy boost, the LC and DSS rates were 56% and 44%, respectively, with $p=0.0001$, as shown in Table 10.13.

TABLE 10.13   Five-Year Actuarial Rates After Radiation Therapy for NPC Related to Boost Techniques. Comparison of LC Rates With and Without Brachytherapy: 1970–1994

	n	LC (%)	DSS (%)
T1–2			
Brachytherapy	92	82	78
No brachytherapy	56	55	43
		$p = 0.0001$	$p = 0.0001$
T3			
Brachytherapy	20	74	74
No brachytherapy	26	60	46
		$p = 0.25$	$p = 0.08$
T1–3			
Brachytherapy	112	81	78
No brachytherapy	82	56	44
		$p = 0.0001$	$p = 0.0001$

SUMMARY

Carcinoma of the nasopharynx is uncommon in the United States. Its management is primarily with high-dose, precision radiation therapy. The role of surgery is limited to biopsy of the primary lesion for histologic confirmation and for dealing with residual lymph node disease after radical radiation therapy. Because of the adjacent vital structures, such as the pituitary gland, brain stem, temporal lobes, eyes, optic nerves, and temporomandibular joint, radiation therapy calls for careful treatment planning with multiportal techniques through the use of high-energy radiation or intracavitary implant.

Concurrently, all cervical lymph nodes, including Rouviere's node, should be irradiated electively, even in patients without palpable nodes. Although neck failure alone is uncommon, occasionally residual node disease after radiation therapy can be treated with neck dissection if the primary lesion is controlled.

Nasopharyngeal carcinoma may be considered one of the radiocurable malignant tumors, along with cancer of the skin, larynx, cervix, and uterus. In early lesions, the 5-year survival rate following careful high-dose radiation therapy is high, approximately 80%. Unfortunately, these tumors tend to develop distant metastases. Their incidence is related to the extent of the primary and the status of the neck nodes (i.e., 20% in the MGH series); this certainly affects the overall survival of patients.

The nasopharynx is not easily examined by most physicians, and such early lesions are rarely discovered. Not infrequently, the disease can be diagnosed only after onset of massive adenopathy in the neck or cranial nerve paralysis, and such extensive lesions generally compromise survival.

Bone and cranial nerve involvement do not necessarily preclude the possibility of cure; 40–50% of patients with T4 lesions survived 5 or more years after high-dose radiation therapy, although a few had persistent disease without symptoms. With the advent of twice-daily radiation therapy, the local control rates for nasopharyngeal carcinoma have been further improved, with acceptable late radiation sequelae.

Carcinoma of the nasopharynx is one of the few malignant lesions in the head and neck in which reirradiation can be carried out, with careful technique (combined external radiation therapy and intracavitary implant), with occasional success. Reirradiation dosage must be radical if lasting cure is the aim; low-dose retreatment generally is ineffective.

With the availability of fiberscopes, the nasopharynx can be examined by direct vision, which is much more satisfactory than indirect nasopharyngoscopy. Careful evaluation of the primary lesion affords the physician better insight into the response of the primary lesion and radiation therapy can be better planned. This may, in turn, be associated with improved therapeutic results.

Of the entire group of patients treated primarily with radiation therapy *de novo* initially, none developed serious radiation therapy complications or transverse myelitis. Minor sequelae of radiation therapy, such as xerostomia and dental caries, were common but generally well tolerated by most patients. One patient developed temporary pituitary dysfunction.

REFERENCES

1. Last RJ: *Anatomy—regional and applied.* Boston: Little, Brown, 1954.
2. Lederman M: *Cancer of the nasopharynx: its natural history and treatment.* Springfield, IL: C Thomas, 1961.
3. Rouviere H (Tobias MJ, translator): *Anatomy of the human lymphatic system.* Ann Arbor, MI: JW Edwards, 1938.
4. Shanmugaratnam K: Histopathology of nasopharyngeal carcinoma. Correlations with epidemiology, survival rates and other biological characteristics. *Cancer* 1979;44(3):1029–1044.
5. Teoh TB: Epidermoid carcinoma of the nasopharynx among Chinese: a study of 31 necropsies. *J Pathol Bacteriol* 1957;73:451.
6. Goldman JM, Goodman ML, Miller D: Antibody to Epstein–Barr virus in American patients with carcinoma of the nasopharynx. *JAMA* 1971;216:1618–1622.
7. de-Vathaire F, Sancho-Garnier H, de-The H, et al: Prognostic value of EBV markers in the clinical management of nasopharyngeal carcinoma (NPC): a multicenter follow-up study. *Int J Cancer* 1988;42(2):176–181.
8. Lynn TC, Tu SM, Kawamura A Jr: Long-term follow-up of IgG and IgA antibodies against viral capsid antigens of Epstein–Barr virus in nasopharyngeal carcinoma. *J Laryngol Otol* 1985;99(6):567–572.
9. Ho HC: An epidemiologic and clinical study of nasopharyngeal carcinoma. *Int J Radiat Oncol Biol Phys* 1978;4:181–198.

10. Wang CC, Little JB, Schulz MD: Cancer of the nasopharynx: its clinical and radiotherapeutic considerations. *Cancer* 1962;15:921–926.

11. Godtfredsen E: Ophthalmologic and neurologic symptoms of malignant nasopharyngeal tumors: a clinical study comprising 454 cases; with special reference to histopathology and the possibility of earlier recognition. *Acta Psychiatr Scand (Suppl)* 1944;34:1–323.

12. Perez CA, Devineni VR, Marcial-Vega V, Marks JE, Simpson JR, Kucik N: Carcinoma of the nasopharynx: factors affecting prognosis. *Int J Radiat Oncol Biol Phys* 1992; 23(2):271–280.

13. Dillon WP, Harnsberger HR: The impact of radiologic imaging on staging of cancer of the head and neck. *Semin Oncol* 1991;18:64–79.

14. American Joint Committee on Cancer: *Manual for staging of cancer*, 3rd ed. Philadelphia: Lippincott, 1992.

15. Kutcher GJ, Fuks Z, Brenner H, et al: Three-dimensional photon treatment planning for carcinoma of the nasopharynx. *Int J Radiat Oncol Biol Phys* 1991;21:169–182.

16. Leibel SA, Kutcher GJ, Harrison LB, et al: Improved dose distributions for 3D conformal boost treatments in carcinoma of the nasopharynx. *Int J Radiat Oncol Biol Phys* 1991;20:823–833.

17. Lam KS, Ho JH, Lee AW, et al: Symptomatic hypothalamic-pituitary dysfunction in nasopharyngeal carcinoma patients following radiation therapy: a retrospective study. *Int J Radiat Oncol Biol Phys* 1987;13(9):1343–1350.

18. Lee AW, Law SC, Ng SH, et al: Retrospective analysis of nasopharyngeal carcinoma treated during 1976–1985: late complications following megavoltage irradiation. *Br J Radiol* 1992;65(778):918–928.

19. Wang CC: Improved local control of nasopharyngeal carcinoma after intracavitary brachytherapy boost. *Am J Clin Oncol* 1991;14(1):5–8.

20. Wang CC: Re-irradiation of recurrent nasopharyngeal carcinoma—treatment techniques and results. *Int J Radiat Oncol Biol Phys* 1987;13(7):953–956.

21. Vaeth JM: Radiation therapy of locally recurrent nasopharyngeal cancer. *Radiol Clin North Am* 1964;33:72–76.

22. Feehan PE, Castro JR, Phillips TL, et al: Recurrent locally advanced nasopharyngeal carcinoma treated with heavy charged particle irradiation. *Int J Radiat Oncol Biol Phys* 1992;23(4):881–884.

23. Pryzant RM, Wendt CD, Delclos L, Peters LJ: Re-treatment of nasopharyngeal carcinoma in 53 patients. *Int J Radiat Oncol Biol Phys* 1992;22(5):941–947.

24. Yan JH, Hu YH, Gu XZ: Radiation therapy of recurrent nasopharyngeal carcinoma. Report on 219 patients. *Acta Radiol Oncol* 1983;22(1):23–28.

25. Vikram V: Permanent iodine-125 implants for recurrent carcinoma of the nasopharynx: early results. *Endocurie Hyperth [Oncol]* 1986;2:83–85.

26. Hoppe RT, Goffinet DR, Bagshaw MA: Carcinoma of the nasopharynx: eighteen years' experience with megavoltage radiation therapy. *Cancer* 1976;37:2605–2612.

27. Bedwinek JM, Perez CA, Keys DJ: Analysis of failures after definitive irradiation for epidermoid carcinoma of the nasopharynx. *Cancer* 1980;45:2725–2729.

28. Mesic JB, Fletcher GH, Goepfert H: Megavoltage irradiation of epithelial tumors of the nasopharynx. *Int J Radiat Oncol Biol Phys* 1981;7(4):447–453.

29. Walsh CS, McIntyre JF, Okunieff P, Wang CC: Control of cervical lymph node disease

in carcinoma of the Waldyer's ring: results and complications following twice-a-day radiotherapy. *Int J Radiat Oncol Biol Phys* 1988; 15(suppl 1), abstr.

30. Moench HC, Phillips TL: Carcinoma of the nasopharynx: review of 146 patients with emphasis on radiation dose and time factors. *Am J Surg* 1972;124:515–518.

31. Wang CC, Busse J, Gitterman M: A simple afterloading applicator for intracavitary irradiation for carcinoma of the nasopharynx. *Radiology* 1975;115:737–738.

32. Bailet JW, Mark RJ, Abemayor E, et al: Nasopharyngeal carcinoma: treatment results with primary radiation therapy. Laryngoscope 1992;102(9):965–972.

33. Neel HB: Nasopharyngeal carcinoma: diagnosis, staging, and management. *Oncology* 1992;6(2):87–95.

34. Frezza G, Barbieri E, Emiliani E, Silvano M, Babini L: Patterns of failure in nasopharyngeal cancer treated with megavoltage irradiation. *Radiother Oncol* 1986;5:287–294.

35. Fandi A, Altun M, Azli N, Armand JP, Cvitkovic E: Nasopharyngeal cancer: epidemiology, staging, and treatment. *Semin Oncol* 1994;21:382–397.

36. Fu KK, Newman H, Phillips TL: Treatment of locally recurrent carcinoma of the nasopharynx. *Radiology* 1975;117(2):425–431.

37. Ahmad A, Stefani S: Distant metastases of nasopharyngeal carcinoma: a study of 256 male patients. *J Surg Oncol* 1986;33(3):194–197.

38. Al-Sarraf M, Pajak TF, Cooper JS, Mohiuddin M, Herskovic A, Ager PJ: Chemo-radiotherapy in patients with locally advanced nasopharyngeal carcinoma: a radiation therapy oncology group study. *J Clin Oncol* 1990;8(8):1342–1351.

CHAPTER 11

TUMORS OF THE NASAL CAVITY AND PARANASAL SINUSES

Anatomically, the nasal cavity and paranasal sinuses are complex portions of the head and neck. The ethmoid cells, turbinates, nasal septum, orbits, and maxillary sinuses are closely interrelated and frequently the carcinoma involves multiple sites. These anatomic structures are intricately and closely related, as shown in Figures 11.1a and 11.1b.

The *nasal cavity* is roughly a triangular-shaped space with a narrow roof bordered by the cribriform plate of the ethmoid bone and with a broader floor bordered by the palatine process of the maxillary bones. The cavity is divided by a smooth midline nasal septum. Each lateral wall is bounded by three turbinates and inferiorly by the medial wall of the maxillary sinus and superiorly by the ethmoid sinuses. The nasal cavity is bordered anteriorly by the nasal bones and cartilages of the external nose, columella, and nasal vestibule, while it ends posteriorly at the posterior border of the hard palate and posterior wall of the maxillary antrum, a short distance from the eustachian tube opening at the nasopharynx. The olfactory nerve branches to its receptor cells in the highest part of the nasal cavity; the central processes of the olfactory nerve unite to form bundles of nerve fibers, which penetrate through the cribriform plate to enter the olfactory bulb of the brain. The nasal lacrimal duct drains into the inferior meatus.

The *nasal vestibule* is a pear-shaped dilatation within the aperture of the nostril, bounded laterally by the ala and the lateral crus of the greater alar cartilage, and bounded medially by the medial crus of the same cartilage. The inferior boundary is the intervening portion of the floor of the nose. The squamous epithelium of the skin extends into the vestibule and here has a variable crop of fine hairs. The mucocutaneous junction lies beyond the hair-bearing area.

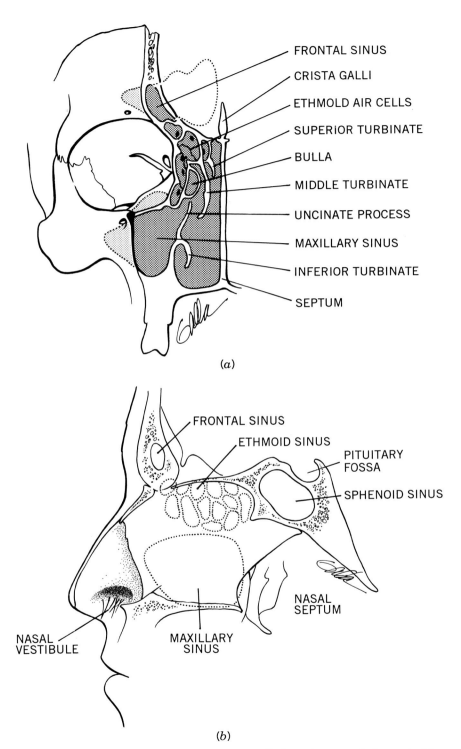

FRONTAL SINUS

CRISTA GALLI

ETHMOLD AIR CELLS

SUPERIOR TURBINATE

BULLA

MIDDLE TURBINATE

UNCINATE PROCESS

MAXILLARY SINUS

INFERIOR TURBINATE

SEPTUM

(a)

FRONTAL SINUS

ETHMOID SINUS

PITUITARY FOSSA

SPHENOID SINUS

NASAL SEPTUM

NASAL VESTIBULE

MAXILLARY SINUS

(b)

FIGURE 11.1 Diagram showing nasal cavity, vestibule, and paranasal sinuses in (a) anteroposterior and (b) lateral view.

ANATOMY OF PARANASAL SINUSES

There are four pairs of hollow cavities scattered in the bones of the skull. The maxillary sinus or antrum of Highmore is the largest. It is roughly pyramidal in shape with the summit of the pyramid pointing toward the malar region. Its anterior wall is the facial surface of the sinus. The posterior wall is intimately related to the infratemporal space and pterygopalatine fossa. The alveolar process of the maxilla forms the floor of the maxillary antrum. The roof makes up most of the orbital floor. The medial wall contributes to the lateral wall of the nasal fossa, often called the antronasal wall, which is divided into two by the insertion of the inferior turbinate. It drains into the middle meatus.

Each ethmoid sinus lies on either side of the nasal cavity and the medial wall of the orbit, being separated by a thin lamina papyracea or "paper plate." Lying anteroposteriorly, there are three groups of ethmoidal air cells—anterior, middle, and posterior—ranging from 3 to 18 cells. The intimate relationships of the ethmoid sinus include the maxillary sinus inferiorly, the nasal fossa medially, the orbit laterally, the optic nerve posteriorly, and the cranial fossa superiorly.

The anterior ethmoid cells drain into the middle meatus, while the middle and posterior ethmoid cells drain into the sphenoethmoidal recess.

The sphenoid sinus lies deep in the head and is related to the nasopharynx inferiorly; the nasal fossa anteriorly; the optic nerve, optic chiasm, and cavernous sinus laterally; and the pituitary gland and the anterior cranial fossa and frontal lobe of the brain superiorly. It drains into the sphenoethmoidal recess.

The frontal sinus lies within the frontal bone and is related to the soft tissues of the forehead anteriorly, the anterior cranial fossa posteriorly, and the orbit inferiorly. It has its separate osteum and drains into the middle meatus.

The paranasal sinuses are lined by ciliated columnar epithelium.

The Lymphatics

The mucosa of the paranasal sinuses and nasal cavity has sparse capillary lymphatics and therefore metastases from carcinoma arising from these tumor sites are uncommon even though lesions are often quite advanced. It is therefore most unusual for a small asymptomatic primary in the paranasal sinus to manifest an occult cervical metastasis. Anatomically, the lymphatics occur in two directions. A small number of lymphatics of the lower anterior nasal mucosa drain to the submandibular and/or parotid nodes and the superior jugular and subdigastric nodes, as shown in Figure 11.2a. The lymphatics of the middle and inferior turbinates and the septum, including the anteroethmoid complex, drain posteriorly toward the nasopharynx, converging at the pretubal plexus just anterior to the eustachian tube opening. From the pretubal plexus, the pattern of spread follows that of the nasopharynx onto the

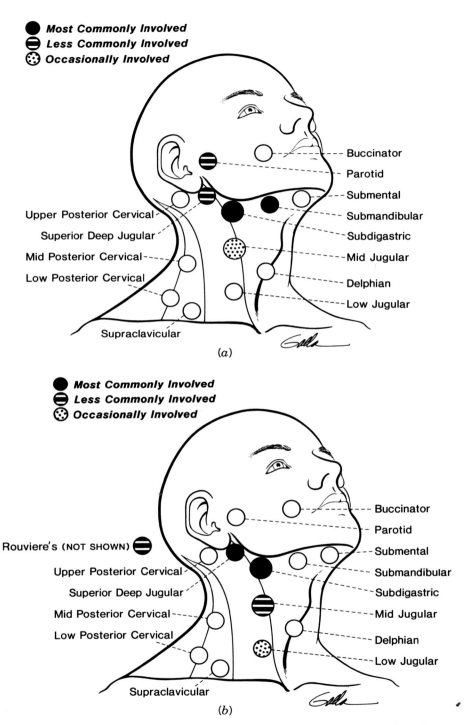

FIGURE 11.2 Diagram showing involvement of lymph nodes by squamous cell carcinoma of (a) anterior and (b) posterior nasal cavities.

retropharyngeal nodes (Rouviere's node) and/or to the deep superior jugular nodes and subdigastric nodes, as shown in Figure 11.2b.

The incidence of metastases is low, especially for early lesions, approximately 10–15% at the time of diagnosis. Less than 10% of the patients with N0 neck develop metastases, if the neck is not treated. In late stages of the disease, the rates range approximately from 25% to 35%. However, for advanced lesions with involvement of the oral cavity, orbit, or soft tissues of the cheek, the incidence of metastases may be as high as 50%. Distant metastases are uncommon and generally occur in the late stages of uncontrolled disease, approximately 10%.

The lymphatic drainage of the nasal vestibule, as shown in Figure 11.3, is predominantly to the submandibular and subdigastric nodes and occasionally to the submental, buccinator, and preauricular nodes. Bilateral involvement is not unusual. The incidence of regional metastases is low, ranging from 10% to 15%.

The most common cell types are squamous cell carcinoma of varying degree of cell differentiation. Other cell types include adenocarcinoma or adenoid cystic carcinoma, melanoma and malignant mesenchymal tumors, and the radioresponsive tumors, that is, lymphomas and plasmacytomas.

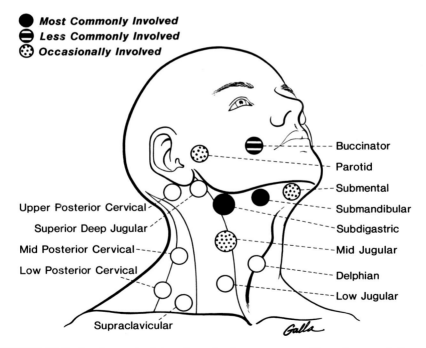

FIGURE 11.3   Involvement of lymph nodes in squamous cell carcinoma of the nasal vestibule.

A. CARCINOMA OF THE NASAL VESTIBULE

Malignant tumors arising from the nasal vestibule are quite uncommon and include squamous cell carcinoma, basal cell carcinoma, and rarely soft tissues sarcomas. Of these, squamous cell carcinoma is the most common cell type and is generally well differentiated and rarely metastasizes.

STAGING

There is no official staging system for squamous cell carcinoma of the nasal vestibule. For the purpose of review of radiation therapy results, the following staging system has been developed at the Massachusetts General Hospital (MGH)[1]:

T1   Lesion is limited to the nasal vestibule and is relatively superficial, involving one or more sites within the vestibule

T2   The lesion has extended from the nasal vestibule to its adjacent structures such as the upper nasal septum, upper lip, philtrum, skin of the nose, and/or nasolabial fold but is not fixed to the underlying bone.

T3   The lesion has become massive with extension to the hard palate, buccogingival sulcus, a large portion of the upper lip, upper nasal septum, turbinate, and/or adjacent paranasal sinuses and is fixed, with deep muscle and bone involvement.

SELECTION OF THERAPY

Small T1 and T2 squamous cell carcinomas can be treated either by surgery or by radiation therapy alone with a satisfactory cure rate.[2,3] The choice of treatment modality for such lesions depends on the cosmetic result following the procedure. If significant deformity will result following surgery, radiation therapy should be the treatment of choice. For extensive T3 lesions with bone involvement, radical surgery in the form of nosectomy with postoperative radiation therapy is preferred. Nodal metastases, though rare in occurrence, are treated by neck dissection and radiation therapy. Buccinator nodal disease may be managed by lumpectomy to be followed by electron beam RT and interstitial implant. Because of the relatively low incidence of occult metastases for T1N0 and T2N0 lesions, elective neck dissection or nodal irradiation is not indicated.

RADIOTHERAPEUTIC MANAGEMENT

Most lesions are relatively superficially situated and may be managed by 4 MV photons, electron beam, or implant. The small T1 and T2 lesions can be treated by ipsilateral appositional electron beam technique, as shown in Figure 11.4, with

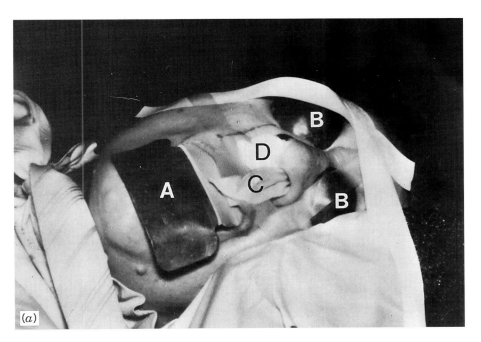

(a)

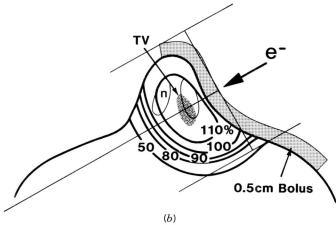

(b)

FIGURE 11.4 (a) Photograph of patient receiving electron beam radiation therapy for carcinoma of the nasal vestibule (T1). Lead shields are placed beneath the lip (A) to protect underlying gum and teeth, in the contralateral nostril (C), and over the eyes (B). Vaseline gauze is inserted in the nostril as a bolus (D). (b) Isodoses in the treated volume.

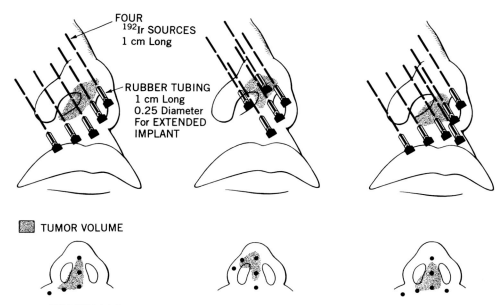

FIGURE 11.5   Patterns of interstitial implant for carcinoma of the nasal vestibule.

supplementary interstitial implant.[1] A dose of approximately 30 Gy in 2 weeks is given and this is followed by interstitial iridium-192 implant with a dose of approximately 30–35 Gy in 3–4 days. By using this combined approach, the contralateral nasal vestibule usually is in good condition without excessive postradiation dryness or crusting. Various implant geometries have been devised to accommodate the extent of the lesions, as shown in Figure 11.5. Generally, needles are inserted into the nasal septum and/or floor of the nasal cavity and/or nasal ala with dose reference at 0.5 cm from the implanted plane. An afterloading technique using blind-end needles with iridium-192 sources has been found useful for most of the lesions in this area. Extensive lesions (T3) are treated by external beam with low megavoltage external irradiation with anterior oblique wedge pair portals for a total dose of approximately 65–70 Gy in 6 weeks, as shown in Figure 11.6.

Technical Pointers

1. When an anteroposterior appositional electron beam is employed, a wax mold to accommodate the curvature of the nasal ala and bridge is required to create inhomogeneity.
2. When using a photon beam, the superior borders of the two anterior oblique wedge pairs are placed below the eyes.
3. Lesions high up in the nasal septum are best treated with a three-field technique, like that employed for nasal cavity carcinoma.

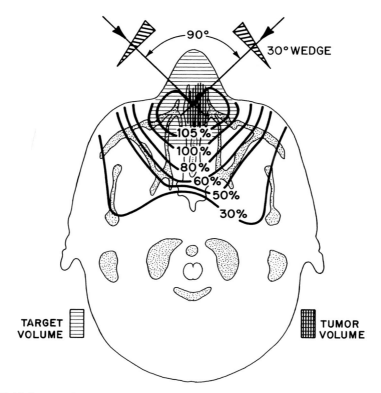

FIGURE 11.6   Anterior oblique wedge pair technique, with 90° hinge angle 30% wedges, for treatment of advanced carcinoma of the nasal vestibule.

4. Metastatic nodes to the buccinator and subdigastric areas are treated with a separate beam, that is, electrons plus implant and photons.

RADIOTHERAPEUTIC RESULTS

The radiation therapy results for early lesions generally are extremely satisfactory, with 3-year NED rates ranging from 80% to 90%.[2-4] Advanced disease, often associated with lymph node metastases, is less curable by radiation therapy alone, with local control rates of approximately 40%.[2,3]

MGH EXPERIENCE

From 1960 to 1985, a total of 54 patients with squamous cell carcinoma of the nasal vestibule were treated by radiation therapy alone. Of these, 34 patients had T1 lesions, 16 had T2 lesions, and 4 had T3 lesions. The incidence of lymph node metas-

TABLE 11.1   Five-Year Actuarial LC and DSS Rates
After Radiation Therapy for Carcinoma of the Nasal
Vestibule: MGH Experience, 1960–1994

Stage	n	LC (%)	DSS (%)
T1	34	81	93
T2	16	79	92
T3	4	53	40

tases in the group was low. Of 54 patients, an initial diagnosis only six presented with nodal disease; four of these patients had N2–3 disease, associated with T3 lesions.

Of 34 patients with T1 lesions, 81% achieved local control; of 14 patients with T2 lesions 79% had local control, while of 4 patients with T3 disease 53% were without disease after radiation therapy. The disease-specific survival rates for T1, T2, and T3 lesions were 93%, 92%, and 40%, respectively, as shown in Table 11.1. Of six patients with metastatic disease in the neck, only one was salvaged.

B. CARCINOMAS OF THE NASAL SEPTUM AND TURBINATES

Squamous cell carcinomas arising from the high nasal septum, anteroethmoid complex, and posterior nasal cavity generally are biologically aggressive, and the lesions tend to be more undifferentiated than the ones located at the inferior and anterior nasal cavity, with higher incidence of metastases.

Owing to the adherence of the mucous membrane to the periosteum and perichondrium, carcinomas arising from the nasal cavity tend to invade the bone and cartilage early and therefore are not readily curable either by surgery or by radiation therapy alone. Treatment varies with cell types and tumor location. Although biopsy through the nares may be possible to obtain tissue for examination, lateral rhinotomy is often necessary for adequate exposure and surgical evaluation of the extent and diagnosis and resection of the lesions, even for small T1 lesions. For inoperable lesions, external beam radiation therapy is given first, followed by resection if made operable by the radiation therapy.

There is no acceptable staging system for carcinoma of the nasal cavity.

RADIOTHERAPEUTIC MANAGEMENT

For lesions high in the nasal cavity and septum, postoperative radiation therapy of 55–60 Gy in 6–7 weeks is given. Because of the possibility of radiation injury to the eyes, any lesions involving the roof of the nasal cavity or ethmoid sinuses cannot be adequately treated by the anterior and lateral wedge pair technique. Such lesions are best managed with a radiation therapy technique similar to that used for carcinoma of the paranasal sinuses, that is, a three-field technique, as shown in Fig-

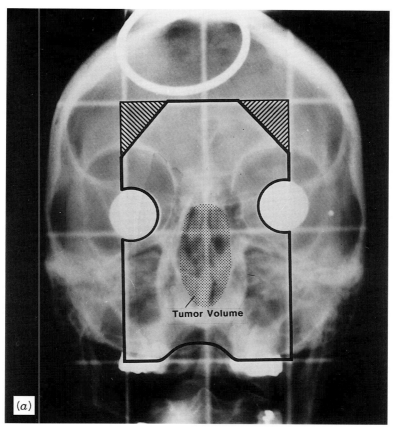

FIGURE 11.7   (a) Simulation film showing anteroposterior portal for treatment of nasal cavity carcinoma.

ure 11.7. Because of the low incidence of nodal metastases in early lesions, approximately 10%, elective neck dissection or neck irradiation is not indicated. For clinically positive nodes after the primary is controlled, the treatment of choice is a combination of radiation therapy and neck dissection.

Technical Pointers

1. Patient is to lie supine and be immobilized with a face mask.
2. A bite block is used to depress and immobilize the tongue to prevent radiation therapy of the dorsum of the tongue.
3. The superior border of the portal includes the bregma, with both eyes protected.
4. The bridge of the nose is placed in a horizontal position, thus sparing the brain from radiation.

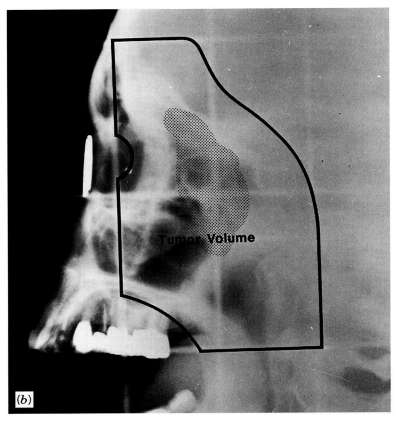

FIGURE 11.7   (b) Simulation film showing lateral portals for treatment of nasal cavity carcinoma.

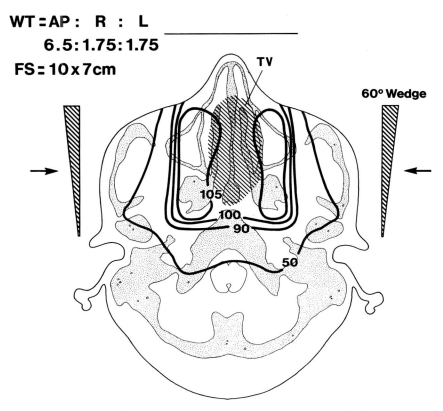

FIGURE 11.8   Isodose distribution to the target volume using a three-field treatment technique for carcinoma of the nasal cavity. (Care must be taken to adjust dosage for air cavity effect.)

5. The lateral portals are shaped to include the soft palate but spare the tongue. The anterior border of portal is at the lateral canthus but spares the lens.
6. Most radiation therapy is given through an anterior portal, right and left portals and boosted through with wedges. The loading is 6.5:1.75:1.75. The isodose distribution is shown in Figure 11.8.

RADIOTHERAPEUTIC RESULTS

Since squamous cell carcinomas of the nasal septum and turbinates uncommon malignancies, the results of radiotherapy are scarce. Most reports[5,6] indicate local control rates ranging from 40% to 60%. Bosch and associates[7] showed a 5-year LC rate of 49% in a group of 40 patients treated by radiation therapy alone.

MGH EXPERIENCE

From 1960 to 1985, a total of 19 patients with "localized" squamous cell carcinoma arising from the nasal septum and/or turbinates received radiation therapy or combined radiotherapy and surgery. Of 10 patients who were treated by radiation therapy alone after biopsy of the lesion or for recurrences, five or 50% were NED. Nine patients were treated by combined surgery and radiation therapy, and of these, seven or 78% were NED at 3 years. All treatment failures were due to uncontrolled primary lesions with or without disease in the neck. Three patients with adenoid cystic carcinoma were treated and all were NED after combined surgery and postoperative radiotherapy. One patient with malignant melanoma was managed by a combined approach and was NED at 5 years.

C. CARCINOMA OF THE PARANASAL SINUSES

Carcinoma arising from the paranasal sinuses generally is a silent tumor. The early symptoms and signs of such lesions mimic those of inflammatory disease[8,9] and most lesions, when first diagnosed, already present evidence of bone destruction and often have extended to the adjacent sinuses, orbit, and/or base of the skull. These signs and symptoms vary with the site of involvement. Approximately 80% of the lesions originate in the maxillary sinuses and 10–15% in the ethmoid sinuses; 80% are squamous cell carcinoma. Tumor arising from the sphenoid or frontal sinuses alone is rare.

The stage, spread, and treatment results of the disease are discussed separately.

Carcinoma of the Maxillary Sinuses

The clinical symptoms and signs, such as a tissue mass that is palpable or visible in the oral or nasal cavity, are readily recognized but unfortunately represent far advanced disease and become incurable. Only by recognizing subtle findings and changes can an early diagnosis be made. These may manifest in a variety of ways as the following categories:

1. *Oral.* When the tumor arises from the floor of the antrum, there is localized or referred pain in the upper molar and premolar region and/or loosening of teeth, dentures become ill-fitting due to swelling of the palate, alveolar ridge, or buccogingival sulcus from tumor, or there is poor healing of tooth sockets. When the tumor extends to the pterygoid fossa, trismus results. These symptoms occur in one-quarter of patients, and 15% at initial presentation.

2. *Nasal.* The nasal symptoms are due to medial spread of the tumor into the nasal cavity with resulting unilateral nasal stuffiness, watery or bloody discharge, and intermittent epistaxis. The tumor may be visible through the nares.

3. *Ocular.* Ocular findings occur in approximately 25% of patients and 5% at presentation. There is displacement of the eyeball and diplopia due to tumor extension through the floor of the orbit. Sometimes a soft tissue mass may be palpated behind the lower eyelid.

4. *Facial.* With the tumor extending through the anterior wall of the antrum, there may be a soft tissue mass visible or palpable on the cheek, filling the nasolabial fold with facial asymmetry. In an advanced stage, the skin may be ulcerated. Invasion of the infraorbital nerve, causing numbness or paresthesia of the skin of the cheek and upper lip, is not uncommon.

5. *Neurologic.* Tumor can involve cranial nerves VII and VIII, resulting in unilateral facial paralysis and deafness.

Carcinoma of the Ethmoid, Sphenoid, and Frontal Sinuses

Nasal obstruction with or without bloody discharge is the most frequent symptom of ethmoidal carcinoma. Advanced lesions may present with visible bone expansion, producing a characteristic broadening of the nasal region or tumefaction between the inner canthus of the eye and bridge of the nose. A unilateral anosmia may result from tumor extending through the cribriform plate. Tumor of the sphenoid sinus may present as deep-seated retro-orbital headache and in advanced stage, signs and symptoms of cranial nerve compression are related to invasion of the orbit and base of the skull. It often is confused with carcinoma of the nasopharynx. Carcinoma of the frontal sinuses is rare and may present as tumefaction over the glabella with signs and symptoms of sinusitis; with tumor extension to the adjacent orbit, there is displacement of the eyeball laterally and inferiorly.

STAGING

Staging of paranasal sinus carcinoma is not well established. The American Joint Committee recommends staging of maxillary sinus lesions based on involvement of the suprastructure or infrastructure and bone involvement. Öhngren's line, as shown in Figure 11.9, represents a theoretical plane joining the medial canthus of the eye with the angle of the mandible. This line is used to divide the maxillary antrum into the anteroinferior portion (the infrastructure) and the superoposterior portion (the suprastructure).

The T staging system is as follows[10]:

T1   Tumor limited to the astral mucosa with no erosion or destruction of bone
T2   Tumor with erosion or destruction of the infrastructure (see anatomic division above), including the hard palate and/or middle nasal meatus
T3   Tumor invades any of the following: skin of cheek, posterior wall of maxillary sinus, floor or medial wall of orbit, or anterior ethmoid sinus
T4   Tumor invades orbital contents and/or any of the following: cribriform plate, posterior ethmoid or sphenoid sinuses, nasopharynx, soft palate, pterygomaxillary or temporal fossae, or base of skull

The TNM Staging System applies only to squamous cell carcinoma.

No official staging system for carcinoma of the frontal, sphenoid, and ethmoid sinuses has been developed.

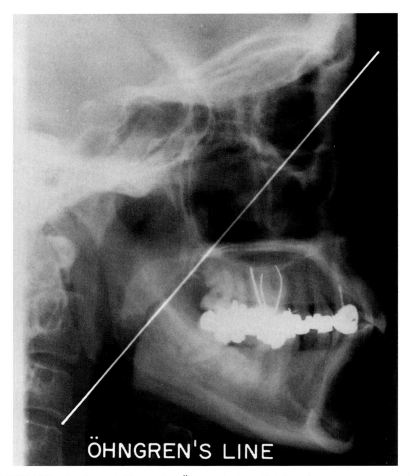

ÖHNGREN'S LINE

FIGURE 11.9   Radiograph illustrating Öhngren's line, dividing the suprastructure and infrastructure of the paranasal sinuses.

Squamous cell carcinoma of varying degree of aggressiveness is the predominant cell type, over 80% of the group. In general, like carcinoma of the nasal cavity, the well differentiated squamous cell carcinoma occurs in the anterior maxillary antrum; the more undifferentiated squamous cell carcinoma arises in the posterior ethmoid adjacent to the nasopharynx. The lesions tend to spread by local extension. Histologic diagnosis can only be made by biopsy of the presenting mass in the nostril, via the Caldwell–Luc procedure, or through an anteronasal window.

Evaluation of tumors of the paranasal sinuses is by careful physical examination, including transillumination of the sinuses and indirect nasopharyngoscopic and fiberoptiscopic inspection of the nasal cavity and nasopharynx. Because of the intricate anatomy and disease process of carcinoma of the paranasal sinuses, detailed radiographic examinations, chiefly AP and lateral CT and MR scans in sagittal and coronal views, are invaluable for assessment of the extent of the tumor, presence or absence of bone involvement or pterygoid invasion,[11] and cervical nodel status. In instances in which orbital spread is suspected, careful evaluation of the orbital contents and its bony wall must be carried out prior to final decision regarding selection of treatment.[11]

SELECTION OF THERAPY

Treatment of squamous cell carcinoma of the paranasal sinuses may be by radiation therapy alone, or surgical resection, or a combination of these two methods. The selection of the treatment depends on the extent of the lesion and the preference of the surgeon and radiation oncologist. Our policy for treating this condition is a combination of radiotherapy and surgery if the lesion is operable.[9,12] Since the incidence of lymph node metastases is quite low in carcinomas, being approximately 20% of all cases, routine radical neck dissection or elective neck irradiation is not recommended in patients with N0 necks.[13] For most operable cases, radical surgery is performed first to remove the bulk of the tumor and to establish drainage of the infected sinuses, to be followed by postoperative radiation therapy. For extensive, inoperable lesions, radiation therapy is generally given first, followed by an attempt at surgical extirpation of the disease (i.e., maxillectomy and ethmoidectomy) in approximately one month if the lesions have been made operable. Radiation therapy may be given postoperatively to any area of residual disease with a boost technique. Orbital exenteration is usually advised for massive tumor involvement of the orbit. On the other hand, with modern radiation therapy techniques,[14,15] the eye can be spared from radiation therapy damage during orbital irradiation of minimal disease, and orbital exenteration may not be necessary.

Primary surgery consists of either partial or total maxillectomy, ethmoidectomy, and/or sphenoidectomy if indicated through a lateral rhinotomy approach. Radical surgery, however, should not be considered for patients with advanced disease with extension to the nasopharynx, base of the skull, or pterygoid fossa, or in patients with distant metastases. For inoperable lesions, high-dose radiation therapy presently given by a BID scheme may offer this unfortunate group of patients some degree of palliation and occasionally local control.

RADIOTHERAPEUTIC MANAGEMENT

Radiation therapy is generally delivered to the hemiparanasal sinuses through a three-field technique, that is, anterior, right, and left laterals. Inoperable advanced disease of the paranasal sinuses is rarely curable by present treatment modalities. High-dose radiation therapy with a BID technique may offer this unfortunate group of patients some palliation and occasionally cure.

Since the lesions may spread along the mucosa into various adjacent sinuses, and synchronous involvement of the antrum and ethmoid sinuses is common, the general principles of radiation therapy are routine coverage of the ipsilateral or hemiparanasal sinuses even in lesions seemingly limited to one sinus. This is particularly true for lesions involving the maxilloethmoid complex. Generally a three-field technique is used to deliver a relatively uniform dose to the maxillary sinus, nasal cavity, and ethmoid and sphenoid sinuses, as shown in Figure 11.10. The dis-

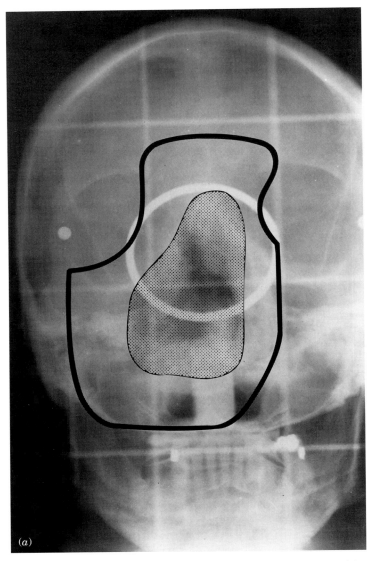

(a)

FIGURE 11.10 Simulation films showing a three-field portal arrangement (a) anteroposterior and (b) opposing lateral wedge portals for treatment of carcinoma of the paranasal sinus. The bulk of the treatment is given though the anterior portal and the laterals are used to boost the posterior volume. (Keep in mind the postoperative cavity effect in determining dosage, and be careful to shield the optic nerve.)

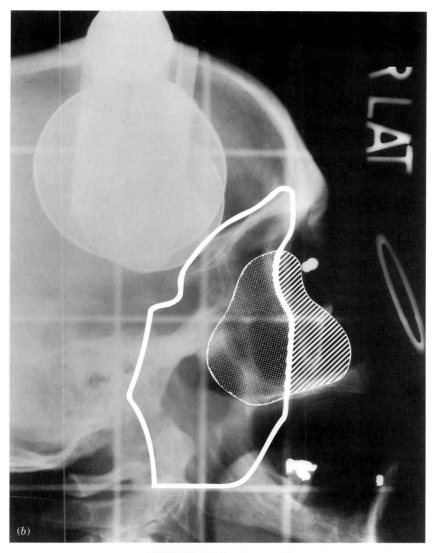

(b)

FIGURE 11.10 *Continued*

tribution of isodoses to the hemiparanasal sinuses with the three-field technique is shown in Figure 11.11. Other techniques using ipsilateral and anterior 45° wedge pairs with 90° angle may be used for the small carcinoma arising from the infrastructures of the maxillary sinus, provided *no* tumor extension is found in the remaining sinuses by CT scan or by surgical exploration. Examples of portal placement and isodose distribution are shown in the treatment planning section of Chapter 2. Owing to the low incidence of occult metastases, elective neck irradiation for patients with N0 neck is not given.

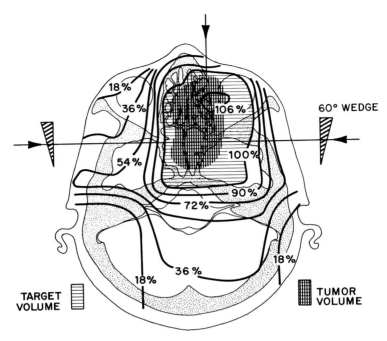

FIGURE 11.11 Diagram showing isodose distribution in the target volume using a three-field technique. Loading: ANT:R:L = 7:2:1

For advanced lesions, often with extensive bone involvement, postoperative radiation therapy is given with 50–55 Gy in 6 weeks. If neck disease is present, ipsilateral neck radiation therapy of 60 Gy is given as a preoperative or postoperative procedure.

For inoperable lesions, high-dose radiation therapy with a BID technique may offer this unfortunate group of patients some palliation and occasionally cure with a dose of 60–65 Gy in 6 weeks. Because of the adjacent organs and the radiosensitive tissues around the paranasal sinuses, such as the globe, optic nerve, and optic chiasm, radiation therapy calls for a careful treatment technique with moderation of total dose and fraction size; otherwise, radiation-induced blindness may ensue.[16] Care is taken to spare the cornea and lens of the eye, the lacrimal gland, and most of the frontal lobe of the brain. No "hot spot" should exceed more than 10–15% of the total dose over the target volume.

Since 1979, most patients with carcinoma of the paranasal sinuses have been treated with the BID program with 1.6 Gy/f for approximately 60 Gy. Because the oropharyngeal mucosa is mostly outside the treatment fields, the patients generally do not experience severe symptomatic mucosal reaction. The "break period" after 38.4 Gy generally is rather short, that is, 7–10 days.

Technical Pointers

1. Patient is to lie supine and be immobilized with a modified face mask, and the tongue should be depressed and immobilized with a bite block.

2. Although the AP and ipsilateral wedge pair technique may be used to irradiate an early lesion of the infrastructures of the maxillary sinus only, its use for treatment of the entire ethmoid sinuses is ill-advised, because the anterior and middle ethmoid air cells, which are located between the eyes, cannot be irradiated fully without damaging the eyes.

3. For the AP portal setup of the three-field technique, the face and chin are placed parallel to the treatment table or perpendicular to the beam.

4. For radiation therapy of the paranasal sinuses, dose inhomogeneity must be kept in mind. A large surgical defect, such as a cavity after orbital exenteration, must be packed with wet gauze, or a cavity created after inferior maxillectomy must be filled with an obturator during irradiation.

5. A contoured Cerrobend cutout is used to protect the lacrimal gland, both eyes, and the adjacent brain.

6. Lateral portals include the nasopharyngeal vault, the sphenoid sinuses, the posterior ethmoid air cells, and Rouviere's node. The anterior and middle ethmoid air cells and frontal sinuses are treated primarily by AP portal.

7. When the entire orbit, including the eye, is irradiated due to tumor invasion using either a 90° wedge pair with the lateral portal slightly tilted posteriorly to avoid the contralateral eye, or with a three-field technique, the irradiated eye should be opened or "looking at the beam" during irradiation. This avoids a dose maximum at the cornea and prevents symptomatic radiation keratitis.

8. When the frontal lobe or brain tissue is largely included with the BID radiation therapy scheme, the interfraction time is 6 hours or longer.

RADIOTHERAPEUTIC RESULTS

Owing to the locally advanced stages of carcinoma of the paranasal sinuses, the therapeutic results following either radiation therapy alone or combined radiation therapy and surgery are poor. In a series of unselected cases, the combined therapies yielded a 5-year survival of about 25%, while in operable cases the rate is nearly 45–50%. Generally, carcinomas of the antrum arising from the infrastructure have somewhat higher survivorship than suprastructure lesions. In carcinoma of the ethmoid sinuses, the survival data following various forms of therapy are scarce and vary considerably. The crude overall 5-year survival is about 20–25%. No meaningful data are available for carcinoma of the sphenoid or frontal sinuses due to rarity of the disease. Radical neck dissection is indicated only when metastatic nodes in the neck become apparent, although the survival patients with cervical disease is poor due to propensity for distant metastases.

MGH EXPERIENCE

From 1970 to 1994, a total of 74 patients with squamous cell carcinoma of the paranasal sinuses received radiation therapy. Of these, 66 patients had lesions arising from the maxillary and/or ethmoid sinuses and 8 had lesions arising from the sphenoid and/or frontal sinuses.

Of 66 patients with carcinoma of the maxillary/ethmoid sinus, 27 or 40% were treated by definitive irradiation; 39 or 60% received combined surgery and radiation therapy. Most of these patients had advanced disease (T3–4) or inoperable lesions. The 5-year actuarial local control (LC) rate after radiation therapy only was 49% and the disease-specific survival (DSS) rate was 42%, as compared to the combined surgery and radiation therapy group with 57% and 67%, respectively, as shown in Table 11.2.

TABLE 11.2 Five-Year Actuarial LC and DSS Rates After Radiation Therapy Only and Combined Surgery and Radiation Therapy

Treatment Method	n	LC (%)	DSS (%)
Radiation therapy	27	49	42
Surgery and radiation therapy	39	57	67
		$p = 0.05$	$p = 0.05$

The difference between the radiation only and combination therapy groups was insignificant in LC ($p=0.5$) but was significant in DSS ($p=0.05$).

As expected, most patients with T4 disease failed at the primary sites. Of four patients with nodal metastases in the neck, three died of locoregional disease and distant metastases and only one was NED. Of eight patients with squamous cell carcinoma of the sphenoid/or frontal sinus, five patients were treated by radiation therapy only and three were treated by combined surgery and radiation therapy. The 5-year actuarial local control and disease-specific survival rates were both 100%.

RESULTS OF BID RADIATION THERAPY

From 1979 through 1994, 42 patients (shown in Table 11.3) with carcinoma of the paranasal sinuses were treated with a BID radiation program. The 5-year actuarial LC and DSS rates were 52% and 69% as compared to 32 patients treated by a QD program from 1970 to 1979, who had LC and DSS rate of 67% and 54%, respectively. The difference, however, is not statistically significant ($p=0.3$), as shown in Table 11.3.

TABLE 11.3 Five-Year Actuarial Rates After BID and QD Radiation Therapy for Squamous Cell Carcinoma of the Paranasal Sinuses: 1970–1994

Treatment Program	n	LC (%)	DSS (%)
BID (1979–1994)	42	52	69
QD (1970–1994)	32	67	54
		$p = 0.3$	$p = 0.2$

SUMMARY

1. Squamous cell carcinoma arising from the nasal vestibule is relatively rare and is often referred to as "nose picker's" cancer. Small lesions (T1 and T2) are highly curable by radiation therapy alone with good functional and cosmetic results. Advanced lesions (T3) with bone destruction and/or metastases are best treated by combined therapies, that is, radical surgery in the form of nosectomy and/or palatectomy and postoperative irradiation, if the lesions are resectable. For inoperable tumors, high-dose megavoltage irradiation may offer palliation and occasionally an unexpected cure.

2. Cancers of the nasal cavity are rare. For lesions invading the adjacent bone and cartilage, the therapeutic choice is combined surgery and postoperative radiation therapy. Although the early mucosal lesions can be controlled by radiation therapy alone, such lesions are not readily identifiable without lateral rhinotomy and resection.

3. Squamous cell carcinoma of the paranasal sinus is a relatively uncommon lesion of the head and neck; approximately 3% of cancers involve the upper air and food passages. Early lesions are relatively silent, mimicking inflammatory disease, and most cases when recognized show evidence of bone destruction. The tumors tend to involve the anteroethmoid complex and spread locally to the adjacent sinuses, orbit, or neighboring soft tissues. It is therefore important to consider the hemiparanasal sinuses as having a high risk of involvement, although the lesion may appear localized. Except for rare mucosal tumors (which are rarely diagnosable), the treatment of choice is a combination of surgery and radiation therapy. Surgery is preferred initially with the idea of removing the gross disease, evaluating the extent of spread, and establishing drainage of infected sinuses, to be followed by high-dose postoperative radiation therapy.

D. INVERTED PAPILLOMA

Inverted papilloma is an infrequent lesion arising from the mucosa of the sinonasal tract. It is a histologically benign tumor but biologically may be very aggressive, with extensive bone destruction and/or intracranial extension. It tends to occur in the nasal cavity and maxilloethmoid complex area and may have a prolonged clinical course with a tendency toward local recurrence. The histologic picture is that of a papilloma that is growing into the stroma rather than outward from it. In approximately 5–10% of patients, the tumor is associated with invasive squamous cell carcinoma or adenocarcinoma, concurrently or sequentially during the course of the disease.[17] The squamous cell component is frequently present at initial diagnosis and may be low or high grade. The lesion occurs more frequently in males, predominantly over 40 years of age. The etiology is unknown. Allergens, chronic inflammation, extrinsic environmental carcinogens, and viral infections have all been suggested as possible contributors.

For inverted papilloma, wide local resection is the treatment of choice. If the resection margins are free from disease, no adjuvant therapy is considered. On the other hand, the rate of recurrence following limited surgical procedure was reported to range from 40% to 80%. With improvement in the surgical techniques of radical resections, the incidence of recurrence has been reduced to less than 10%. Radiation therapy may be considered as an adjuvant therapy for incompletely resected, recurrent, or unresectable lesions or in cases of associated invasive squamous cell carcinoma.

MGH EXPERIENCE

Between 1979 and 1990, 25 patients were treated with radiation therapy. Of these, five of seven patients (A group) with inverted papilla only (A group) and four of 18 with inverted papilla associated with squamous cell carcinoma of the nasal cavity and paranasal sinuses, B group had previous limited resections only. The remaining 16 patients underwent radiation therapy following gross total resection. Radiation therapy for this disease was given with a dose of approximately 50 Gy, commonly a three-field treatment technique.

RESULTS OF TREATMENT

Local control of inverted papillomas of the paranasal sinuses is exceedingly satisfactory after combined surgery and radiation therapy. For Group A, the 5-year actuarial local control was 86%. For Group B, the corresponding rate was 89% after radiation therapy; one of the long-term survivors developed recurrence with sarcoma 17 years after treatment. No regional lymph nodes or distant metastases were observed. Two patients in Group B died of their disease.

E. OLFACTORY NEUROBLASTOMA

Olfactory neuroblastoma or esthesioneuroblastoma arising from olfactory epithelium is a rare disease.[18,19] Its clinical presentation is similar to most malignant nasal tumors with nasal obstruction, epistaxis, and anosmia. The tumor may spread to and/or occur in the antrum and ethmoid sinus. With intraorbital extension, there is pain and proptosis of the eye.[20,21] Intracranial spread of tumor may result in positive tumor cytology in the cerebrospinal fluid (CSF). This disease is more common in young females and affects all ages from 3 to 80.

Olfactory neuroblastoma varies in its aggressiveness and may recur locally and develop distant metastases late in the course of the disease. The incidence of cervical lymph node metastases is approximately 20%, although bilateral involvement is infrequent.

Evaluation of the extent of the lesion calls for careful radiographic examination, including polytomes and CT and MR scans of the paranasal sinuses, skull, and brain. Occasionally, angiographic studies may reveal the detailed vascular pattern of the lesion. CSF cytology is used to detect the possibility of intracranial extension and/or meningeal involvement by tumor.

No official staging system has been accepted for this disease. A staging system based on the clinical and radiographic findings as devised at the MGH is as follows[22]:

Group A   Tumor confined to nasal cavity
Group B   Tumor extending beyond the nasal cavity and into paranasal sinus
Group C   Tumor spreading beyond the nasal cavity and paranasal sinus

The above clinical staging has significant connotation regarding the prognosis and survival after appropriate therapy.

SELECTION OF THERAPY

Surgery, radiation therapy, or a combination of these two are employed in the treatment of this disease.[18,22–24] The data that follow suggest that a combination of surgery and radiation therapy is the therapeutic modality of choice. After biopsy confirmation of the disease, a patient is generally considered according to the extent and location of the lesion for surgical removal of tumor. For adequate exposure of the tumor, lateral rhinotomy is used followed by medial maxillectomy and/or ethmoidectomy, sphenoidectomy, and excision of the lesion. Because of the inaccessible location of most lesions, surgery is rarely adequate. After removal of the gross tumor, the patient should be considered for postoperative radiation therapy. Although the metastatic nodes in the neck should be dealt with by combined radiation therapy and surgery, routing elective neck dissection or irradiation is not indicated for N0 neck due to the low incidence of cervical lymph node metastases.

RADIOTHERAPEUTIC MANAGEMENT

The technique for radiation therapy of olfactory neuroblastoma is similar to radiation therapy for paranasal sinus carcinoma using an anterior and bilateral wedge technique with heavy loading through the anterior portal. If tumor extends to the orbit, the cornea and lens should be protected during radiation therapy by placing a "pencil" lead block over the cornea. For tumor extension to the brain with positive cytological CSF, cerebrospinal axis irradiation is used, or whole brain irradiation with intrathecal chemotherapy. Although, in general, neuroblastomas are considered radiosensitive tumors, for olfactory neuroblastoma a high dose is required for permanent local control of the disease. The radiation therapy dose level would be quite similar to that for control of epitheliomas in general, that is, 55–60 Gy in 6–7 weeks.

Technical Pointers

1. For most lesions high up in the nasal cavity, use a three-field technique similar to that used for the paranasal sinus or nasal cavity.
2. The anterior cranial fossa and cribriform plate and a strip of the base of the brain are included in the treatment portal.
3. A Cerrobend cutoff excludes the pituitary gland and optic chiasm.
4. Dose per fraction is kept below 1.8 Gy per fraction.
5. If a BID scheme is used, 6 hours is the time period between fractions.

RADIOTHERAPEUTIC RESULTS

Because of the rarity of the disease, the survival rates as reported in the literature generally consist of a small number of patients treated a couple of decades ago. The staging and treatment methods are less than ideal. The survival rates after various treatment techniques are approximately 50–80%, depending on the stages of the disease. For Group A lesions, the local control and survival rates are extremely satisfactory. Elkon and associates,[25] in a literature review, indicated NED rates of 96% (23/24) for Group A, 83% for Group B, and 53% for Group C lesions, emphasizing the importance of combined surgery and radiation therapy for this disease. Tables 11.4 and 11.5 summarize the cases as reported in the literature related to the treatment methods and stages. These historical data suggest that surgery with and with-

TABLE 11.4 Five-Year Survival of Patients with Olfactory Neuroblastoma Related to Treatment Methods[a]

Treatment Method	n	Survival (%)
Radiation therapy	14/35	40
Surgery	28/35	77
Surg and radiation therapy	41/73	56

[a]Data collected from Refs. 18, 19, 20, 21, 23, 24. et al.[xx]

TABLE 11.5   Five-Year Survival of Patients with Olfactory Neuroblastoma Related to Treatment Methods and Stages

Treatment Method	Group A	Group B	Group C
Radiation therapy	4/4 (100%)	4/5 (80%)	0/3 (0%)
Surgery	11/11 (100%)	5/8 (63%)	19/23 (83%)
Surg and radiation therapy	10/10 (100%)	19/23 (43%)	5/11 (45%)

Data collected from Refs. 25 and 22.

out radiation therapy achieved somewhat higher cure rates than single modality treatment alone especially for advanced lesions, as shown in Tables 11.4 and 11.5.

MGH EXPERIENCE

From 1970 through 1994, a total of 18 patients with olfactory neuroblastoma were treated by radiation therapy. The majority of the patients were treated by combined surgery and radiation therapy. Only three patients were treated by radiation therapy alone. The 5-year actuarial LC and DSS rates were 56% and 68%, respectively, as shown in Figure 11.12.

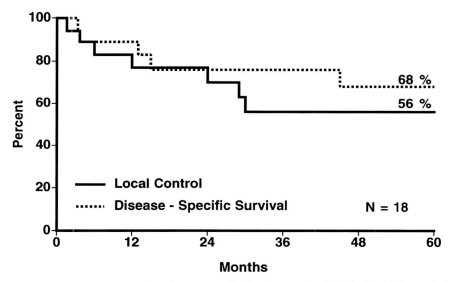

FIGURE 11.12   Graph showing 5-year actuarial local control and disease-specific survival in 18 patients with olfactory neuroblastoma after treatment: MGH experience, 1970–1994.

SUMMARY

Olfactory neuroblastoma is a rare tumor originating in the olfactory epithelium in the roof of the nasal cavity. It may cause death by local invasion and/or distant metastases. In the localized disease, the treatment of choice is a combination of surgery and radiation therapy. Except for extremely early lesions without bone invasion or paranasal spread, primary radiation therapy is rarely successful and is therefore not recommended. Because of the low incidence of cervical nodal metastases, elective neck dissection or irradiation is not indicated.

REFERENCES

1. Wang CC: Treatment of carcinoma of the nasal vestibule by irradiation. *Cancer* 1976; 38:100–106.
2. Goepfert H, Guillamondegui OM, Jesse RH, Lindberg RD. Squamous cell carcinoma of nasal vestibule. *Arch Otolaryngol* 1974;100:8–10.
3. Haynes WD, Tapley NV: Radiation treatment of carcinoma of the nasal vestibule. *Am J Roentgenol Radium Ther Nucl Med* 1974;120:595–602.
4. Ash JE, Beck MR, Wilkes JD: Tumors of the upper respiratory tract and ear. In: Atlas of tumor pathology, Sect IV, Fasc 12 and 13. Washington DC: Armed Forces Institute of Pathology, 1964; 79.
5. Yarington CT, Jaquiss GW, Sprinkle PM: Carcinoma of the nose and nasal septum: treatment and reconstruction. *Trans Am Acad Ophthalmol Otolaryngol* 1969;73:1178–1183.
6. Young JR: Malignant tumors of nasal septum. *J Laryngol Otol* 1979;93:817–832.
7. Bosch V, Vallecillo L, Frias Z: Cancer of the nasal cavity. *Cancer* 1976;37:1458–1463.
8. Lewis JS, Castro EB: Cancer of the nasal cavity and paranasal sinuses. *J Laryngol Otol* 1972;86:255–262.
9. Hamberger CA, Martensson G: Carcinoma of the paranasal sinuses, combined approach. *Front Radiat Ther Oncol* 1970;5:130–146.
10. American Joint Committee on Cancer: *Manual for staging of cancer*, 4th ed. Philadelphia: Lippincott, 1992.
11. Jesse RH: Pre-operative *versus* post-operative radiation in the treatment of squamous carcinoma of the paranasal sinuses. *Am J Surg* 1965;110:552–556.
12. Cheng VST, Wang CC: Carcinomas of the paranasal sinuses. A study of sixty-six cases. *Cancer* 1977;40:3038–3041.
13. Pezner RD, Moss WT, Tong D, et al: Cervical lymph node metastases in patients with squamous cell carcinoma of the maxillary antrum. *Int J Radiat Oncol Biol Phys* 1979;5: 1977–1980.
14. Bataini JP, Ennuyer A: Advanced carcinoma of the maxillary antrum treated by cobalt therapy and electron beam irradiation. *Br J Radiol* 1971;44:590–598.
15. Boone ML, Harle TS, Higholt HW, et al: Malignant disease of the paranasal sinuses and nasal cavity: importance of precise localization of extent of disease. *AJR Am J Roentgenol* 1968;102:627–636.

16. Shukovsky LJ, Fletcher GH: Retinal and optic nerve complications in a high dose irradiation technique of ethmoid sinus and nasal cavity. *Radiology* 1972;104:629–634.

17. Batsakis JG, Rice DH, Solomon AR: The pathology of head and neck tumors: squamous and mucous gland carcinomas of the nasal cavity, paranasal sinuses and larynx. *Head Neck Surg* 1980;2:497–508.

18. Baker DC, Perzin KH, Conley J: Olfactory neuroblastoma. *Otolaryngol Head Neck Surg* 1979;87:279–283.

19. Skolnick EM, Massari FS, Tenta LT: Olfactory neuroepithelioma: review of the world literature and presentation of two cases. *Arch Otolaryngol* 1966;84:644–653.

20. Dibble PA, Brown AK: Esthesioneuroepithelioma. *Laryngoscope* 1965;71:192–199.

21. Schenk NL, Ogura JH: Esthesioneuroblastoma: an enigma in diagnosis, a dilemma in treatment. *Arch Otolaryngol* 1972;96:322–324.

22. Kadish S, Goodman M, Wang CC: Olfactory neuroblastoma. *Cancer* 1976;37:1571–1576.

23. Robinson F, Solitare GB: Olfactory neuroblastoma: neurosurgical implications of an intranasal tumor. *J Neurosurg* 1966;25:133–139.

24. Bailey BJ, Barton S: Olfactory neuroblastoma: management and prognosis. *Arch Otolaryngol* 1975;101:1–5.

25. Elkon D, Hightower SI, Lim ML, et al: Esthesioblastoma. *Cancer* 1979;44:1087–1094.

CHAPTER 12

TUMORS OF THE SALIVARY GLANDS

ANATOMIC CONSIDERATION

The major salivary glands consist of paired parotid, submandibular, and sublingual glands and are serous, seromucous, and mucous, respectively. The parotid gland is the largest salivary gland and anatomically is grooved by the ascending ramus of the mandible and lies anterior and inferior to the cartilaginous external auditory canal, and posterior to the mastoid process and posterior belly of the digastric and sternomastoid muscle. Anteriorly, the parotid gland wraps around the ramus of the mandible and extends to the masseter muscle, superiorly the gland abuts the zygoma at the level of the temporomandibular joint, and medially the gland borders the parapharyngeal space and base of the skull. Stensen's duct emerges into the oral cavity adjacent to the upper second molar. Figure 12.1 shows the anatomic relationship of a normal parotid gland (outlined by sialogram) to the bony landmarks of the mandible and spine.

The parotid gland is arbitrarily divided into superficial (80%) and deep (20%) lobes by the facial nerve, which exits from the skull through the stylomastoid foramen and loops immediately around the external auditory meatus inferiorly. The deep lobe of the parotid gland lies along the medial aspect of the angle of the mandible and connects to the superficial lobe by an isthmus.[1]

The submandibular gland is approximately one-quarter the size of the parotid gland and lies in the upper anterior triangle of the neck, adjacent to the body of the mandible, and is in close proximity to the lower portion of the parotid gland at the angle of the jaw. Wharton's duct exits through the gap between the mylohyoid and hyoglossus muscles anteriorly to the floor of the mouth, as shown in Figure 12.2.

The sublingual gland is approximately one-tenth the size of the parotid gland

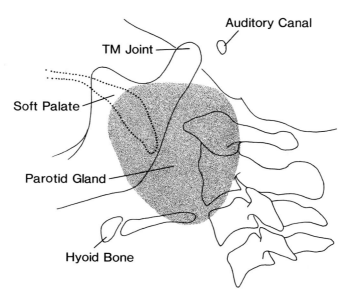

FIGURE 12.1 Diagram showing anatomic position of a normal parotid gland from a sialogram related to the bony landmarks of the mandible and skull base. The contralateral normal parotid gland should be spared if possible during irradiation.

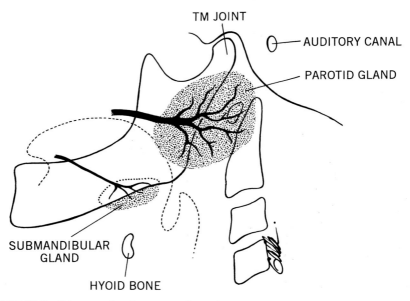

FIGURE 12.2 Diagram showing anatomic position of a normal parotid gland and submandibular gland related to the angle of the jaw, hyoid bone and cervical spine.

and lies in the anterior floor of the mouth and relates laterally to the mandible. The excretory ducts empty into the floor of the mouth.

The minor salivary glands include mucus-secreting glands in the lining membrane of the upper aerodigestive tract.

The AJC staging system for salivary gland cancer is as follows[2]:

Primary Tumor (T)

T1	Tumor 2 cm or less in greatest dimension
T2	Tumor more than 2 cm but not more than 4 cm in greatest dimension
T3	Tumor more than 4 cm but not more than 6 cm in greatest dimension
T4	Tumor more than 6 cm in greatest dimension
Note:	All categories are subdivided: (a) no local extension and (b) local extension. Local extension is clinical or macroscopic evidence of invasion of skin, soft tissue, bone, or nerve. Microscopic evidence alone is not local extension for classification purposes.

Neck Node (N) Status

N0	No regional lymph node metastasis
N1	Metastasis in a single ipsilateral lymph node, 3 cm or less in greatest dimension
N2	Metastasis in a single ipsilateral lymph node, more than 3 cm but not more than 6 cm in greatest dimension; or in multiple ipsilateral lymph nodes, none more than 6 cm in greatest dimension; or in bilateral or contralateral lymph nodes, none more than 6 cm in greatest dimension
N2a	Metastasis in a single ipsilateral lymph node, more than 3 cm but not more than 6 cm in greatest dimension
N2b	Metastasis in multiple ipsilateral lymph nodes, none more than 6 cm in greatest dimension
N2c	Metastasis in bilateral or contralateral lymph nodes, none more than 6 cm in greatest dimension
N3	Metastasis in a lymph node, more than 6 cm in greatest dimension

Metastases (M) Status

M0	No distant metastasis
M1	Distant metastasis

CLINICOPATHOLOGIC CONSIDERATION

The pathologic aspects of malignant tumors of the salivary glands were extensively discussed by Batsakis[3] and are comprised of (1) mucoepidermoid carcinoma, (2) adenoid cystic carcinoma, (3) adenocarcinoma, (4) squamous cell carcinoma, (5) acinic cell carcinoma, (6) malignant mixed tumor, (7) undifferentiated carcinoma, and (8) others including lymphoma, melanoma, and some soft tissue sarcomas.

Salivary gland tumors are uncommon and account for approximately 5–7% of all head and neck epithelial tumors. Because of the difference in sizes of the glands, approximately 80–90% of salivary gland tumors occur in the parotid glands. It is estimated[4] that for every 100 neoplasms of the parotid gland, there are 10 in the submandibular gland, 1 in the sublingual gland, and 10 in the minor salivary gland. Of the parotid gland tumors, approximately 80% are benign, mostly pleomorphic adenomas (mixed tumors). Approximately one of two intraoral minor salivary gland tumors occurs in the hard palate.

Approximately one of five parotid gland tumors is malignant, while more than half of submandibular tumors are malignant. Most sublingual gland tumors, although extremely rare (less than 1%), are cancerous.[5]

Malignant tumors of the minor salivary gland are rare; common sites are the oral cavity, tongue, cheek, lip, floor of the mouth, nasal cavity, paranasal sinuses, larynx, and trachea.

Salivary gland cancers are seldom symptomatic and usually manifest as a painless swelling or lump. Episodic pain occasionally occurs in 10–20% of patients with parotid and submandibular tumors. In advanced stages these lesions may rapidly increase in size and be associated with constant pain or, in the parotid region, facial nerve paralysis. These tumors are marked by their unpredictable clinical course and are characterized by chronicity and tendency to multiple recurrences.

The spread of most malignant salivary gland tumors is by local infiltration, perineural extension, and hematogenous and, less commonly, lymphatic routes. The lymphatics of the parotid gland drain to the intra- or paraparotid, submandibular, superior jugular, and subdigastric nodes. Unlike the parotid gland, the submandibular gland does not have intraglandular parenchymal lymph nodes, and its lymphatics drain to the adjacent submandibular and subdigastric nodes. Distant metastases are mostly to lung, bone, and liver.[6,7]

The incidence of regional lymph node and distant metastases depends on the cell types of the tumors and their stage at presentation. Table 12.1 shows the incidence of overt and occult regional metastases in parotid carcinoma. The mucoepidermoid

TABLE 12.1   Metastases in Cancer of the Parotid Gland: 96 Patients

Tumor Types	Overt (%)	Occult (%)
Mucoepidermoid (High grade)	44	16
Acinic cell	13	6
Adenoid cystic	5	0
Adenocarcinoma	26	9
Malignant mixed	21	0
Squamous cell	37	40
Undifferentiated	23	0

Source: Johns and Kaplan.[8]

TABLE 12.2   Metastatic Patterns of Salivary Gland Tumors

Tumor Types	Local Nodes (%)	Distant Metastases (%)
Adenoid cystic		
Spiro et al.	15	3
Conley	16	34
Blanck et al.	20	34
Malignant mixed		
Spiro et al.	25	32
Eneroth et al.	24	24
Mucoepidermoid (all grade)		
Spiro et al.	29	15

Source: Johns and Kaplan.[8]

carcinoma, squamous cell carcinoma, and undifferentiated carcinoma presented with high incidence of overt and occult metastases.

The incidence of local and distant spread of parotid carcinomas is shown in Table 12.2. The adenoid cystic tumor, malignant mixed tumor, and mucoepidermoid carcinomas had a propensity to distant and local metastases, ranging from 25% to 35%. Metastases from minor salivary carcinomas are infrequent and often indicate advanced disease.

Patients with salivary gland malignant tumors should be fully evaluated by careful physical examination to delineate the extent of the primary growth and nodal status, including inspection, palpation, neurologic evaluation of the 7th cranial nerve or other nerves, and radiological studies, including radiographs of the mandible and CT and MR scans. Sialograms are used less frequently, unlike for benign conditions. The final diagnosis should be made by histologic examination of the excised specimen, commonly superficial parotidectomy.

ADJUVANT RADIATION THERAPY

Treatment of salivary gland carcinoma has been and probably will continue to be by surgical removal if the lesions are operable.[5,6] Radiation therapy is primarily adjuvant, occasionally curative and frequently palliative in nature. The beneficial effects of adjuvant radiation therapy after surgery in the management of salivary gland carcinomas were extensively published in the literature.[9-12]

Table 12.3 illustrates local control of salivary gland malignancies. The data clearly indicate improvement of local control after combined therapies, especially for T3–4 and high grade tumors, but less so for early and low grade lesions.

**TABLE 12.3   Local Control of Salivary Gland
Carcinoma Related to Stages and Tumor Grades:
Surgery Versus Combined Surgery and RT**

Lesions	Surgery (%)	Surg and RT (%)
Stages		
1 and 2	100 ($n = 23$)	97 ($n = 37$)
3 and 4	42 ($n = 26$)	73 ($n = 22$)
Grades		
Low	92 ($n = 38$)	90 ($n = 49$)
HIgh	43 ($n = 21$)	80 ($n = 10$)

Source: Borthne et al.[12]

Indications for Adjuvant Postoperative Radiation Therapy

1. Incomplete surgical removal with known residual disease.
2. Tumor extension beyond the capsule and/or at the resection margin.
3. Extensive perineural involvement and/or lymph node metastases.
4. High grade malignant tumors.
5. Facial nerve sparing procedure with close tumor margins.
6. Large tumors requiring radical resection of facial nerve, mandible, temporal bone, and so on.
7. Parotid tumors of deep lobe origin with inadequate resection margins.
8. Tumors with one or more local recurrences after previous surgical procedures.
9. Inoperable lesions.

RADIOTHERAPEUTIC MANAGEMENT

Carcinomas of the salivary glands, although they are slow to respond and regress following radiation therapy, are erroneously considered radioresistant. Such a misconception has repeatedly been refuted by modern radiation therapy with satisfactory local control and marked reduction of local recurrence after radiation therapy.

Since the incidence of nodal metastases in patients with low grade localized lesions is low, the management of these lesions does not include treatment of neck disease. For undifferentiated and high grade mucoepidermoid carcinomas or in patients with palpable metastatic disease in the neck, neck treatment either by neck dissection or radiation therapy is indicated.

RADIATION DOSES AND TECHNIQUES

Generally, a dose of 65–70 Gy in 7 weeks is given for lesions with known residual disease or inoperable lesions. For microscopic disease, with close or positive margin, a dose of 55–60 Gy in 5–6 weeks is given. For parotid and submandibular tumors, radiation therapy is delivered by a combination of external photon beam with

ISODOSE FOR PAROTID TUMORS
4500 RAD ^{60}Co WEDGE PAIR
1000 RAD 90% 15 MeV ELECTRONS

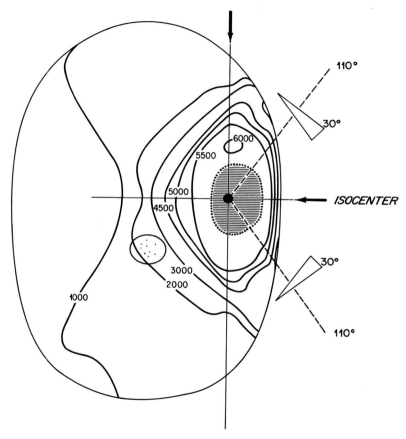

FIGURE 12.3   Diagram showing composite isodose for irradiating parotid tumor, using 45 Gy ipsilateral oblique wedge pair and 10 Gy appositional 15 MeV electron beam boost (90% isodose line).

wedge pair technique for about 40 Gy and *en face* electron beam boost for an additional 15–20 Gy. Figure 12.3 illustrates the composite isodoses for treatment of parotid tumor by such combined modalities. Interstitial implant is not suitable for lesions situated in the deep lobe of the parotid gland.

For undifferentiated carcinoma of the parotid glands with or without node involvement, the primary lesion and neck can be irradiated in continuity with AP and PA portals, that is, with the hemi-neck portals shown in Figure 12.4a and the composite isodoses shown in Figure 12.4b. After a dose of 40 Gy photons in 4 weeks, the primary site is boosted to bring the total dose to the primary site up to 55–60 Gy in 6 weeks

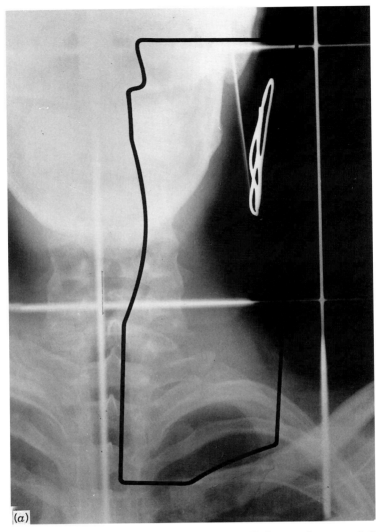

(a)

FIGURE 12.4 (a) Simulation film showing AP–PA radiotherapeutic approach for extensive carcinoma of the parotid gland with nodal disease; portals include the primary site and ipsilateral neck. (b) diagram showing composite isodoses after AP–PA portals with 40 Gy and appositional electron beam boost to the parotid with 20 Gy (15 MeV electrons).

Technical Pointers

A. For Treatment of Parotid Gland Tumor (Tumor Bed Only)

1. Patient is in a supine position and the chin is hyperextended and immobilized with a face mask.

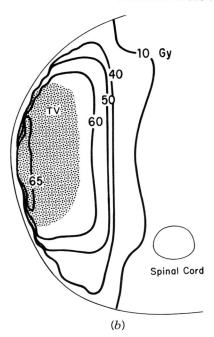

(b)

FIGURE 12.4 *Continued*

2. The superior border clears the lateral canthus of the eye, 1–1.5 cm superior to the TMJ (temporomandibular joint); the eyes are avoided.
3. The inferior border is 3–4 cm below the angle of the jaw or at the thyroid notch.
4. The posterior border includes the mastoid process.
5. Use 110° hinge angle with isocenter 2–2.5 cm below the surface, and use an anterior and posterior oblique wedge pair, with 30° wedges. Cobalt-60 or 4× radiation therapy is employed.
6. For *en face* electron beam boost use an "ear plug" (Figure 12.5) to protect the middle and inner ear.

B. *For Treatment of Submandibular Gland Tumor (Tumor Bed Only)*

1. Use an AP and ipsilateral wedge pair technique with photons.
2. Use a bite block to separate the upper and lower jaws.
3. Portal should include the submandibular triangle, the angle of the mandible, and the subdigastric and submandibular lymph nodes.

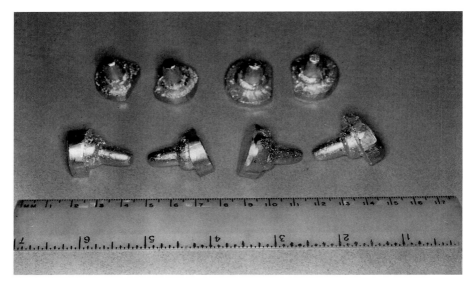

FIGURE 12.5 Ear plugs are used to protect the tympanic membrane, middle ear, and concha of the ear during electron beam irradiation. Two sizes, made of Cerrobend, are available.

4. For adenoid cystic carcinoma with perineural spread, the portals should cover the adjacent base of the skull comprehensively for 40 Gy, to be followed by appositional electron boost to the primary site for 15–20 Gy.

C. *For Treatment of Tumor Bed and the Cervical Lymphatics (Hemi-neck and Tumor Bed)*

1. Patient is to be in a supine position with the chin hyperextended.
2. For parotid lesions, the superior border is below the canthus of the eye or at the top of the auricle.
3. A Cerrobend cutout is used to shield the tongue inside the commissure of the mouth.
4. Calculate the various thicknesses of the jaw level and the low neck; keep a record of doses and/or use a tissue compensator.
5. After 40 Gy, discontinue low neck irradiation and continue RT to the primary site with either an oblique wedge pair or *en face* electron boost to a total dose of 60–65 Gy.
6. For adenoid cystic carcinoma, the top field is at the TMJ or trachus.

RADIOTHERAPEUTIC RESULTS

The prognosis of malignant salivary gland tumors is closely related to the histologic type and grade, tumor size (T), status of nodal disease (N), location, and resection margin. In general, small tumors, low grade mucoepidermoid carcinoma, malignant mixed tumors, and acinic cell tumors have favorable biologic behavior. On the other hand, large tumors, adenocarcinoma, adenoid cystic carcinoma, high grade mucoepidermoid carcinoma, poorly differentiated carcinoma, and squamous cell carcinoma are generally aggressive in nature, with poor prognosis. Younger patients, less than 40 years of age, generally fare better than those of advanced age (more than 60 years old); for example, survival is 58% for younger patients versus 30% for the older group.[5] Female patients have a better survival rate than male patients (i.e., 50% versus 30%). If the lesion is totally resected, the patient's chance of survival is reasonably good, with 5-year survival rates of 85% and 67% for T1 and T2 lesions, respectively. Tumors located in the parotid gland have a better outlook than those in the submandibular or sublingual glands (46% versus 19%). Since most major salivary gland malignant tumors are treated by surgery, the results of primary radiation therapy are scarce, but scattered reports suggest that irradiation plays an important role for local control.[9-11] Postoperative radiation therapy for high grade malignancies has reduced the local failure rates following resection. Fu et al.[9] reported 35 patients with known microscopic tumor at or close to surgical margins following curative surgery; 14% (3/22) developed recurrence after postoperative radiation therapy as compared to 54% (7/13) in the nonirradiated group ($p > 0.05$). The radiotherapeutic results for inoperable salivary gland malignant tumors are poor, with local control rates ranging from 20% to 40% after conventional radiation therapy. Catterell et al. and others[13-15] reported significant improvement in local control rates of various parotid malignancies after neutron irradiation although there were increased radiation complications. Of 65 patients with locally advanced or recurrent parotid tumors, local control was achieved by fast neutron therapy in 72%, with a 5-year survival rate of 50%.

MGH EXPERIENCE

Our experience in treatment of salivary glands tumors were published in detail elsewhere[16] and updated recently. For T1−2 carcinomas ($n = 64$) the 5- and 10-year actuarial local control (LC) rates were 92% and 87%, respectively. For T3−4 tumors, both rates were 90%. The disease-free survival (DSS) rates were 89% and 82% for T1−2, and 68% and 60% for T3−4 lesions, respectively, as shown in Table 12.4.

Most of the treatment failures were due to local and distant spread, particularly for T3−4 squamous cell carcinoma, adenocarcinoma, undifferentiated carcinoma, and adenoid cystic carcinoma with an incidence ranging from one-quarter to one-half, as shown in Table 12.5.

TABLE 12.4   Actuarial Rates of Parotid Carcinoma After Combined Surgery and Radiation Therapy: MGH Experience, 1975–1994

	T1–2 ($n = 64$)	T3–4 ($n = 37$)
LC		
5 years	92	90
10 years	87	90
	$p = $ NS	
DSS		
5 years	89	82
10 years	68	60
	$p = 0.0007$	

TABLE 12.5   Patterns of Treatment Failure of Parotid Gland Carcinomas Related to Histology[16]

Tumor Types	Local (%)	Nodal (%)	Distant Metastases (%)
Mucoepidermoid (High grade)	6	0	6
Squamous cell	50	0	50
Adenocarcinoma	0	14	53
Undifferentiated	0	33	33
Adenoid cystic	19	0	25
Acinic cell	0	0	11

BID Radiation Therapy

For the past 15 years, accelerated hyperfractionated radiation therapy with two daily fractions of 1.6 Gy each (BID) has been used at the MGH for treatment of inoperable or advanced salivary gland malignant tumors, and the short-term local control has been extremely satisfactory. The results previously published elsewhere indicate good local control of most unresectable carcinomas.[17]

SPECIAL SITUATIONS

Adenoid Cystic Carcinoma

Adenoid cystic carcinoma is a relatively common subtype of salivary gland carcinomas and is characterized by chronicity and high incidence of distant spread. Its management is by combined surgery and radiation therapy. Eighty-four patients with such lesions were treated at the MGH. Sixty-four received combined surgery and radiation therapy and the 5- and 10-year actuarial local control (LC) rates were 87% and 78%, respectively; the corresponding disease-specific survival (DSS) rates were 93% and 82%, respectively.

TABLE 12.6 Actuarial LC and DSS Rates of Adenoid Cystic Carcinoma Related to Treatment Methods: 1975–1994

	S&RT ($n = 64$)	RT($n = 20$)	Total
LC			
5 years	87%	66%	82%
10 years	78%	66%	75%
			$p = 0.049$
DSS			
5 years	93%	85%	92%
10 years	82%	66%	78%

S&RT, surgery and radiation therapy; RT, radiation therapy.

Twenty patients were treated by radiation alone and the 5-year and 10-year local control rates were both 66%; the corresponding disease-specific survival rates were 85% and 66%, respectively as shown in Table 12.6.

Mucoepidermoid Carcinoma

Mucoepidermoid carcinomas comprise approximately 10% of all salivary gland tumors. The parotid gland is most commonly involved by the neoplasms. Next to the parotid gland, the palate is a common site of involvement. These tumors may have various degrees of biologic aggressiveness. The high grade lesions may invade the adjacent structures and/or spread distantly and become unresectable. Treatment therefore calls for radical surgery and postoperative radiation therapy. The low grade lesions generally carry a relatively favorable prognosis and do not require postoperative radiation therapy if the resection margins are free from involvement. Table 12.7 shows the local control of mucoepidermoid carcinomas treated at the MGH, mostly by combined surgery and radiation therapy.

TABLE 12.7 Five-Year Actuarial LC and DSS Rates of Mucoepidermoid Carcinoma Related to Grades Treated by Combined Radiation Therapy and Surgery or Radiation Therapy Alone: MGH Experience, 1970–1994

	High Grade		Low Grade	
	S&RT	RT	S&RT	RT
T1–2	$n = 26$	$n = 1$	$n = 7$	$n = 1$
LC	95%	100%	100%	100%
DSS	91%	100%	100%	100%
T3–4	$n = 10$	$n = 9$	$n = 2$	$n = 2$
LC	100%	42%	100%	50%
DSS	100%	53%	100%	0%

Unresectable Salivary Gland Carcinoma

Our experience with photon irradiation of unresectable salivary gland carcinoma was published elsewhere.[17] A total of 14 patients with unresectable parotid carcinomas received full-course radiation therapy, and the 5-year actuarial local control rate was 82% while the disease-specific survival rate was 55%. Twenty-seven patients with inoperable oral and oropharyngeal minor salivary gland carcinoma had a local control rate of 75% and disease-specific survival rate of 85%, after definitive radiation therapy. Of a total of 41 patients with unresectable salivary gland carcinoma, the LC and DSS rates were 77% and 75%, respectively, as shown in Table 12.8.

TABLE 12.8   Five-Year Actuarial LC and DSS Rates of Unresectable Salivary Carcinoma After Radiation Therapy: MGH Experience, 1975–1994

Parotid gland	$n = 14$	
LC		82%
DSS		55%
Oral and oropharyngeal	$n = 27$	
LC		75%
DSS		85%
Total	$n = 41$	
LC		77%
DSS		75%

Recurrent Pleomorphic Adenomas

From 1975 through 1994, 39 patients with recurrent pleomorphic adenomas received irradiation with or without debulking and enjoyed a 10-year actuarial local control rate of 91%, and disease-specific survival rate of 100%, as shown in Figure 12.6.

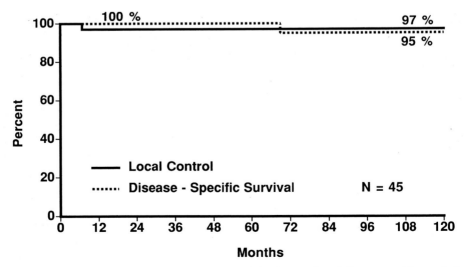

FIGURE 12.6   Graph showing 10-year actuarial local control and disease-specific survival rates in patients with pleomorphic adenoma, treated by combined surgery and radiation therapy.

SUMMARY

Malignant tumors arising from the salivary glands are uncommon lesions. These tumors have varied biologic and clinical unpredictability. Their primary treatment is surgical resection. Radiation therapy is used as an adjuvant, either before or after surgery, or sandwiched for unresectable tumors. The radiation techniques should be individualized according to the size and site of the lesion. For the small lesion arising from the oral cavity, local control can be achieved by combined external radiation and intersitital implant with good functional and cosmetic results.

Recurrent pleomorphic adenomas are treated by debulking surgery and postoperative radiation. Meticulous evaluation of the disease process, careful RT techniques, and combined efforts among surgeons, radiation oncologists, and pathologists yield good local control and survival. These tumors tend to late recurrences. Therefore long-term follow-up is required.

Management of salivary gland malignancies has traditionally been within the province of surgeons. In the past decade, significant progress in radiation oncology has been made in the management of this disease. In order to achieve maximal cure rate and preservation of functions and cosmesis, radiation oncologists must come be able to offer patients the utmost benefits in terms of adjuvant or curative endeavors.

REFERENCES

1. Paff GH: *Anatomy of the head and neck.* Philadelphia: Saunders, 1973.
2. American Joint Committee on *Cancer. Manual for staging of cancer*, 4th ed. Philadelphia: Lippincott, 1992.
3. Batsakis JG: *Tumors of the head and neck. Clinical and pathological considerations,* 2nd ed. Baltimore: Williams & Wilkins, 1979.
4. Gates GA: Current concepts in otolaryngology: malignant neoplasms of the minor salivary glands. *N Engl J Med* 1982;306:718–722.
5. Frazell EL: Clinical aspects of tumors of the major salivary glands. *Cancer* 1954;7: 637–659.
6. Eneroth CM: Salivary gland tumors in the parotid gland, submandibular gland and the palate region. *Cancer* 1971;27:1415.
7. Spiro RH, Huvos AG, Strong EW: Cancer of the parotid gland: a clinicopathologic study of 289 primary cases. *Am J Surg* 1975;130:452–459.
8. Johns ME, Kaplan MJ: Surgical therapy of tumors of the salivary gland. In: *Comprehensive management of head and neck tumors.* X, eds. Thawley SE, Panje WR, Batsakis JG, Lindberg RD: Philadelphia, WB SAunders 1987; 1122.
9. Fu KK, Leibel SA, Levine ML, et al: Carcinoma of the major and minor salivary glands. *Cancer* 1977;40:2882–2890.
10. Shidnia H, Hornback NB, Hamaker R, et al: Carcinoma of the major salivary glands. *Cancer* 1980;45:693–697.
11. McNaney D, McNeese MD, Guillamondegui OM, et al: Postoperative irradiation in malignant epithelial tumors of the parotid. *Int J Radiat Oncol Biol Phys* 1983;9: 1289–1295.

12. Borthne A, Kjellevoid K, Kaalhus O, et al. Salivary gland malignant neoplasms: treatment and prognosis. *Int J Radiat Oncol Biol Phys* 1986;12:747–754.

13. Griffin TW, Pajak TF, Laramore GE, et al: Neutron versus photon irradiation of inoperable salivary gland tumors: results of an RTOG-MRC cooperative randomized study. *Int J Radiat Oncol Biol Phys* 1988;15:1085–1090.

14. Duncan W, Orr JA, Amott SJ, et al: Neutrol therapy for malignant tumors of the salivary gland. *Radiother Oncol* 1987;8:97–104.

15. Cattrerall M, Errington RD, Bewley DK: A comparison of clinical and laboratory data on neutron therapy for locally advanced tumors. *Int J Radiat Oncol Biol Phys* 1987;13:1783–1791.

16. Spiro IJ, Wang CC, Montgomery WW: Carcinoma of the parotid gland. *Cancer* 1993;71:2699–2705.

17. Wang CC, Goodman M: Photon irradiation of unresectable carcinomas of salivary glands. *Int J Radiat Oncol Biol Phys* 1991;21:569–576.

CHAPTER 13

CARCINOMA IN CERVICAL NODE WITH UNKNOWN PRIMARY

A lump in the neck or enlarged cervical lymph node in an adult presents a challenge to diagnostic acumen and therapeutic skills.[1] Although some of the adenopathy is benign, most lesions in adults should be considered malignant until proved otherwise. This is particularly true in patients older than 40 years with a history of heavy tobacco and alcohol consumption.

An enlarged cervical lymph node calls for careful general evaluation before a biopsy is performed. In the parotid area, careful examination should be done for a primary lesion in the skin of the face or scalp or inquiry should be made regarding previous history of removal of a skin lesion in a private office. When a patient presents with cervical adenopathy, a complete head and neck examination is mandatory to exclude the possibility of primary carcinoma arising from the upper air and food passages with cervical metastasis. This should include careful inspection and palpation, if feasible, of the oral cavity, oropharynx, hypopharynx, and larynx by gloved finger and indirect laryngoscopy. Examination of the nasopharynx by indirect nasopharyngoscopy is a casual procedure at best; direct fiberoptiscopy through the nares is preferred.

Radiographic studies including CT, MR, and contrast studies of the suspicious site and the neck nodes may yield information of abnormalities that may exist in the head and neck regions, which are not revealed by clinical examination. If no primary lesion is found after these procedures are performed, fine needle aspiration may yield invaluable information as to the lesions histologic cell type. Should the needling procedure be unrevealing, incisional or excisional biopsy of the lymph node may reveal the histologic diagnosis (i.e., epithelial versus lymphomatous cancer).

There are two manageable therapeutic options after the histologic nature of the cervical lymph node is known. First, if it is lymphoma, the patient should have a "lymphoma work-up" to exclude the possibility of systemic disease. Treatment by localized radiation therapy versus systemic chemotherapy will be determined. Second, if it is carcinoma, a further search for the primary site by mapping and multiple biopsies of Waldeyer's ring (nasopharynx, tonsil, base of the tongue) as well as the hypopharynx and supraglottis should be considered. Again, if multiple biopsies reveal no pathologic lesion, the diagnosis of carcinoma in the neck with "unknown primary" is made. The primary lesion is occult and may or may not become apparent, depending on the treatment procedure used.

Squamous cell carcinoma arising from a branchial cleft is extremely rare. Therefore any carcinoma in the cervical lymph node must be considered to represent metastasis from a primary lesion either in the head and neck region (thyroid included) or below the clavicle (lung or gastrointestinal tract). The cervical lesion is staged according to the AJC (N) classification.[2]

Since the pattern of spread is reasonably predictable,[3,4] knowledge of (1) cell type, (2) location of the node, and (3) associated symptoms may provide the clues to search for the primary lesion.

1. *Cell Type*   Carcinomas arising from various anatomic sites of the head and neck have different cell types and degrees of differentiation. Undifferentiated carcinomas or lymphoepitheliomas most likely arise from Waldeyer's ring. Carcinomas of the oral cavity tend to be well differentiated, whereas lesions arising from the hypopharynx and supraglottis are moderately to poorly differentiated.

2. *Location of Node*   The pattern of spread of carcinoma of the head and neck generally is specific and predictable. The location of the metastatic lymph nodes in the neck may reveal a clue as to the primary site. Carcinoma of the nasopharynx, for instance, commonly metastasizes to the upper neck between the angle of the jaw and the mastoid tip (i.e., superior deep jugular, submastoid, and subdigastric lymph nodes and posterior cervical triangle) and is most unlikely to spread to the submandibular or midjugular lymph nodes. Carcinomas of the faucial tonsil or base of the tongue commonly metastasize to the subdigastric (tonsil) lymph node. Likewise, carcinomas of the supraglottis and pyriform sinus usually spread to the subdigastric and midjugular lymph nodes. On the contrary, solitary metastatic carcinoma to the posterior cervical lymph nodes from the anterior oral cavity and supraglottic larynx almost never occurs. Identification of the site of nodal involvement allows the clinician to proceed with inspection and biopsy of the suspected or most likely site of the primary lesion. The location of various groups of lymph nodes in the head and neck area are shown in Figure 13.1. The following list is a general summary of the location of lymph node disease related to possible sites of primary lesions:

Level 1	Submental nodes — skin of nose, nasal vestibule, lip, anterior floor of the mouth
	Submandibular nodes — skin of the face, lips, oral cavity
Level 2	Upper deep jugular nodes — nasopharynx, oropharynx, soft palate

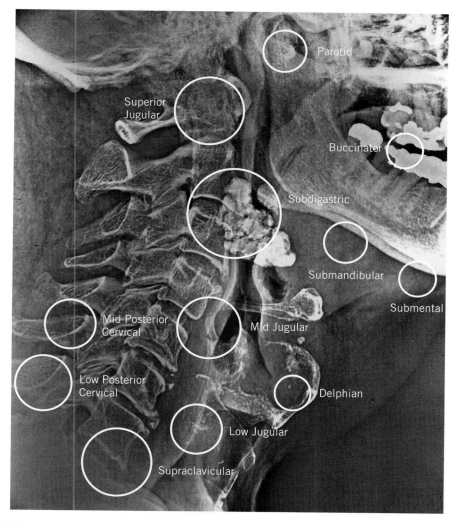

FIGURE 13.1   Location of various cervical lymph nodes relevant to management of cancer of the head and neck.

Subdiagastric nodes—Waldeyer's ring, that is nasopharynx, tonsil, base of tongue, hypopharynx, posterior oral cavity, soft palate.

Level 3   Midjugular nodes—anterior oral tongue, hypopharynx, supraglottis, thyroid

Level 4   Inferior jugular nodes—glottis, subglottis, thyroid, cervical esophagus

Delphian node—Larynx, thyroid

Level 5	Posterior cervical triangle nodes—skin of posterior neck, scalp, subocciput
Rouviere's node	Nasopharynx, pharyngeal wall, hypopharynx
Parotid node	Skin of face, eyelid, scalp, anterior auricle, upper lip, parotid gland
Supraclavicular nodes	Thyroid, cervical esophagus, infraclavicular (i.e., lung, esophagus) and infradiaphragmatic primaries

3. *Symptoms* Most metastatic lymph nodes are painless and rarely produce any symptoms locally. Careful evaluation of the patient's discomfort or symptoms and signs in the head and neck regions may give a clue to the site of the primary lesion. For example, the following associations can be made:

Earache	Faucial tonsil, floor of mouth, tongue, hypopharynx, supraglottis, glottis
Sore throat or odynophagia	Soft palate, tonsil, base of tongue, hypopharynx, supraglottis
Hoarseness	Larynx, pyriform sinus, supraglottis, thyroid, mediastinum
Nasal obstruction	Nasopharynx, paranasal sinus, nasal vestibule and cavity
Cranial nerve paralysis and facial pain	Nasopharynx, paranasal sinus, deep lobe of parotid gland, jugular foramen
Impaired hearing and otitis media	Nasopharynx, middle and inner ear, petrous apex, internal auditory meatus

Pain in the ear is a common complaint in the patient with head and neck carcinoma. It is the referred earache from advanced ulcerative and infiltrative lesions. Knowledge of the origin of the earache, or otalgia, and of the nerve pathways may aid in the search for the primary lesion. Figure 13.2 illustrates anatomic pathways of referred earache from various sites.

After patients are carefully examined by indirect and direct laryngoscopy, nasopharyngoscopy, and fiberoptiscopy, biopsy of the suspected sites is indicated, and, in most instances, the primary lesion can be found. Therapeutic management should be guided accordingly, as discussed in other chapters.

SELECTION OF THERAPY

The selection of therapeutic options is difficult and varies with the skill, experience, and attitude of the surgeon or radiation oncologist. Because most malignant neck lymph nodes represent metastatic disease from a head and neck primary lesion, comprehensive radiation therapy to the suspected primary site and the neck appears to be the appropriate therapeutic option.

Other conservative options include neck dissection followed by a "wait-and-see" policy for the manifestation of the primary lesion.[5] This policy may be suitable for

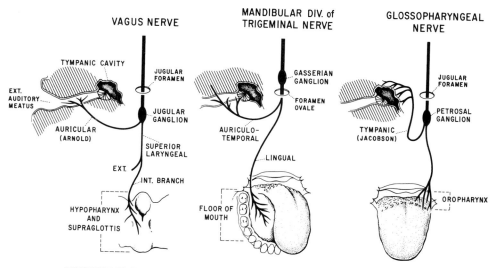

FIGURE 13.2   Pathways of referred otalgia related to various tumor sites.

well differentiated lesions in Level I location, in which the occult lesion most likely is in the oral cavity and easily detected and treated. For undifferentiated lesions involving multiple levels (i.e., N2–3), a combination of radiation therapy and surgery is indicated. Radiation therapy is effective not only in improving local control but also in preventing contralateral neck metastases.[6,7]

The following management policies for occult primaries are used at the MGH:

N1 lesion (small node)

   Surgery   Lumpectomy or limited neck dissection to be followed by "wait-and-see" program for Level I lesions

              or

   Radiation therapy   60 Gy to suspicious sites; 50 Gy to whole neck; 10–15 Gy to lumpectomy site

N2a,b,c lesions (large or multiple nodes)

   Surgery   Radical or functional neck dissection, followed by 60 Gy postoperatively to the neck and suspicious primary sites

              or

   Radiation therapy   60 Gy preoperatively to whole neck, suspicious site boosted to 65 Gy, followed by RND or functional neck dissection

N3 lesions (large nodes or fixed nodes)—most likely inoperable

   Radiation therapy   60 Gy to whole neck and suspicious site and 10–15 Gy boost to bulky nodes preoperatively

   Surgery   Postradiation neck dissection, if operable; if inoperable, consider chemotherapy

RADIOTHERAPEUTIC MANAGEMENT

Radiation therapy for an occult primary lesion with metastatic disease in the neck calls for careful treatment planning to prevent xerostomia. If the neck disease is high in the neck and poorly differentiated, the entire Waldeyer's ring and lymph node disease are treated in continuity on the presumption that the primary lesion arises either in the nasopharynx, base of the tongue, or faucial tonsil. In such instances, the parotid glands must be included within the beam, resulting in marked xerostomia. On the other hand, if the subdigastric or midjugular lymph nodes only are affected and the high jugular and submastoid lymph nodes are uninvolved, the probability of nasopharyngeal carcinoma is low, and therefore the nasopharynx and part of the parotid glands can be excluded from the high-dose volume and the resulting xerostomia can be lessened. For carcinoma located in the submandibular area or low jugular lymph nodes, the probability of a nasopharyngeal or oropharyngeal primary lesion is exceedingly low, and therefore these sites and the parotid glands need not be irradiated.

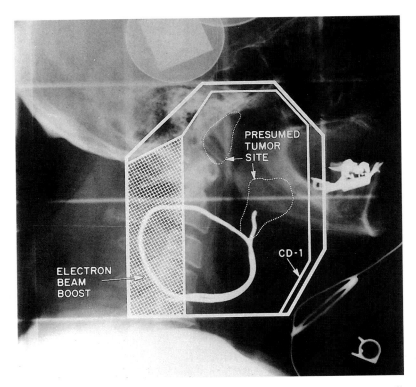

FIGURE 13.3 Simulation film showing portal arrangement for large squamous cell carcinoma in the neck with an occult primary, presumably in Waldeyer's ring. The patient is NED 25 years after treatment but developed a second primary in the lung.

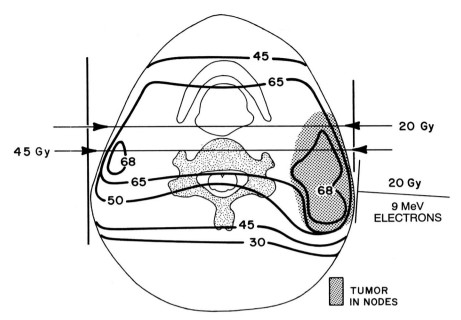

FIGURE 13.4 Composite isodoses of external photons through opposing lateral portals and electron boost to the node.

Technical Pointers

1. Patient is to lie supine with the head immobilized.

2. Exploit the concept of tumoritis and deliver 20 Gy in 2 weeks, with 1.8–2 Gy/f initially through large portals, to the nasopharynx, oropharynx, and hypopharynx. Look for tumoritis, which may indicate the primary site. If the primary lesion is detected, revise the portals and continue comprehensive radiation therapy to the known primary site and neck nodes for a dose of 50 Gy.

3. If the lesion is ipsilateral, a wedge pair technique or electron beam is used to boost the primary toward the completion of radiation therapy.

4. If no primary site is found, use a large off-cord field to deliver a total dose of 60 Gy to the neck and suspicious site (Figures 13.3, 13.4). Continue to monitor and search for the primary.

5. It is important to irradiate both sides of the neck to prevent contralateral nodal recurrence even in patients with ipsilateral neck nodes.

6. For metastatic nodes in the submandibular triangle, use an ipsilateral and AP wedge pair technique to deliver approximately 50 Gy, followed by electron beam boost. Concurrently, irradiate the ipsilateral low neck for 45 Gy electively. The parotid gland and the posterior cervical lymph nodes need not be included within the treatment portals.

RESULTS OF THERAPY

Radical neck dissection alone is effective in controlling carcinoma in the neck with unknown primary. If the neck is treated by surgery without adjuvant mucosal irradiation to the primary, 20–30% of the patients may subsequently develop primary lesions in the head and neck region.[8] Survival in the patients is decreased compared with that in patients whose primary lesion remained occult (30% versus 60%, respectively).[8–10]

Most reported series indicate that surgery or radiation therapy yield 3-year survival of 40–50% and 5-year survival of 25–50%.[9,11] Results after combined therapies (i.e., surgery and radiation therapy) generally show somewhat higher survival rates.[8] Most series indicate overall survival results without subdivision of the stages of the disease. These data, however, can only be used as a general guideline in the management of this disease.

Recent publications indicate that local control rates range from 70% to 80% at 5 years, with corresponding survival rates of 30–60%. The prognosis is influenced by the N stage, number of positive nodes, fixation of node, extracapsular tumor spread, probably cell types, and level of the nodes in the neck.[5,12–14] The incidence of development of primaries range from 20% to 30% without irradiation; contralateral neck metastases occur in 15% of cases if the contralateral neck did not receive either irradiation or surgical treatment.[7]

MGH EXPERIENCE

From 1970 through 1994, 88 patients received radiation therapy for squamous cell carcinoma in the neck with unknown primary. All lesions were staged according to the AJC N stage[2] classification, and all patients received, high-dose radiation therapy with or without radical neck dissection (RND). The 5-year actuarial local control (LC) and disease-specific survival (DSS) rates after treatment are shown in Table 13.1.

Of 20 patients with N1 disease, the LC and DSS rates were 88% and 89%, respectively. Of 47 patients with N2 disease the LC and DSS rates were 58% and 57%, respectively. There were 21 patients with N3 disease, and the corresponding rates were 81% and 65%, respectively. Thus, of a total of 88 patients, the LC and DSS rates were 74% and 68%, respectively, after radiation therapy with or without surgery. Those patients who required radical neck dissection generally had more advanced disease, with poor prognosis. Fourteen patients in the N1 group had lumpectomy (excision of the

TABLE 13.1 Five-Year Actuarial LC and DSS Rates After Treatment of Occult Primary with or Without RND: MGH Experience, 1970–1994

Stage	n	LC (%)	DSS (%)
N1	20	88	89
N2	47	58	57
N3	21	81	65
Total	88	74	68

TABLE 13.2 Five-Year LC and DSS Rates After Treatment of Squamous Cell Carcinoma in the Neck with Occult Primary, Related to Cell Types

Cell Type	n	LC (%)	DSS (%)
Lymphoepithelioma	7	60	80
Squamous cell carcinoma	78	76	67
Undifferentiated carcinoma	1	100	100

node) and postoperative radiation therapy; all remained free of disease. Of six patients with N1 disease having RND, only 63% achieved local control while the DSS rate for this group was 80%. Of 53 patients with N2 and N3 disease combined, who were treated with radiation therapy alone, 74% had no evidence of disease, while of 15 patients who had undergone RND, only 47% were NED.

Cell types did not appear to affect local control and survival. For all tumor types, the LC and DSS rates ranged from 70% to 80%, as shown in Table 13.2.

The numbers of patients having the diagnosis of lymphoepithelioma and undifferentiated carcinoma are small, and most patients with such initial diagnoses had their primaries discovered in Waldeyer's ring. The data therefore showed no significant difference among various cell types.

Results of Twice-Daily Radiation Therapy

From 1979 through 1994, 46 patients received twice-daily radiation therapy for occult primary with metastases to the neck. Of these, 7 had N1 disease and 39 had N2–3 lesions treated either with lumpectomy or neck dissection. Of the entire group, the 5-year actuarial LC rate of neck disease without manifestation of a primary lesion was 77% and the DSS rate was 70%, as shown in Table 13.3. These results were not significantly different from the results for the once-daily group treated from 1970 to 1978.

TABLE 13.3 Five-Year Actuarial Rates After Treatment of Occult Primary with or Without RND: QD versus BID RT

	n	LC	DSS
N1			
BID	7	100%	100%
QD	13	83%	84%
		$p = 0.32$	$p = 0.28$
N2–3			
BID	39	71%	63%
QD	29	67%	56%
		$p = 0.6$	$p = 0.6$
Total			
BID	46	77%	70%
QD	42	72%	67%
		$p = 0.6$	$p = 0.6$

SUMMARY

Squamous cell carcinoma in the cervical lymph nodes is not a disease per se but represents a variety of malignancies arising from different anatomic sites of the head and neck. The most common sites of occult primary lesions are within Waldeyer's ring, the hypopharynx, and supraglottis; and the least common sites are the oral cavity, nasal cavity, and paranasal sinuses. Therefore these probable tumor sites must be targeted for intensive investigation before a diagnosis of metastatic carcinoma in the neck with an "unknown primary" can be made. Detailed treatment depends on the location, size, number of lymph nodes, extranodal spread, bilaterality, and cell type.

The prognosis depends on the radiosensitivity of the lymph nodes and the extent of neck involvement. Most therapeutic failures are due to inability to control the disease in the neck and/or development of contralateral neck nodes if only one side of the diseased neck is treated either by surgery or radiation therapy in appropriate patients. Generally, a dose of 60 Gy to the occult site can sterilize the microscopic primary lesion satisfactorily.

For N1 lesions diagnosed with either lympectomy or incisional biopsy, neck dissection alone may be adequate in highly selected patients, preferably with easily observed presumed primary sites. Since radiation therapy to the suspected primary site and the neck can achieve a high cure rate without the necessity of neck dissection, radiation therapy is a good alternative treatment method. For N2 lesions, the management should be combined therapies, that is, neck dissection with either preoperative or postoperative radiation therapy to both sides of the neck. For N3 disease, local control is poor, management should be combined preoperative radiation therapy and (if operable) radical neck dissection. Survival of the patient is dismal due to the failure to control the neck disease and the development of distant metastases.

The present data indicate that twice-daily (BID) radiation therapy is not more effective than once-daily (QD) radiation therapy, although the number of patients in the two groups was small for meaningful analysis.

REFERENCES

1. Greenberg BE: Cervical lymph node metastasis from unknown primary sites: unresolved problem in management. *Cancer* 1966;19:1091–1095.
2. American Joint Committee on Cancer: *Manual for staging of cancer.* Philadelphia: Lippincott, 1992.
3. Shear M, Hawkins DM, Farr HW: The prediction of lymph node metastases from oral squamous carcinoma. *Cancer* 1976;37:1901–1907.
4. Lindberg RD: Distribution of cervical lymph node metastasis from squamous cell carcinoma of the upper respiratory and digestive tracts. *Cancer* 1972;29:1446.
5. Coster JR, Foote RL, Olsen KD, et al: Cervical nodal metastases of squamous cell carcinoma of unknown origin: indications for withholding radiation therapy. *Int J Radiat Oncol Biol Phys* 1992;23:743–749.

6. Glynne-Jones RGT, Anand AK, Young TE, Berry RJ: Metastatic carcinoma in the cervical lymph nodes from an occult primary: a conservative approach to the role of radiotherapy. *Int J Radiat Oncol Biol Phys* 1990;18:289–294.

7. Carlson LS, Fletcher GH, Oswald MJ: Guidelines for radiotherapeutic techniques for cervical metastases from an unknown primary. *Int J Radiat Oncol Biol Phys* 1986; 12:2101–2110.

8. Fletcher GH: Elective irradiation of subclinical disease in cancers of the head and neck. *Cancer* 1972;29:1450–1454.

9. Coker DD, Casterline PF, Chambers RG, et al: Metastases to lymph nodes of the head and neck from an unknown primary site. *Am J Surg* 1977;134:517–522.

10. Jesse RH, Perez CA, Fletcher GH: Cervical lymph node metastases: with an unknown primary cancer. *Cancer* 1973;31:854–859.

11. Barrie JR, Knapper, WH, Strong EW: Cervical nodal metastases of unknown origin. *Cancer* 1971;21:112–119.

12. Stell PM, Morton RP, Singh SD: Cervical lymph node metastases: the significance of the level of the lymph node. *Clin Oncol* 1983;9:101–107.

13. Maulard C, Housset M, Brunel P, et al: Postoperative radiation therapy for cervical lymph node metastases from an occult squamous cell carcinoma. *Laryngoscope* 1992; 102:884–890.

14. Dickson R, Vargas DR: Occult primary of the head and neck. *J Otolaryngol* 1979;8: 427–434.

CHAPTER 14

TUMORS OF THE TEMPORAL BONE AND SKULL BASE

Of radiotherapeutic interest, tumors of the temporal bone and skull base area consist of carcinoma and glomus tumor. These tumors are uncommon and will be discussed in separate categories.

A. CARCINOMAS

Carcinoma arising from the temporal bone is extremely rare. Its incidence is estimated to be one case in 10,000 to 20,000 otologic pathologic conditions.[1] Chronic otitis externa and otorrhea are often associated with carcinoma of the external auditory canal. About one-quarter of these cases arising from the middle ear and mastoid exhibit, in addition, cholesteatoma.[2] This disease affects the middle-aged population with a slight female predominance. Because of the rarity of this disease, there is a lack of awareness on the part of general physicians to suspect a malignancy being present in the ear canal or its adjacent part. Therefore early diagnosis is rarely made, and in most cases when first seen the lesions are often associated with bone involvement, thus rendering a marked decrease of curability.

To evaluate the extent of the disease, careful physical examination must include inspection of the external auditory canal and palpation of the adjacent parotid gland and the regional lymphatic area for adenopathy. Cranial nerves VII and VIII and the last four cranial nerves should carefully be evaluated. Radiographic examination includes CT and MR scans with or without supplemental angiography. If accessible, the lesion should be biopsied for histologic confirmation of cell type prior to definitive therapies.

SELECTION OF THERAPY

Because of the rarity of this disease, treatments vary greatly in various institutions and include radical surgery, radiation therapy alone,[3,4] and a combination of surgery and radiation therapy,[5-7] with local control rates ranging from 10% to 50%.[6,8-12] Without an established acceptable staging system, it is impossible to compare treatment results from various institutions or treatment modalities.

The present treatment policy for temporal bone malignancies is a combination of surgery and radiation therapy. It is desirable that radical surgery be performed first with removal of the bulk of the lesion, evaluation of the extent of the disease, establishment of drainage and control of the suppurative process, and resurfacing of the exposed bone by skin or fat grafts, to be followed by postoperative radiation therapy. Except in early lesions without evidence of bone destruction, primary radiation therapy for this disease is rarely successful and therefore is not advised. The incidence of regional lymph node metastases is low, approximately 10%, and elective treatment is not indicated in patients with no neck disease.

RADIOTHERAPEUTIC MANAGEMENT

Radiation therapy of this disease calls for meticulous technique. Ipsilateral wedge paired portals with megavoltage radiations combined with electrons are used. Generally, 40 Gy with photons and 20 Gy with electrons are well tolerated. There is a delicate balance between permanent local control of the malignant process in the temporal bone achieved by high doses of radiation therapy and the increased incidence of osteoradionecrosis. The radiation dosage is limited to 60 Gy with 1.8–2 Gy/fraction in 6–7 weeks, 5 fractions per week. No portion of the temporal bone should receive radiation therapy dosages in excess of 70 Gy, if osteoradionecrosis is to be avoided.[13] Figure 14.1a illustrates the wedge-shaped isodose distributions in the treatment of temporal bone tumors. Figure 14.1b shows a modified form, combining wedge pair photon and appositional electron beams in a 2:1 ratio, with "brick-shaped" isodose distributions for larger lesions.

Technical Pointers

1. Patient is to lie supine, with chin hyperextended, and is immobilized with a face mask.
2. Do not begin radiation therapy until the surgical wound is completely healed. Exposed bone is prone to develop osteoradionecrosis.
3. If the lesion is limited within the temporal bone, use an ipsilateral oblique wedge pair technique. Be certain that the exit beam of the posterior oblique portal does not include the contralateral eye.

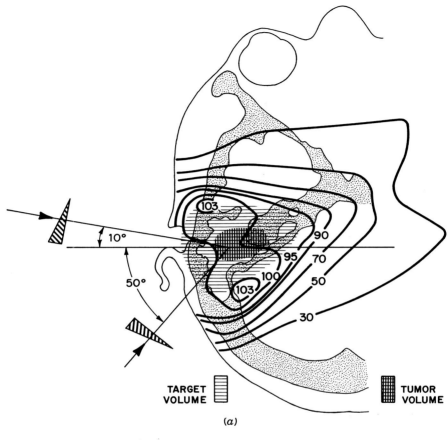

WEDGE PAIR TECHNIQUE

60° HINGE ANGLE
45° WEDGES : 60° WEDGES   1:1 RATIO

FIGURE 14.1   Diagrams showing isodose distributions: (a) using ipsilateral oblique wedge pair portal technique for tumors arising within the temporal bone for 50 Gy and supplemented by electron beam to higher dose as needed, and (b) using a combination of oblique wedge pair and appositional electron boost technique, in a 2:1 ratio, with "brick-shaped" composite isodoses.

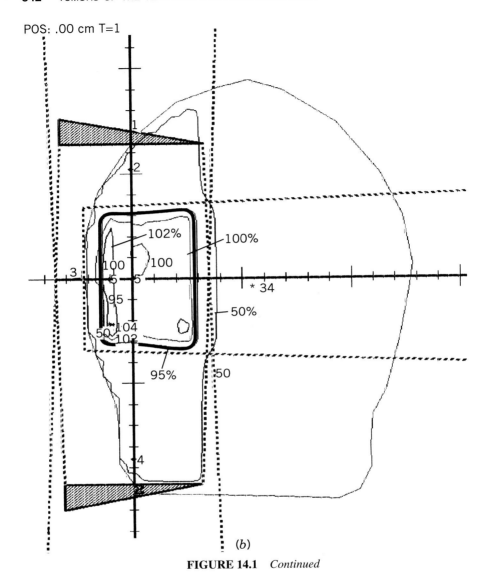

FIGURE 14.1 *Continued*

4. In order to reduce the "hot spot" behind the wedge, mix with an appositional electron beam technique in a 2:1 ratio if more than 60 Gy is planned.

5. For the extensive lesion involving the parotid gland with nodal disease, use an anteroposterior approach to include the temporal bone, parotid gland, and entire ipsilateral neck for approximately 40 Gy, to be followed by either wedge pair photon or appositional electrons for an additional 20 Gy. (See Chapter 12 for discussion of parotid gland tumors.)

MGH AND MEEI EXPERIENCE

From 1956 through 1994 inclusive, a total of 63 patients with carcinoma of the temporal bone region received radiation therapy; and of these 59 had combined surgery and radiation therapy and four had radiation therapy alone due to inoperable lesions. Thirty-four patients had carcinoma arising from the external auditory canal, and 29 had tumors involving the middle ear and mastoid. Various cell types included 51 squamous cell carcinomas, six adenocysticcarcinomas, two adenocarcinomas, two basal cell carcinomas, and one myoepithelioma, and one poorly differentiated carcinoma. The female to male ratio was 1.4:1. Surgical procedures included excisional resection, radical mastoidectomy, and/or temporal bone resection with or without parotidectomy or mandibulectomy. Some procedures were considered as palliative due to the presence of gross residual disease after surgery. All patients were treated with megavoltage radiations.

Figure 14.2 shows the 5- and 10-year actuarial local control rates for these two groups of patients following treatment by combined surgery and radiation therapy. Of 34 patients with carcinoma of the external auditory canal, the local control rates for 5 and 10 years were 64% and 60%, respectively. For the 29 patients with middle ear and mastoid carcinomas, the corresponding rates were 48% and 48%.

Six patients with adenoid cystic carcinoma and two with adenocarcinoma had 100% survival, except for one whose tumor recurred at the sixth year after treatment. One patient with myoepithelioma was free of disease 5 years after undergo-

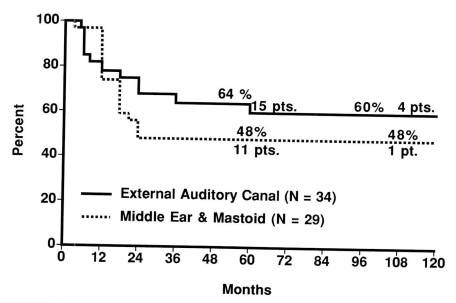

FIGURE 14.2   Diagram showing 5- and 10-year actuarial local control rates in patients with carcinoma of the external auditory canal and the middle ear and mastoid sinus.

ing combined therapies. Four patients received radiation therapy alone because of inoperability of the lesion and died within 2 years.

Six patients developed osteoradionecrosis of the temporal bone. Of these, three were free of cancer and three died with malignant disease. All patients with osteoradionecrosis were treated by excessively high doses of radiation therapy, exceeding the limits of tolerance as previously reported.[13]

B. PARAGANGLIOMA

Glomus tumors or chemodectomas arising from the jugular bulb, nerve of Jacobson, and nerve of Arnold are uncommon tumors. These vascular lesions are now commonly termed, according to site of origin, as glomus jugulare, glomus tympanicum, and glomus vagale, respectively, and pathologically are best described under the common category of paraganglioma. The great majority of glomus tumors are benign, slowly growing and spreading by local extension.[14] Owing to lack of significant symptoms, the tumors tend to be diagnosed late in the course of the disease. Metastases to the regional nodes and distant sites are extremely rare.

The frequent otologic symptoms and signs of these tumors originating or extending into the middle ear are pressure sensation in the ear, the presence of an aural polyp, progressive loss of hearing, a sensation of fullness, or pulsating tinnitus. Patients with extensive disease extending to the middle cranial fossa may experience vertigo, temporoparietal headache, retro-orbital pain, proptosis, and paresis of cranial nerves V and VI. Other symptoms and signs include dysphagia, occipital headache, ataxia, and hoarseness of voice; paralysis of cranial nerves IX to XII may occur if the tumor reaches the posterior cranial fossa and nerves V to VII, while invasion of the jugular foramen causes paralysis.

Glomus tumor may secrete norepinephrine and epinephrine, producing symptoms similar to pheochromocytoma. The catecholamines are rapidly inactivated and their urinary metabolites vanillylmandelic acid can be measured and used as a guide to the success of therapies.

Evaluation of the extent of these lesions is based on careful analysis of the symptoms and neurologic signs and detailed radiological examinations, including CT and MR scans of the temporal bone and brain in appropriate projections. Angiography is a useful radiographic technique for assessment of intracranial extension of the disease, or possible second or third tumors, and as a vehicle for embolization. Biopsy is rarely required and in fact is quite risky if the angiogram is positive.

SELECTION OF THERAPY

For small tumors limited to the middle ear, surgical excision may be undertaken. This is in the form of hypotympanectomy or radical mastoidectomy and temporal bone resection. Because of the intricate anatomy of the temporal bone, the surgical removal of extensive glomus tumors arising from the jugular bulb is often incomplete and followed by postoperative local recurrence.[15] Large tumors with intracranial extension are rarely amenable to treatment by surgical removal. Since these tumors are generally extremely vascular, radical surgery is difficult and dangerous, and the surgical advocates frequently recommend radiation therapy.

Intra-arterial embolization of glomus tumors may be carried out either as a preoperative procedure or for palliation. Since most of these tumors are extremely vascular, embolization is seldom complete, and therefore the procedure may be considered prior to radiation therapy during angiographic study. Radiation therapy is used for residual or recurrent disease after radical mastoidectomy and/or temporal resection or for inoperable lesions as a growth restraint procedure.[14,16-20]

RADIOTHERAPEUTIC MANAGEMENT

For glomus tumors eccentrically situated in the temporal bone and skull base, the radiation therapy technique consists of ipsilateral wedge pair photons and appositional electrons for a dose of 45 Gy in 4.5–5 weeks with a daily fraction of 1.8 Gy.[21] For inoperable lesions, a dose of 50 Gy in 5–5.5 weeks should suffice to stop further progression of the disease. An extra high dose (i.e., 70 Gy) of radiation therapy for a benign chemodectoma is rarely justified.

RADIOTHERAPEUTIC RESULTS

Because of the indolent nature of most glomus tumors, it is difficult to assess and/or compare the results of various forms of therapy. The reported series have shown that results after combined surgery and radiation therapy for the lesion in the temporal bone were superior to surgery alone. Local recurrence can be reduced with postoperative radiation therapy.[15]

MGH EXPERIENCE

From 1958 through 1994, a total of 58 patients with glomus jugulare, glomus tympanicum, and glomus vagale were treated by radiation therapy. Of these, 23 received postoperative radiation therapy for residual disease preceded by radical mastoidectomy and/or temporal bone resection. Twenty-six patients received radiation therapy alone for inoperable tumors. Nine patients with gross recurrence after previous surgery had radiation therapy as a salvage procedure.

Figure 14.3 shows the results of treatment after radiation therapy. The 5- and 10-year actuarial progression-free survival rates of the entire group of patients, ranging from 1 to 25 years, were 98% and 87%, respectively.

Two patients had osteoradionecrosis: one died at 5½ years post-treatment and one was living at 6 years. One patient suffered recurrence (after treatment with 30

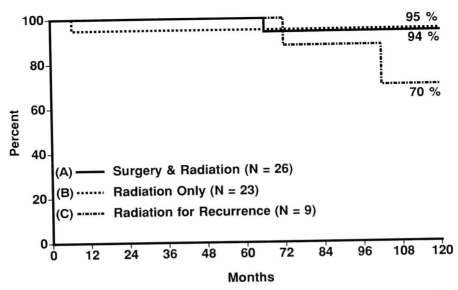

FIGURE 14.3 Diagram showing 5- and 10-year actuarial tumor progression-free survival of patients with glomus tumor after radiation therapy for various conditions: (A) after surgery for residual disease, (B) for gross recurrence after surgery, and (C) for inoperable tumor.

Gy) at 11 years. Of nine patients with gross recurrences after surgical resection, six were salvaged with no visible growth, one had a persistent but smaller growth, and two died of the disease with persistent tumor. Of nine patients receiving radiation therapy alone for unresectable tumors, six were living without progressive tumor, and one had persistent but smaller tumors of the glomus vagale, and two died of local disease.

SUMMARY

Carcinoma arising from or adjacent to the temporal bone is rare. The treatment of choice of this disease is a combination of surgery and radiation therapy. More than one-half of the patients so treated had survivorship of 5 or more years. Except in extremely early lesions without bony involvement, treatment by radiation therapy alone is rarely successful and therefore is not recommended. Likewise, patients with gross residual disease or postoperative recurrence are rarely salvageable by radiation therapy. Whether multidrug chemotherapy would alter such a dismal outlook remains to be seen.

Paragangliomas of the temporal bone or near the skull base area, including glomus lesions arising from the jugular bulb, nerve of Jacobson, and nerve of Arnold, are uncommon tumors and are treated by a combination of surgical resection (if the lesions are operable) and postoperative radiation therapy, which is effective in reducing the incidence of local recurrence. For inoperable glomus tumors, radiation therapy alone is the preferred treatment modality; it results in satisfactory local control and can provide patients with tumor progression-free survival. For patients with poor health and short-term prospect of survival, no treatment of a benign paraganglioma is appropriate.

The most serious complication of radiation therapy is osteoradionecrosis of the temporal bone; such complication is often due to an excessively high dose of radiation therapy but can be minimized by improvement of radiotherapeutic and surgical techniques. Treatment of benign paraganglioma, either by surgical or radiotherapeutic techniques, must be tempered with conservatism. Aggressive radiation therapy with excessively high dose is a disservice to patients with this disease.[13,22]

REFERENCES

1. Lewis JS: Cancer of the external auditory canal, middle ear and mastoid. In: Suen JY, Myers EN, eds. *Cancer of the head and neck.* New York: Churchill Livingstone, 1981; 561–562.

2. Lewis JS: Squamous cell carcinoma of the ear. *Arch Otolaryngol* 1973;97:41–42.

3. Boland J: The management of carcinoma of the middle ear. *Radiology* 1963;80:285.

4. Lederman M: Malignant tumors of the ear. *J Laryngol Otol* 1965;79:85–119.

5. Conley JJ, Schuller DE: Reconstruction following temporal bone resection. *Arch Otolaryngol* 1977;103:34–37.

6. Johns ME, Headington JT: Squamous cell carcinoma of the external auditory canal. A clinicopathologic study of 20 cases. *Arch Otolaryngol* 1974;100:45–49.

7. Lewis JS: Cancer of the ear: a report of 100 cases. *Laryngoscope* 1966;70:551–579.

8. Sinha PP, Aziz HI: Treatment of carcinoma of the middle ear. *Radiology* 1978;126:485–487.

9. Sorenson H: Cancer of the middle ear and mastoid. *Acta Radiol* 1960;54:460–468.

10. Tucker WN: Cancer of the middle ear. A review of 89 cases. *Cancer* 1965;18:642–650.

11. Wang CC: Radiation therapy in the management of carcinoma of the external auditory canal, middle ear or mastoid. *Radiology* 1975;116:713–715.

12. Kinney SE: Squamous cell carcinoma of the external auditory canal. *Am J Otol* 1989;10:111–116.

13. Wang CC, Doppke K: Osteoradionecrosis of the temporal bone: consideration of Nominal Standard Dose. *Int J Radiat Oncol Biol Phys* 1976;1:881–883.

14. Fuller AM, Brown HA, Harrison EG, et al: Chemodectomas of the glomus jugulare tumors. *Laryngoscope* 1967;77:218–238.

15. Hatfield PM, James AE, Schulz MD: Chemodectomas of the glomus jugulare. *Cancer* 1972;30:1164–1168.

16. Bradshaw JD: Radiotherapy in glomus jugulare tumors. *Clin Radiol* 1961;12:227–234.

17. Hudgins PT: Radiotherapy for extensive glomus jugulare tumors. *Radiology* 1972;103:427–429.

18. Maruyama Y, Gold LH, Kieffer SA: Radioactive cobalt treatment of glomus jugulare tumors. *Acta Radiol* 1971;10:239–247.

19. Simko TG, Griffin TW, Gerdes AJ, et al: The role of radiation therapy in the treatment of glomus jugulare tumors. *Cancer* 1978;42:104–106.

20. Spector GJ, Compagno J, Perez CA, et al: Glomus jugulare tumors: effects of radiotherapy. *Cancer* 1975;35:1316–1321.

21. Wang CC: What is the optimum dose of radiation therapy for glomus jugulare? (editorial) *Int J Radiat Oncol Biol Phys* 1980;6:945–946.

22. Schuknecht HF, Karmody CS: Radionecrosis of the temporal bone. *Laryngoscope* 1966;76:1416–1428.

MISCELLANEOUS TUMORS

A. MALIGNANT LYMPHOMA

Malignant lymphoma, other than Hodgkin's disease, may arise from the oral cavity, Waldeyer's ring, paranasal sinuses, larynx, parotid gland, and thyroid. These tumors, so-called extranodal lymphomas, tend to involve multiple adjacent sites. If localized, they are highly curable by radiation therapy. Such extranodal lymphomas must be evaluated appropriately from the standpoint of systemic disease by CT scans, bipedal lymphograms, bone marrow biopsy, blood and liver profiles, and soon. If the disease is localized, Stages I and II, radiation therapy is the preferred treatment. On the other hand, if the disease is found to be generalized in nature, chemotherapy will have to be the treatment of choice and radiation therapy is reserved for relief of localized symptoms.

The classification of head and neck lymphoma is the same as for lymphoma in general and is as follows[1]:

Stage I Involvement of a single lymph node region (I) or localized involvement of a single extralymphatic organ or site $(I_E)^*$

Stage II Involvement of two or more lymph node regions on the same side of the diaphragm (II), or localized involvement of a single associated extralymphatic organ or site and its regional nodes with or without other lymph node regions on the same side of the diaphragm (II_E)

Stage III Involvement of lymph node regions on both sides of the diaphragm (III) that may also be accompanied by localized involvement of an extralymphatic organ or site (III_E) or involvement of the spleen (III_S) or both $III_{E+S})$

The number of lymph node regions involved may be indicated by a subscript (e.g., II_3).

Stage IV   Disseminated (multifocal) involvement of one or more extralymphatic organs with or without associated lymph node involvement,
or isolated extralymphatic organ involvement with distant (nonre-
gional) nodal involvement

Extranodal lymphomas in the head and neck region commonly involve
Waldeyer's ring,[2,3] that is faucial, lingual, and nasopharyngeal tonsils. Other sites
include the parotid gland and thyroid. Radiation therapy for the localized lymphoma, Stages I and II, consists of 45–50 Gy to the primary site and cervical
nodes. Elective irradiation to the low neck and supraclavicular area is also given
with 45 Gy in 1 month. For lymphomas arising from the oral cavity, localized irradiation with generous margins is necessary.[4] Lymphoma of the paranasal sinuses requires large-field irradiation covering the entire paranasal sinuses with a total dose
of 45 Gy in 5–6 weeks, generally using a three-field technique.[5] Lymphomas of the
parotid gland and thyroid gland are uncommon. When the disease is diagnosed, not
infrequently the lesion has become widespread. In a small number of patients, the
process may be localized and curable.

Extranodal lymphomas tend to develop, concurrently or sequentially, multiple
extranodal lesions, particularly in the gastrointestinal tract. Therefore routine contrast studies of the alimentary tract should be part of the clinical evaluation. If a
separate extranodal lymphoma is found, the condition does not always mean systemic disease and the lesion should therefore be managed as a localized process
(i.e., Stage I), and in some instances local treatment, either by radiation therapy or
surgery, has resulted in permanent freedom from disease.

Stage II extranodal lymphomas with bilateral cervical metastases represent advanced disease. Chemotherapy may be considered initially, to be followed by local
irradiation. Some data indicate improved survival rates following the combined approach.

MGH EXPERIENCE

The results of treatment of Stage I and Stage II extranodal lymphomas of
Waldeyer's ring show 3/4 and 1/2 patients being cured following radical radiation
therapy.[2] For lesions arising from the oral cavity and paranasal sinuses, the 5-year
survival rate is approximately 65% for Stage I and 33% for Stage II lesions following radiation therapy.[6] No long-term survivors with lesions spreading below the
clavicle are recorded. Those results were not associated with adjuvant chemotherapy. Results of radiation therapy of Waldeyer's ring were updated by Shimm et al.,[3]
indicating acturial 5-year survival of 53%, disease-free survival of 48%, and local
control of 98%.

Non-Hodgkin's lymphoma of the nasoparansal sinuses is not a common tumor. The
MGH experiences were recently updated[5] and consists of 24 patients with Stage I and
8 patients with Stage II disease. Twenty-nine patients were treated by radiation therapy
alone and three also received combined chemotherapy and radiation therapy. The actuarial 5-year survival rate was 62%. For Stage I and Stage II disease, the corresponding

rates were 67% and 50%, with relapse-free rates of 65% and 38%, respectively. Most radiation failures were due to distant disease. Because of the high rate of distant failure, adjuvant chemotherapy is advised after primary radiation therapy.

B. EXTRAMEDULLARY PLASMACYTOMA

Extramedullary plasmacytoma is a rare tumor. Approximately 80% occur in the head and neck region. The nasopharynx, nasal cavity, paranasal sinuses, orbit, and tonsil are the sites of common involvement. In the upper air passages the majority of the lesions are solitary and approximately 10% are in the form of multiple lesions. The male/female patient ratio is 4:1 and three-fourths of the patients present between 40 and 70 years of age. Solitary extramedullary plasmacytoma is generally not a manifestation or herald of multiple myeloma. If systemic disease does develop in a patient with soft tissue plasmacytoma, it may occur years later and run a prolonged course. This is in contrast to the course of this disease in patients who develop multiple myeloma de novo and usually die within 2–3 years.

Recurrence of tumors may occur as late as 10 years after treatment and is compatible with long-term survival. Treatment of this disease is by radiation therapy. Primary radical surgery is not justified in light of the radioresponsiveness and radiocurability of this tumor. Surgery may be used in the management of small lesions easily excised without morbidity or recurrences after irradiation, however. For localized solitary tumor, a dose of 45–50 Gy in 5 weeks is adequate. No elective neck irradiation is advised. The MGH radiotherapeutic results indicate that approximately one out of two patients is free of disease for 5 or more years after adequate irradiation.[6]

C. MIDLINE "LETHAL" GRANULOMA AND PLEOMORPHIC RETICULOSIS

Pleomorphic reticulosis represents a form of "lethal" midline granuloma that involves the upper airway with destruction of nasal and paranasal sinus structures. It may produce necrosis, ulceration of the palate, and loss of soft tissues of the face. Histologically, the condition is characterized by angiocentric lymphoid infiltration with extensive vascular thrombosis and secondary infection. The condition cannot be easily diagnosed because superficial biopsies often show nonspecific inflammatory reaction. The clinical course is prolonged and the ulcerations often are refractory to antibiotic treatment, which should alert the physician to consider this rare entity.

Radiation therapy is effective in promoting healing of the lesion and, not infrequently, in achieving permanent local control of the disease, although patients often develop regional and distant lesions, biopsy of which often discloses non-Hodgkin's lymphoma. For the localized disease, a dose of 45–50 Gy should suffice.[7]

The following case is reported to show the prompt response of the lesion to radiation therapy.

Case E.R. #297-52-74

This 77-year-old caucasian woman had a gradual progression of a destructive lesion on her right cheek; initially she presented in 1986 with nostril itching. The lesion progressed and destroyed the right upper lip, extending to the nasal septum and adjacent buccogingival sulcus and palate (Figure 15.1a). CT scan on 7/28/88 showed

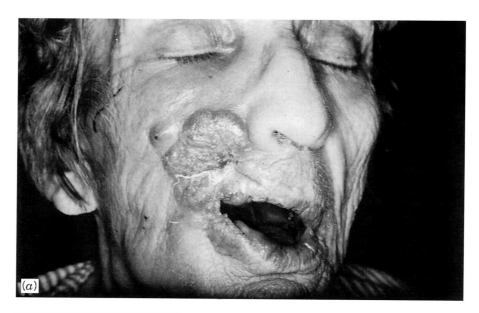

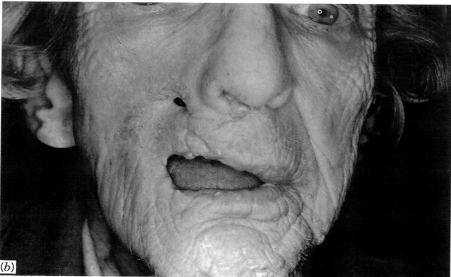

FIGURE 15.1   (a) Pretreatment appearance of lesion. (b) Post-treatment photograph.

destruction of the anteroinferior wall of the maxillary sinus and alveloar ridge with opacity of the antrum. Other paranasal sinuses were clear. A few enlarged lymph nodes were palpable in the subdigastric and submandibular regions. Multiple biopsies showed acute and chronic inflammatory changes without evidence of malignancy.

On the basis of these findings and chronicity of the disease process, a diagnosis of midline granuloma was made and she was accepted for radiation therapy. From 8/15/88 to 9/9/88 she was treated with BID radiation therapy for a total dose of 44.8 Gy in 28 elapsed days. The lesion regressed rapidly and patient's well-being improved remarkably (Figure 15.1b). She was seen on 1/23/89 and was found to have no evidence of recurrence.

D. JUVENILE ANGIOFIBROMA

Juvenile angiofibroma may arise in the nasopharynx and postnasal cavity, mostly in adolescent males, and is a highly vascular, benign tumor.[8] The tumor may produce nasal obstruction and epistaxis, invading the nasopharynx and its adjacent structures along the suture lines of the skull. The extent of the tumor should be delineated by careful radiographic studies, including polytomes and CT scans of the nasopharynx and paranasal sinuses. Angiograms may outline the exact extent of the tumor and its blood supply pattern and help in the diagnosis of the disease.

Treatment of juvenile angiofibroma is preoperative vascular embolization followed by surgical removal. Results have been satisfactory. For patients in whom surgical resection is impossible and/or in patients with multiple recurrences after repeated surgical attempts, a course of radiation therapy may be considered and has been found to be effective in controlling the disease. The dose of radiation therapy for this disease is in the neighborhood of 35–40 Gy with megavoltage radiations,[8] for a local control rate over 75%.[9] There is always a risk of malignant degeneration in young individuals following radiation therapy for benign conditions, but such risks are extremely low. In a large series of cases with long-term follow-up up to 40 years after treatment, none developed secondary malignancies.[9]

E. AMELOBLASTOMA

Ameloblastoma is a rare benign tumor[10] that may occur at any age, although the average age of onset is about 40 years. Approximately 80% arise in the molar ramus of the mandible. In the maxilla (20%) the third molar region is also a common site. When present in the maxilla, the tumor may extend into the maxillary sinus, nasal cavity, orbit, or pterygoid fossa or even the base of the skull. Despite the lack of cellular malignant characteristics, ameloblastoma has a tendency to continuously grow and invade surrounding tissues. Distant metastases occur in patients with a tumor of long duration, with multiple recurrences after repeated surgical procedures or radiation therapy. Treatment of this disease is by wide surgical resection with clean resection margins. For the lesion with multiple recurrences after attempts at surgery, radiation therapy is indicated and is effective in controlling the disease, particularly aggressive lesions with malignant degeneration.[4] A tumor dose of 60 Gy in 6–7 weeks should suffice for this disease.[11]

F. GIANT CELL REPARATIVE GRANULOMA

Giant cell reparative granuloma occurs predominantly in adolescents and young adult females, usually under 21 years of age.[12] Histologically, it is identical to brown tumor (osteoclastoma) of hyperparathyroidism but differs by clinical data. It involves the mandible more frequently than the maxilla and paranasal sinuses. Occasionally, the tumor may extend through the bone to involve soft tissue. The lesion may be self-limited, seldom recurs, and never metastasizes. Local curettage or excision is usually curative, but in some inoperable or recurrent lesions, a modest dose of radiation therapy—45–50 Gy—may be employed for control of the recent disease or inoperable tumors.

The following case is presented to illustrate the response of this tumor to radiation therapy.

Case S.S. #252-65-28

This 13-year-old Caucasian girl with a 5-year history of rhinorrhea and partial nasal obstruction, in 1981 developed swelling around her right eye. Radiographs revealed opacification of the right maxillary sinus, ethmoid cells, and sphenoid sinus and a soft tissue mass in the nasal cavity. The floor of the orbit was pushed upward, as shown in Figure 15.2a.

On 1/19/82, a limited Caldwell–Luc procedure with biopsy revealed a giant cell reparative granuloma. One month later further removal of the growth was carried out through a right Caldwell–Luc approach with an estimated blood loss of 1300 cc. There was tumor left at the floor and posterior wall of the orbit and the postero-superior antrum.

Approximately 6 months after surgery, CT scan showed recurrent tumor in the nasal cavity extending into the medial apex of the orbit, maxillary sinus, and ethmoid cells. No further surgery was possible and the patient was referred for radiation therapy.

From 10/1/82 through 11/16/82, in a total period of 45 elapsed days, the right hemiparanasal sinuses were irradiated on a cobalt-60 machine for a total of 54 Gy using a standard three-field technique (eyes excluded). There was slow regression of the tumor with subsequent reossification of the lesion during subsequent years, as shown in Figure 15.2b. She was seen in 1995, approximately 12 years after radiation therapy, and found to be free of disease and happily married.

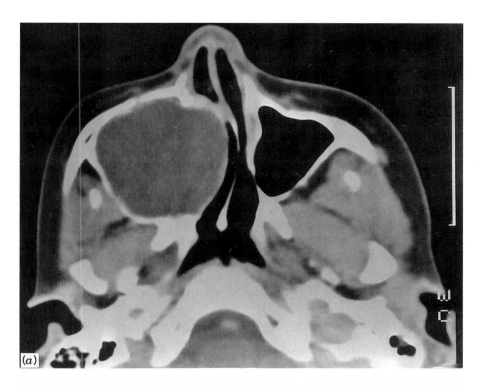

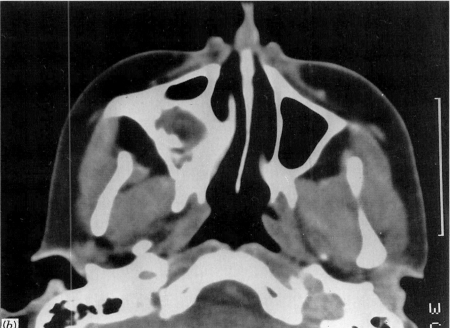

FIGURE 15.2 (a) CT scan showing expanding lesion in the maxillary sinus. (b) CT scan showing excellent response to radiation therapy.

G. GIANT CELL TUMOR OF THE BONE

Giant cell tumors may occur in the head and neck region. In contrast to giant cell reparative granuloma, a giant cell tumor of bone usually occurs in patients over 20 years of age.[12] The lesions are aggressive without spontaneous regression and recur often and occasionally metastasize. Recurrences occur often if the tumors are not completely resected.

For inoperable lesions, radiation therapy may be used with a dose of about 50 Gy in 5 weeks.

H. FIBROMYXOMA OF OROPHARYNX

Although fibromyxoma is not a malignant tumor, its location in the oropharynx makes it unresectable. The role of radiation therapy has not been established. The following case is reported, illustrating the unexpected radiation response.

Case R. B. #273-47-19

This 59-year-old Caucasian woman noted a mass in her throat associated with left-sided dysphagia, odynophagia, and otalgia for 5–6 months. She was seen by a head and neck surgeon who palpated a mass in the left oropharyngeal wall. Biopsy showed an unusual benign tumor, which was sent to the Armed Forces Institute of Pathology, and a diagnosis of fibromyxoma was made.

Physical examination was unremarkable except for the presence of an oropharyngeal mass, mostly submucosal, in the left lateral and posterior pharyngeal wall, extending from the base of the tonsillar fossa to the left hypopharynx at the level of the epiglottis. The tumor did not extend to the apex of the pyriform sinus or across the midline.

CT scan showed a left parapharyngeal mass contiguous with the great vessels of the neck. Surgical removal of the lesion according to our head and neck surgeon would most certainly result in severe and crippling cranial nerve deficits and radiation therapy was recommended as the preferred treatment.

In spite of the benign nature of the lesion, she was accepted for radiation therapy as an alternative treatment option. From 9/19/84 through 10/26/84, in a total period of 37 elapsed days, the tumor was treated for a total dose of 67.2 Gy using the BID scheme with 1.6 Gy/fraction on the cobalt 60 unit through 9×5 cm^2 parallel opposing portals. Treatment was concluded without difficulty with slow shrinkage of the lesion.

On 5/10/85, slightly over 6 months after radiation therapy, examination showed marked regression of the soft tissue mass with a slit-like ulceration in the midportion of the tumor. Six months later, the ulceration healed with complete disappearance of the tumor and the patient was completely asymptomatic. She was seen on 11/22/88 and remained free from evidence of recurrence.

Note: The response of fibromyxoma to radiation therapy certainly was surprisingly gratifying. This is the only case treated by radiation therapy with the BID scheme and hopefully this anecdotal experience will serve as an example for future treatment of this disease.

I. SOFT TISSUE SARCOMAS OF THE HEAD AND NECK

Malignant tumors of mesenchymal origin may arise from various sites of the head and neck and include malignant fibrohistiocytoma, hemangiopericytoma, liposarcoma, and neurofibrosarcoma, among others. These tumors present with a nontender, enlarging mass, causing unsightliness and interfering with respiratory and swallowing functions. The first step in management should probably be an incisional biopsy. After the biopsy specimen is carefully reviewed as to the cell type and grade, definitive therapy should be carefully planned and carried out. If the lesions are small and encompassible by excision, surgery may be considered the preferred procedure.

Although radiation therapy has not been found effective in controlling large soft tissue sarcomas in general, it is used in combination with other treatment modalities as an adjunct to enhance local control. In the head and neck areas, the soft tissue sarcomas tend to infiltrate the adjacent structures extensively, thus making surgical dissection difficult, resulting in marginal recurrence.[13] Under such circumstances, adjuvent radiation therapy is effective in enhancing local regional control.[14] If the lesions are too extensive for resection due to strategic location, high-dose radiation therapy should be offered to patients, employing a combination of external radiations and interstitial implant with a dose generally in the range of 70–75 Gy in 7–8 weeks.[15]

Occasionally, residual tumor remains after high-dose radiation therapy and this would better be treated by limited surgical removal than by an ultrahigh radiation therapy boost. The latter may entail a higher incidence of radiation necrosis.

Because soft tissue sarcomas are uncommon tumors, their management would best be carried out in a cancer center by a special team with specific interest in such tumors. No meaningful survival data pertaining to the head and neck region have been accumulated. A few cases treated by radiation therapy alone and/or by combined surgery and radiation therapy apparently did well for 5 or more years.

REFERENCES

1. American Joint Committee on Cancer: *Manual for staging of cancer*, 4th ed. Philadelphia: Lippincott, 1992.
2. Wang CC: Malignant lymphoma of Waldeyer's ring. *Radiology* 1969;92:1335–1339.
3. Shimm D, Dosoretz D, Harris N, et al: Radiation therapy of Waldeyer's ring lymphoma. *Cancer* 1984;54:426–431.

4. Wang CC: Primary malignant lymphoma of the oral cavity and paranasal sinuses. *Radiology* 1971;100:151–154.

5. Khil SU, Wang CC, Harris N: Treatment of non-Hodgkin's lymphoma in the nasal cavity and paranasal sinuses. (*Unpublished data.*)

6. Kotner L, Wang CC: Plasmacytoma of the upper air and food passages. *Cancer* 1972;30:414–418.

7. Halperin EC, Dosoretz DE, Goodman M, et al: Radiotherapy of polymorphic reticulosis. *Br J Radiol* 1982;55:645–649.

8. Briant TDR, Fitzpatrick PJ, Berman J: Nasopharyngeal angiofibroma: a twenty year study. *Laryngoscope* 1978;88:1247–1251.

9. Jereb B, Anggard A, Baryds I: Juvenile nasopharyngeal angiofibroma: a disease study of 69 cases. *Acta Radiol Ther* 1970;9:302–310.

10. Batsakis JG: *Tumors of the head and neck*, 2nd ed. Baltimore: Williams & Wilkins, 1979;531–536.

11. Singleton J: Malignant ameloblastoma. *Br J Oral Surg* 1970;8:154–158.

12. Goodman ML, Domanowski GP: *Guide to dental problems for physicians and surgeons.* In: Neoplasms, Thaller SR, Montgomery WW, eds. Baltimore, Williams & Wilkins Co, 1988.

13. Goepfert H, Lindberg RD, Sinkovics JG: Soft-tissue sarcoma of the head and neck after puberty. *Arch Otol* 1977;103:365–368.

14. Suit HD, Mankin HJ, Wood WC, et al: Radiation and surgery in the treatment of primary sarcoma of soft tissue: pre-operative, intra-operative and post-operative. *Cancer* 1985;55:2659–2667.

15. Tepper JE, Suit HD: Radiation therapy alone for sarcoma of soft tissue. *Cancer* 1985;56:475–479.

CHAPTER 16

TUMORS OF THE EYE

The eye and its adjacent soft tissue and bony part may be the sites of many neoplasms. Of these tumors, basal cell carcinoma of the eyelid is the most common and frequently seen by the radiation oncologist for consultation and treatment. Other cancers arising from the lacrimal gland, conjunctiva, and orbit constitute a small bulk of the clinical experience in most general hospitals. Basal cell carcinoma of the eyelid has been discussed in detail previously (see Chapter 5).

A. CANCER OF THE CONJUNCTIVA

Cancer of the conjunctiva is a rare disease and includes Bowen's disease, squamous cell carcinoma, lymphoma, and melanoma. Bowen's disease is an intraepithelial carcinoma and is noninvasive, but if untreated it may develop into invasive carcinoma. Conjunctival or episcleral lymphoma is a rare, infiltrative process, which histologically is indistinguishable from other varieties of malignant lymphomas. Some of these lymphomatous infiltrations are primary and are unassociated with lymphomatous disease elsewhere and are characterized by long periods of freedom from disease following removal. These tumors respond exceedingly well to radiation therapy and involute after a small dose of radiation.[1] If the infiltration is unassociated with generalized lymphoma, the patient may be expected to do well. Conjunctival melanoma, unlike cutaneous melanoma, is radiosensitive and radiocurable. According to Lederman,[2] the closer the melanoma is to the limbus of the eye, the more radiosensitive is the tumor.

RADIOTHERAPEUTIC MANAGEMENT

Radiation therapy for conjunctival cancers requires special technique for protection of the underlying radiosensitive structures. Selection of appropriate energies of x-rays or electron beam according to the depth of the lesions, or the use of an isotopic beta-ray applicator such as ^{32}P or ^{90}Sr sources is necessary for optimal irradiation.[3,4] If the cornea is not involved by the malignant process, a specially made lead contact lens may be used to shield the cornea and lens from irradiation of the conjunctival lesion by low megavoltage electron beam. This has been found to be highly effective without resulting in radiation damage to the cornea and/or the lens (Figure 16.1). The dosimetry of the lead contact lens is shown in Figure 16.2.

Radiation dose varies with the nature of the growth. In general, for lymphoma of the conjunctiva, a dose of 24 Gy in 8 daily fractions should suffice. For conjunctival melanoma, squamous cell carcinoma, or Bowen's disease, a dose of 60 Gy in 5 weeks is required. Such high radiation dose may damage the underlying globe, cornea, and lens and requires extreme technical sophistication if lasting injuries are to be avoided.

Although pterygium is not a malignant disorder, it is often referred for radiation therapy. Our policy is to excise the lesion as much as possible to be followed immediately by postoperative beta irradiation with a strontium 90 applicator. A surface dose of 20 Gy in one application is found to be effective in preventing further recurrence in a high percentage of patients.

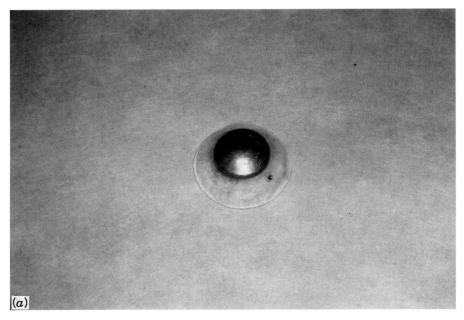

(a)

FIGURE 16.1 (a) Lead contact lens for shielding of cornea and lens in treatment of conjunctival lymphoma. (b) Lead contact lens in place during irradiation.

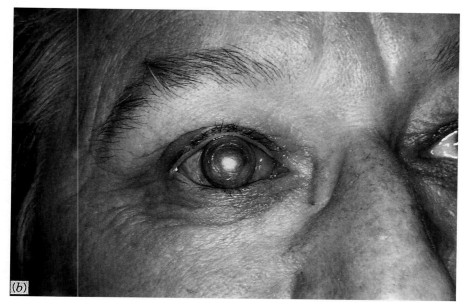

FIGURE 16.1   *Continued*

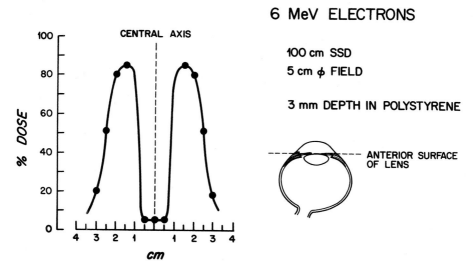

FIGURE 16.2   Percent depth dose to the anterior surface of the lens using lead contact lens shield (1.3 cm in diameter) by thermal luminescent dosimeter (TLD) measurement.

RADIATION THERAPY RESULTS—MGH EXPERIENCE

Our experience in treating conjunctival malignant lymphoma[5] ($n=12$) indicates that local control was achieved in all patients with a follow-up of up to 10 years. With the use of a specially made lead contact lens during radiation therapy, no patients developed cataract from the treatment.

B. LYMPHOMA OF THE ORBIT

Orbital tumors of radiotherapeutic interest include lymphoma, plasmacytoma, rhabdomyosarcoma, carcinoma of the lacrimal gland, retinoblastoma,[6-8] choroidal melanoma,[9] and optic glioma,[10] among others. Lymphoma of the orbit is relatively common and may occur in the orbit de novo or may arise in association with a generalized systemic lymphoma. It frequently occurs in the anterior part of the orbit, displacing the eyeball, and is most common in middle-aged and elderly patients. The diagnosis is made by biopsy. Pretreatment evaluation of orbital lymphoma includes sonogram, CT scan, or MRI of the orbit for delineation of the disease. A complete physical examination including liver profile and/or bipedal lymphogram should be performed to exclude systemic lymphoma before treatment is decided.

RADIOTHERAPEUTIC MANAGEMENT

Radiation therapy is directed to the entire orbital contents. Low megavoltage or cobalt-60 radiation is used. Generally, anterior and ipsilateral oblique wedge pair portals are used, as shown in Figure 16.3. This can deliver a relatively homogeneous dose to the entire orbit and yet the dose to the contralateral globe and lens is minimal. In order to avoid full-dose buildup to the cornea, the patient's eye should be widely open and looking at the beam. Because of the likelihood of involvement of the lacrimal gland, no attempt should be made to shield the gland, with the expectation that there will be some dryness of the eye after radiation therapy. A dose of 40 Gy in 4 weeks is planned for localized disease and 25 Gy in 3 weeks for systemic disease, to be followed by chemotherapy.

RADIOTHERAPEUTIC RESULTS

No meaningful data are available due to its uncommon occurrence. The local control of orbital lymphoma by radiation therapy is generally good. Unfortunately, over 50% of patients develop systemic disease with variable clinical course.

C. MISCELLANEOUS TUMORS OF THE ORBIT

Plasmacytoma of the orbit, like lymphoma, may be either a localized lesion or part of systemic disease. It is quite radioresponsive and a localized lesion can be con-

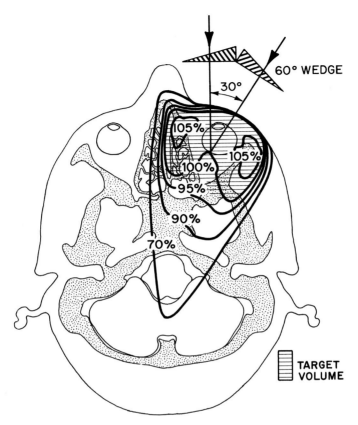

FIGURE 16.3   Diagram showing "ice cream cone" shaped isodose distribution with anterior and ipsilateral oblique wedge pair technique for irradiation of intraorbital tumors.

trolled well by radiation therapy. If the lesion represents a localized process, radiation therapy is the treatment of choice. For systemic disease with secondary involvement of the orbit, chemotherapy is the primary treatment with local radiation therapy to palliate the orbital growths.

Lacrimal gland tumors have histologic characteristics similar to those of tumors of the salivary gland, ranging from completely benign pleomorphic adenoma to highly malignant mucoepidermoid or adenocystic carcinoma, among others. These tumors tend to grow slowly and painlessly for a long time, and when diagnosed, they often have invaded the orbital bone and adjacent organs. The management of these lesions calls for complete surgical removal to be followed by adjuvant radiation therapy. For inoperable or recurrent lesions, radiation therapy may be used and can occasionally produce respite and a prolonged palliation. Rhabdomyosarcomas are common orbital malignant tumors in childhood and are managed by multidrug chemotherapy and radiation therapy with good local control of disease and preservation of vision. Other infrequent tumors include retinoblastoma and choroidal melanoma, which are best managed by a team of specialists at a cancer center. Retinoblastoma[7,8] can be treated by radiation therapy or photocoagulation and/or orbital enucleation, depending on the extent of the tumor or the usefulness of vision after treatment. Choroidal melanomas, at the present time, can be managed by radiation therapy with cobalt-60 plaque or heavy charge particle beams, such as the proton beam from the MGH–Harvard cyclotron, with a high degree of success and tumor control and preservation of vision.[9] Treatment of these tumors requires expensive equipment and a certain level of professional expertise on the part of the physician and is beyond the province of the general radiation oncologist in a general hospital.

D. GRAVES' OPHTHALMOPATHY

Although Graves' ophthalmopathy is not a malignant process, the condition may have a waxing and waning course and can be clinically troublesome, with pain and deterioration of vision.[11] Patients exhibit an inflammatory response in the orbit, which can lead to venous engorgement, resulting in inadequate drainage of interstitial fluid with periorbital edema and proptosis and ultimately compression of the optic nerve. In early stages, the ocular muscles become heavily infiltrated with lymphocytes and become enlarged, as seen by MR or CT scans; in late stages, the muscles are fibrosed with deposition of collagen. The early phase may be self-limited and may resolve in months or years. The condition has been treated with steroids and/or orbital decompression with relief of symptoms. There is increasing evidence in the past decade that a modest dose of radiation therapy can be effective in causing regression of the ocular lesion in the early stage, with improvement in symptoms and regression of exophthalmos, particularly the soft tissue component. A dose of 20–25 Gy in 2 weeks to the entire orbit is used,[11,12] commonly through opposing lateral portals to both orbital contents, sparing the lens. In the late stages of the disease, the changes are rarely reversible and in many patients eventual treatment with surgery will be required, especially in those patients with crippling diplopia.

Technical Pointers

1. Patient is to lie supine and be immobilized with a face mask. Cross-table top 4–6 MV photon beams are used.
2. The anterior border is placed behind the lens of the eye, while the posterior border is at the apex of the orbit or the anterior clinoid process and includes all ocular muscles.
3. Use a split half-beam or 10° posterior tilt to avoid irradiation of the contralateral lens.

4. Be aware of the narrowing of the isodoses at midplane, which may be much smaller than the surface portal sizes indicated, resulting in undercoverage of medial lesions at midline.

E. METASTATIC CHOROIDAL METASTASES

The retina is a frequent site for metastatic disease. The common primary lesions are breast, lung, and malignant melanoma among others. These metastatic lesions present a typical appearance and can be diagnosed by the experienced ophthalmologist with a great deal of certainty. Tissue confirmation is seldom necessary. Radiation therapy is effective in controlling the disease with preservation of vision. A dose of 40 Gy in 3 weeks is planned. This is delivered through an ipsilateral portal limited to the posterior globe. Over 50% of the irradiated eyes will have improved vision or stabilized lesions after radiation therapy.

SUMMARY

Early cancers of the eyelid and conjunctival lymphoma are radiocurable tumors. If adequately irradiated, the cure rates are extremely high, well over 90%. These lesions are best dealt with by radiation therapy first, with surgery being reserved for salvage. Primary orbital tumors are uncommon. Of these, lymphoma and plasmacytoma are highly radiosensitive and radiocurable, and if the lesions are localized, radiation therapy is the treatment of choice. Other orbital tumors are uncommon in a general hospital and their management requires cooperation among surgeons, ophthalmologists, pediatric surgeons, medical oncologists, radiation oncologists, and others, if maximum preservation of vision and good local control of the disease are the goals.

REFERENCES

1. Schulz MD, Heath CG: Lymphoma of the conjunctiva. *Radiology* 1948;50:500–505.
2. Lederman M: Radiotherapy of malignant melanomata of the eye. *Br J Radiol* 1961;34:21–42.
3. Schulz MD, Wipfelder R: Reactor-activated applicators for treatment of conjunctival neoplasms. *Radiology* 1969;92:1553–1556.
4. Lederman M: Some applications of radioactive isotopes in ophthalmology. *Br J Radiol* 1956;29:1–13.
5. Dunbar SF, Linggood RM, Doppke KP, Duby A, Wang CC: Conjunctival lymphoma: results and treatment with a single anterior electron field. A lens sparing approach. *Int J Radiat Oncol Biol Phys* 1990;19:249–257.
6. Bedford MA, Bedotto C, MacFaul PA: Retinoblastoma of 139 cases. *Br J Ophthalmol* 1971;55:19–27.

7. Gaitan-Yanquas M: Retinoblastoma: analysis of 235 cases. *Int J Radiat Oncol Biol Phys* 1978;4:359–365.

8. Tapley N: Retinoblastoma, cancer in childhood. *Pediatr Ann* 1974;2:35–38.

9. Gragoudas ES, Seddon J, Goitein M, et al: Current results of proton beam irradiation of uveal melanomas. *Ophthalmology* 1985;92:284–291.

10. Dosoretz DE, Blitzer PH, Wang CC, et al: Management of glioma of the optic nerve and/or chiasm—an analysis of 20 cases. *Cancer* 1980;45(6):1467–1471.

11. Palmer D, Greenberg P, Cornell P, et al: Radiation therapy for Graves' ophthalmopathy. A retrospective analysis. *Int J Radiat Oncol Biol Phys* 1987;13:1815–1820.

12. Donaldson S, Bagshaw M, Kriss J: Supervoltage orbital radiotherapy for Graves' ophthalmology. *J Clin Endocrinol Metab* 1973;37:276–285.

CHAPTER 17

COMPLICATIONS OF RADIATION THERAPY

Since radiation affects both normal and abnormal tissues, certain effects of radiation therapy are expected. A distinction must be made between side effects or sequelae in the normal tissues, which are produced as a necessity of radiation therapy for malignant disease, though different in degree with outcome of complete or partial recovery over time, and the major complications, often irreversible, requiring surgical intervention or leading to death.

The sequelae of radiation therapy of head and neck tumors are relatively common following curative radiation therapy and at times are severe and unavoidable. These commonly occur in the skin, subcutaneous tissues, and mucous membrane of the upper aerodigestive tract.

With the advent of megavoltage radiation, acute effects in the skin are rarely observed even after a curative dose of radiation therapy for epithelial tumors. Rarely moist desquamation occurs. Temporary epilation usually occurs after a dose of 40–50 Gy, and hair regrowth may be sparse. With further increase of dose in the range of 75–80 Gy, permanent epilation and necrosis with marked subcutaneous fibrosis may develop.

The mucous membrane reacts to radiation in the form of radiation mucositis. In general, symptoms and signs of radiation reaction develop at the end of the second week of radiation therapy, with the mucosa exhibiting erythema. Because of the lapse of 10–14 days required for injured cells to migrate from the active proliferative compartment into the inactive compartment, at this time, the tumor exhibits radiation injury in the form of "mucositis." With further increase in dose, the mucositis fades but is reactivated toward the completion of radiation therapy. The acute symptoms of severe mucositis in the oropharynx are sore throat, dysphagia, dryness of mouth, and loss of taste, which may interfere with nutrition. Excessive radiation may result in serious complications with ulceration of mucous membranes delaying healing after slight trauma.

MAJOR COMPLICATIONS

Major complications in the head and neck area include soft tissue ulceration, orocutaneous fistulas, osteoradionecrosis, and chondronecrosis and are invariably related to curative radiation therapy but may be coincidental to unusually aggressive therapy or faulty treatment technique. Important etiologic factors in such complications include treatment method, time–dose–fraction (TDF) program, size of target volume, fraction size and total dosage, extent of disease and its location, and the patient's age and nutritional status.[1] A large daily fraction tends to exaggerate the development of severe late complications.[2] The incidence is further increased following combined radiation therapy and surgery because of excessive impairment of local blood supply and secondary infection, particularly when curative doses of radiation are given before radical surgery. In such an environment, postoperative morbidity, including delayed wound healing, occasional carotid artery blowout, and mortality can be exceptionally high, and at times unacceptable in the modern practice of oncology.

Osteoradionecrosis of the mandible and temporal bone and necrosis of the larynx or functionless larynx are serious radiation complications and are often the result of high total dose or large daily fraction size of radiation therapy or large irradiated volume. Any treatment program delivering a total dose over 70 Gy with large daily fraction must be looked at with caution. As a general guideline, a total TDF value of 120 with conventional fractionation should not be exceeded. Each of these conditions was discussed in the related chapter of this book.

Radiation neuritis of cranial nerve XII may occur following curative radiation therapy for oropharyngeal cancer.[3] Fortunately, it is infrequent, and its incidence can be markedly reduced if the radiation therapy dosage is kept below 70 Gy in 7 weeks.

Other uncommon radiotherapeutic complications are radiation-induced carotid artery disease,[4] hypopituitarism,[5-7] and hypothyroidism.[8] However, these complications of treatment should be accepted as a risk in the management of extensive head and neck tumors but may be minimized by observing careful radiotherapeutic and surgical principles and techniques.

Radiation brain necrosis[9-11] or radiation-induced transverse myelitis are occasionally seen following treatment of nasopharyngeal carcinoma and paranasal sinus cancers and such complications must be accepted as the possible risk[12] for dealing with a lethal disease. Fortunately, these serious complications are extremely rare and should be avoided by limiting the dose to the brain and spinal cord below 50 Gy in 4½–5 weeks.[13,14] For late-responding tissue, like spinal cord and brain tissues, the increase of fraction size over the conventional radiation may also account for the increase of CNS complications and the fraction sizes therefore should be kept below 2 Gy.[15]

Long-term effects, such as abnormal facial growth or radiation-induced malignancy,[16,17] particularly in childhood, have been observed, but the incidence of malignant transformation is extremely low and should not be taken into serious consideration in the selection of radiation therapy for life-threatening malignant tumors.

RADIATION COMPLICATIONS OF THE SENSORY ORGANS

The side effects of radiation therapy to the salivary glands, taste buds, and teeth, including xerostomia, dental caries, and loss of taste, have been discussed in Chapter 3.

Eye

The eye response to radiation varies greatly in terms of dose and fraction size. The most notable radiation injuries are to the lens, the retina, and the iris.

Glaucoma   With a dose of 50–60 Gy, the flow of aqueous humor into the canal of Schlemm is interfered with or obstructed, resulting in increased intraocular pressure; glaucoma may develop secondary to the inflammation, with vascular congestion and posterior and anterior synechia. In selected patients, surgical intervention may relieve the tension and save the eye and vision.

Radiation Cataract   The dose of radiation required to cause a vision-impairing cataract depends on the total dose, dose rate, and quality of radiation. The threshold dose in humans appears to be about 2 Gy of a single exposure to x-rays and 5 Gy fractionated over 3 months. The higher the dose the shorter the interval and the higher the incidence of progressive opacity. The latent period from time of exposure to cataract appearance may be 6 months to 35 years (average 2–3 years).[18] With fractionated conventional radiation therapy, a dose of 20–40 Gy over 46–85 days resulted in radiation-induced cataract in four (5%) of 85 patients; only two of the four had grossly impaired vision. With a dose of 60 Gy over 6 weeks, approximately 10% of patients develop serious vision-impairing cataract.[19]

Radiation therapy with pterygium with a ^{90}Sr beta-ray applicator may produce localized lenticular changes. A surface dose of 18 Gy may result in a 1% incidence of lenticular change (with a lens dose of 3 mm depth), and with a surface dose of 18–36 Gy there may be a 20% incidence of lenticular change. A dose of more than 70 Gy carries an incidence of more than 40%.[20]

Retinopathy   The mature retina is considered relatively insensitive to the injurious effects of radiation. Radiation retinopathy is the result of pathologic changes in the fine vascular tissues. A dose of more than 40 Gy over 4 weeks may produce changes. A dose of 60 Gy over 6 weeks produces vascular damage, leading to infarction of tissue, with formation of exudate and hemorrhage and decreased vision. In severe cases, changes consist of edema, congestion leading to retinal detachment and subsequent atrophy of the external layers of the retina, constriction of the visual field, and even complete blindness. The changes may mimic diabetic retinopathy. A history of long-standing diabetes mellitus may differentiate the two.

Radiation injuries to the optic nerve and chiasm may occur after a dose of 50–60 Gy over 5 weeks[19] and are related to the high total dose and, more important, the increased fraction size (2.5 Gy/fraction) and may lead to blindness.[21]

Lacrimal Gland   After a dose of 40–50 Gy at conventional fractionation, the secretion of the lacrimal gland is suppressed and dry eye syndrome may develop, with increasing thick mucoid secretion and irritation, leading to secondary infection.

Ear

Information regarding radiation complications on the function of the cochlear and vestibular end organs is sparse.[22,23] It is generally agreed that radiation effects on the middle and inner ear are primarily damage to the capillaries and other fine vasculature, with capillary hyperemia, increased capillary permeability, serous exudation, and edema, leading to the development of acute vasculitis or acute inflammation of the middle ear (otitis media) and inner ear (labyrinthitis).[23] These structures are not likely to be effected by the usual clinical dose of radiation (60 Gy over 6 weeks).[23]

SUMMARY

Radiation complications will continue to accompany curative radiation therapy for malignant disease. Various methods have been devised to decrease the incidence of development, such as the use of altered fractionated radiation therapy, the use of small fraction size with multiple daily treatment, and limitation of the total dose within the range of tolerance of the vasculoconnective tissues.[2,24] For large tumors, programs employing combined surgery and radiation therapy may play a significant part in reducing the risk of radiation complications.

Since the advent of megavoltage radiation and careful radiation therapy planning and techniques with the aid of a dedicated computer, and better understanding of altered fractionation radiobiology and the interaction between radiation and surgical principles, these major complications occur less frequently in the modern practice of radiation oncology.

REFERENCES

1. Delclos L, Lindberg RD, Fletcher GH: Squamous cell carcinoma of the oral tongue and floor of the mouth: evaluation of interstitial radium therapy. *AJR Am J Roentgenol* 1976;126:223–228.

2. Withers HR, Horiot J: *Hyperfractionation in innovations in radiation oncology.* Withers RH, Peters L, eds. New York: Springer-Verlag, 1985;223.

3. Cheng VST, Schulz MD: Unilateral hypoglossal nerve atrophy as a late complication of radiation therapy of head and neck carcinoma: a report of four cases and a review of the literature on peripheral and cranial nerve damages after radiation therapy. *Cancer* 1975;35:1537–1544.

4. Silverberg GD, Britt RH, Goffinet DR: Radiation induced carotid artery disease. *Cancer* 1978;41:130–137.

5. Aristizabal S, Caldwell WL, Avila J: The relationship of time–dose fractionation factors to complications in the treatment of pituitary tumors by irradiation. *Int J Radiat Oncol Biol Phys* 1977;2:667–673.

6. Samaan NA, Bakdash MM, Caderao JB, Cangir A, Jesse RH Jr, Ballantyne AJ: Hypopituitarism after external irradiation. *Ann Intern Med* 1975;83:771–777.

7. Lam KS, Wang C, Yeung RT, et al: Hypothalamic hypopituitarism following cranial irradiation for nasopharyngeal carcinoma. *Clin Endocrinol (Oxf)* 1986;24:643–651.

8. Shafer RB, Nuttall FQ, Pollack K, et al: Thyroid function after radiation and surgery for head and neck cancer. *Arch Intern Med* 1975;135:843–846.

9. Sheline GE, Wara WM, Smith V: Therapeutic irradiation and brain injury. *Int J Radiat Oncol Biol Phys* 1980;6:1215–1228.

10. Marks JE, Baglan JR, Prassad SC, Blank WF: Cerebral radionecrosis: incidence and risk in relation to dose, time, fractionation and volume. *Int J Radiat Oncol Biol Phys* 1981;7:243–252.

11. Lee AW, Ng SH, Ho JH, et al: Clinical diagnosis of late temporal lobe necrosis following radiation therapy for nasopharyngeal carcinoma. *Cancer* 1988;61:1535–1542.

12. Pezner RD, Archambeau JO: Brain tolerance unit: a method to estimate risk of radiation brain injury for various dose schedules. *Int J Radiat Oncol Biol Phys* 1981;7:397–402.

13. Abbatucci JS, Delosier T, Quint R, et al: Radiation myelopathy of the cervical spinal cord: time, dose and volume factors. *Int J Radiat Oncol Biol Phys* 1978;4:239–248.

14. Wara W, Phillips TL, Sheline GE, et al: Radiation tolerance of the spinal cord. *Cancer* 1975;35:1558–1562.

15. Jeremic B, Djuric L, Mijatovic L: Incidence of radiation myelitis of the cervical spinal cord at doses of 5500 cGy or greater. *Cancer* 1991;68:2138–2141.

16. Southwick HW: Radiation-associated head and neck tumors. *Am J Surg* 1977;134:438–443.

17. Mark RJ, Bailet JW, Poen J, et al: Postirradiation sarcoma of the head and neck. *Cancer* 1993;72:887–893.

18. Wang CC, Doppke KP: Osteoradionecrosis of the temporal bone: consideration of nominal standard dose. *In J Radiat Oncol Biol Phys* 1976;1:881–883.

19. Parker RG, Wootton P, Burnett L: Dosage to important sites in radiation therapy of tumors about the head and heck. *AJR Am J Roetgenol* 1963;90:240–245.

20. Merriam GR, Focht EF: Radiation dose to the lens in treatment of tumors of the eye and adjacent structures: possibility of cataract formation. *Radiology* 1958;71:357.

21. Harris JR, Levene MB: Visual complications following irradiation for pituitary adenomas and craniopharyngiomas. *Radiology* 1976;120:167–171.

22. Borsanyi SJ: The effects of radiation therapy on the ear, with particular reference of radiation otitis media. *South Med J* 1962;55:740–743.

23. Berg NO, Lindgren M: Dose factors and morphology of delayed radiation lesions of the internal and middle ear in rabbits. *Acta Radiol* 1961;56:305–319.

24. Wang CC: Accelerated hyperfraction. In: Withers HR, Peters LJ, eds. *Innovations in radiation oncology*. Berlin: Springer-Verlag, 1987.

CHAPTER 18

FUTURE PROSPECTS OF RADIATION THERAPY FOR HEAD AND NECK TUMORS

THE PAST AND THE PRESENT

Squamous cell carcinomas of the head and neck are potentially curable cancers. When the tumor is diagnosed in early stages (T1–2) and treated appropriately, the cure rates achieved with either radiation therapy or surgery are extremely high. For advanced (T3–4) lesions, the cure rates by conventional treatment modalities are low. The choice of treatment modality is extremely complex and demands full knowledge of the biology of tumors, advantages and disadvantages of various disciplines, and expected therapeutic and cosmetic results.

In general, T1–2 tumors are better treated by radiation therapy first, because satisfactory control of the disease can be achieved in better than three of four patients, with preservation of normal function and anatomy; surgery is then reserved as a salvage procedure for radiation failures. If early tumors can be managed by resection without functional and cosmetic mutilation, surgery may be carried out expediently and should be the treatment of choice. Extensive lesions are often associated with deep muscle involvement and cervical lymph node metastasis, and local control requires extremely high doses of radiation, often resulting in radiation complications. For such large tumors, the current treatment is combined surgery and radiation therapy, if the lesion is operable. For inoperable tumors, combined therapies (chemotherapy, surgery, and radiation therapy) may be tried, although the prognosis is dismal.

Metastatic disease to the neck from carcinoma of the head and neck presents a great challenge to both surgeons and radiation oncologists and accounts for a high percentage of treatment failures for these diseases. The management of cervical lymph node metastases depends on the primary site and the size and number of affected nodes. Not all neck nodes should be treated by radical neck dissection. Limited metastatic lymph node disease (N1 and N2b) with the primary site in Waldeyer's ring can be satisfactorily controlled with radiations therapy alone in a high percentage of patients, and the residual disease in the neck can be treated with neck dissection. Large metastatic lymph nodes (N2 and N3) with the primary site in the oral cavity, hypopharynx, or larynx are rarely controllable by radiation therapy alone and are better treated by neck dissection and radiation therapy.

The goal of any treatment program for head and neck tumors should be to offer the patient maximal locoregional control of the disease with a minimum of complications. Modern radiation therapy calls for extreme technical sophistication. For squamous cell carcinomas, high doses are required but are often limited by radiosensitivity of adjacent structures, such as the spinal cord, temporomandibular joint, mandible, teeth, or neighboring brain. To achieve maximal cure rates, various techniques must be used to deliver radiation to the tumor yet spare these structures to avoid irreparable damage. A prime example of this concept is the use of interstitial implant and IOC electron beam radiation therapy for carcinoma of the tongue, floor of the mouth, retromolar trigone, buccal mucosa, or soft palate to boost the dose delivered to the primary sites higher than the dose tolerated by the mandible, thus improving the therapeutic ratio. Various treatment modalities must be available to radiation oncologists in daily clinical practice. If none of these treatment modalities is suitable or possible, a high dose of external beam radiation therapy must be given through progressive field-reduction technique to maximize the tumor control effect and to reduce the damaging effects of large-field irradiation.

It has been apparent for some time that surgery has reached its limit of applicability in the treatment of advanced cancer of the head and neck. On the other hand, radiation therapy with high-energy radiation from a ^{60}Co machine or 4–10 MV linear accelerators has not significantly improved the therapeutic results, although complication rates have reduced considerably. Further improvement in locoregional control of T3 and T4 lesions is much needed. At present, these advance lesions are managed with combined radiation therapy and surgery, with or without chemotherapy.

ADJUVANT CHEMOTHERAPY

Chemotherapy as an adjuvant procedure for management of head and neck carcinoma has been a disappointment. Induction chemotherapy and surgery or radiation therapy showed no improvement in terms of survival or locoregional tumor control or of decreased incidence of distant metastases in patients who achieved a complete remission.[1] The only benefits of induction chemotherapy with 5-fluorouracil and cisplatin in operable cases were that radical resection may be avoided in patients with complete remission and definitive radiation therapy can be offered to patients instead.[2] The long-term survival was not improved with chemotherapy, however.

At present, induction chemotherapy is not advised as a standard treatment procedure prior to definitive surgery or radiation therapy. For inoperable or incurable lesions, chemotherapy may be used for palliation. At the MGH, a protocol of post-treatment adjuvant chemotherapy is available for the T3–4 tumors but no meaningful data are available yet.

INNOVATIVE METHODS WITH POTENTIAL THERAPEUTIC GAINS

Because of the limitations of conventional treatment methods, various innovative modalities are employed, some of which are promising and some not. They are discussed briefly below.

1. In the hope of improving the therapeutic ratio, various methods to alter the radiosensitivity of the cancer cells without significantly affecting the normal cells were available in the past decade, including hyperbaric oxygen therapy,[3,4] hypoxic cell sensitizers,[5–7] and hyperthermia[8,9] with radiation therapy. A great many publications and much enthusiasm were generated, but the results in general have been disappointing and the methods play a very limited role in daily patient care.

2. Neutron beam radiations possess a higher relative biologic effectiveness (RBE) and lower oxygen-enhancement ratio (OER). Because of a lack of repair of sublethal or potentially lethal damage normal cells, neutron beam irradiation has not been found superior to conventional photon irradiation in terms of local control and patient survival in a randomized prospective clinical trial for head and neck tumors. Scattered reports showed good local control of parotid gland tumors and soft tissue sarcomas after neutron therapy.[10–12] This treatment modality is beyond the need of daily treatment for a vast number of cancer patients with head and neck cancer.

3. Proton beams have been used for radiation therapy for over 20 years. These heavy particles are produced from a cyclotron. Although the relative biologic effectiveness (RBE) is similar to that of x-rays, this form of radiation may improve distribution of the physical dose, so that a high dose can be delivered to the target volume and a minimal dose to the adjacent vital organs, in an attempt to increase local tumor control and to decrease radiation complications. This has been used in clinical radiation therapy in the head and neck region by the radiation oncologists at the Massachusetts General Hospital.[13] At present, proton beam radiation therapy is used extensively for treatment of choroidal melanoma, skull based chordoma, and localized chondrosarcoma of the head and neck region,[14,15] with good control and cosmesis.

4. Three-dimensional (3-D) treatment for patients with cancer is rapidly becoming popular. By using sophisticated computers, the tumor volume can be irradiated with a higher dose, but adjacent normal tissues are spared, thus bettering the therapeutic ratio and improving local control. The 3-D treatment has routinely been carried out with proton beam therapy at the MGH for the past 10–15 years. The procedure is time-consuming and costly and should be done on a protocol basis.

5. Traditionally, radiation therapy has been given once-daily, 5 days a week, for a number of weeks. The conventional radiation therapy has been effective in con-

trolling early squamous cell carcinomas of the head and neck; for large tumors, local control is poor. The principles and practice of altered fractionation radiation therapy are discussed in Chapter 4.

Accelerated fractionation and hyperfractionation using smaller fraction size than 2 Gy to a total dose 10–15% greater than conventional radiation therapy have been used for clinical radiation therapy by various radiation therapy centers,[16] with some improvement of local control of head and neck carcinoma.

Twice-daily (BID) radiation therapy with 1.6 Gy/fraction has been carried out at the Massachusetts General Hospital since October 1979 and found effective. It achieves higher local control[17,18,19,20,21] than conventional once-daily radiation therapy, with acceptable complications.

As indicated throughout this text, improved results are particularly pronounced in patients with moderate to advanced squamous cell carcinoma or with lymph node disease. More important is the fact that those lesions arising from Waldeyer's ring and the supraglottic larynx responded to twice-daily radiation therapy exceptionally well. Other tumor sites, such as the oral cavity, hypopharynx, and glottic larynx, also showed moderate improvement. The response of inoperable salivary gland malignancies is also impressive. In general, gray for gray, the twice-daily program is well tolerated, and the associated complications are minimal. The radiation therapy oncology group has initiated a controlled randomized trial with this scheme, and it is hoped the final answer will be known after the study is concluded. At the present time, as for the past 15 years, most patients with advanced carcinoma of the head and neck are managed by the BID program with gratifying results.

Radiation therapy is a fast-evolving, dynamic medical specialty. Progress is being made constantly. Some "newer" treatment methods of the past 10–15 years have not lived up to their expectations and soon become outmoded forms of radiation therapy.

For the immediate future, newer and more effective drugs and better treatment schemes with various drugs are urgently needed if chemotherapy is to play an important role in the management of head and neck carcinomas. Likewise, the schemes of altered fractionation radiation therapy and techniques, the total tumor controlled doses and the treatment time have not been established satisfactorily. Further study is needed in order to achieve the maximum local control and minimum radiation complications.

REFERENCES

1. Hong WK, Bromer HR, Amato DA, et al: Patterns of relapse in locally advanced head and neck cancer patients who achieved complete remission after combined modality therapy. *Cancer* 1985;56:1242–1245.
2. Jacobs C, Goffinet DR, Kohler M, et al: Chemotherapy as a substitute for surgery and in the treatment of advanced resectable head and neck cancer: a report from the Northern California. Oncology Group. *Cancer* 1987;60:1178–1183.

3. Cade IS, McEwen J: Clinical trials of radiotherapy in hyperbaric oxygen at Portsmouth (1964–76). *Clin Radiol* 1978;29:333–338.

4. Henk JM, Smith CW: Radiotherapy and hyperbaric oxygen in head and neck cancer. *Lancet* 1977;1:104–105.

5. Adams GE: Hypoxic cell sensitizers for radiotherapy. *Int J Radiat Oncol Biol Phys* 1978;4:135–141.

6. Karim ABMF: Prolonged metronidazole administration with protracted radiotherapy. *Br J Cancer* 1978;37(suppl):299–301.

7. Dische S: Hypoxic cell sensitizers in radiotherapy. *Int J Radiat Oncol Biol Phys* 1978;4:157–160.

8. Arcanbgeli G, Cevidali A, Nervi C: Tumor control and therapeutic gain with different schedules of combined radiation therapy and local and external hyperthermia in humor cancer. *Int J Radiat Oncol Biol Phys* 1983;9:1125–1134.

9. Overgard J: Hyperthermia modification of the radiation response in solid tumors. In: Flecture G, Neroi C, Withers H, ed. *Biological bases and clinical implications of tumor resistance*. New York: Masson, 1983.

10. Griffin TW, Pajak TF, Laramore LE, et al: Neuron versus photon irradiation of inoperable salivary gland tumors: results of an RTOG-MRC cooperative randomized study. *Int J Radiat Oncol Biol Phys* 1988;15:1085–1090.

11. Catterall M, Errington RD, Bewley DK: A comparison of clinical and laboratory data on neutron therapy for locally advanced tumors. *Int J Radiat Oncol Biol Phys* 1987;13:1783–1791.

12. Henry LW, Blasko JC, Griffin TW: Evaluation of fast neutron teletherapy for advanced carcinomas of the major salivary glands. *Cancer* 1979;44:814–818.

13. Suit HD, Goitein M, Tepper JE, et al: Clinical experience and expectation with protons and heavy ions. *Int J Radiat Oncol Biol Phys* 1977;3:115–125.

14. Brown AP, Urie MM, Chisin R, Suit HD: Proton therapy for carcinoma of the nasopharynx. *Int J Radiat Oncol Biol Phys* 1989;16:1607–1614.

15. Suit HD, Goitein M, Munzenrider J, et al: Definitive radiation therapy for chordoma and chondrosarcoma of base of skull and cervical spine. *J Neurosurg* 1982;56:377–385.

16. Million R: Hyperfractionation in cancer therapy: an overview. Franz Buschke Lecture, University of California at San Francisco, Spring 1989.

17. Wang CC: The enigma of accelerated hyperfractionated radiation therapy for head and neck cancer. *Int J Radiat Oncol Biol Phys* 1987;14:209–210.

18. Wang CC, Blitzer PH, Suit HD: Twice daily radiation therapy for cancer of the head and neck. *Cancer* 1985;55:2100–2104.

19. Wang CC: Accelerated hyperfractionation radiation therapy for head and neck. Franz Buschke Lecture, University of California at San Francisco, Spring 1985.

20. Wang CC, Efind J, Nakfoor B and Martins P: Local control of T3 carcinomas after accelerated fractionation: A look at the "Gap." *Int J Radiat Oncol Biol Phys* 1996;439–441.

21. Brenner DJ and Hall EJ: Alternative fractionation schemes: Is the "Gap" the way? *Int J Radiat Oncol Biol Phys* 1996;629–630.

INDEX